TEXTBOOK OF
GENERAL AND ORAL
SURGERY

Commissioning Editor: Michael Parkinson
Project Development Manager: Hannah Kenner
Project Manager: Nancy Arnott
Designer: Erik Bigland

www.fleshandbones.com

The international community for medical students and instructors. Have you joined?

The great online resource

For students

- Free
- Online favou
- Stude
- Down
- Win and

oks

roducts

ry,

Log on and re

fleshandbones.co
– an online resourc
for medical instruc
and students

nes.com

TEXTBOOK OF GENERAL AND ORAL SURGERY

David Wray, MD, FDS RCS(Ed), FDS RCPS (Glasg), F Med Sci
Dean of the Dental School and Professor of Oral Medicine, University of Glasgow
Honorary Consultant in Oral Medicine, North Glasgow University Hospitals NHS Trust

David Stenhouse, DDS, BDS, FDS RCPS (Glasg)
Senior Lecturer in Oral Surgery, University of Glasgow
Honorary Consultant in Oral Surgery, North Glasgow University Hospitals NHS Trust

David Lee, BSc, MB ChB, FRCS(Ed)
Consultant General and Endocrine Surgeon, Lothian University Hospitals NHS Trust,
Royal Infirmary, Edinburgh
Member of Council, Royal College of Surgeons of Edinburgh

Andrew J E Clark, BSc(Hons), MB ChB MRCS(Ed)
Clinical Research Fellow in General Surgery Western General Hospital, Edinburgh

Illustrations by Ian Ramsden

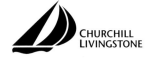
CHURCHILL
LIVINGSTONE

EDINBURGH LONDON NEW YORK PHILADELPHIA ST LOUIS SYDNEY TORONTO 2003

CHURCHILL LIVINGSTONE
An imprint of Elsevier Science Limited

First published 2003

ISBN 0 4430 7083 0

British Library Cataloguing in Publication Data
A catalogue record for this book is available from the British
Library

Library of Congress Cataloging in Publication Data
A catalog record for this book is available from the Library of
Congress

Note
Medical knowledge is constantly changing. As new information
becomes available, changes in treatment, procedures, equipment
and the use of drugs become necessary. The editors and the
publishers have taken care to ensure that the information given in
this text is accurate and up to date. However, readers are strongly
advised to confirm that the information, especially with regard to
drug usage, complies with the latest legislation and standards of
practice.

ELSEVIER SCIENCE
your source for books,
journals and multimedia
in the health sciences
www.elsevierhealth.com

The
publisher's
policy is to use
**paper manufactured
from sustainable forests**

Printed in China

Preface

The scope of dental practice has evolved enormously since the era of the barber surgeon. Oral surgery remains, however, not only a traditional skill in dentistry but also a core skill for all dental surgeons regardless of their area of specialism, and therefore it is an important part of the undergraduate curriculum and general professional training.

Over the years, as the medical status of the population has become more complex and surgical expertise has increased, oral surgery has evolved into identified sub-specialties. These include maxillofacial surgery, which, in the UK, is a specialty of medicine; oral surgery, which embraces maxillofacial trauma and orthognathic surgery; and dentoalveolar surgery, which is designated surgical dentistry by the General Dental Council in the UK. The first two – maxillofacial surgery and oral surgery – are the remit of specialists, whereas all dentists are expected to be competent in dentoalveolar surgery. A sound knowledge of basic surgical principles is a prerequisite to the practice of any of these areas of surgery.

This text includes a consideration of general surgical principles, specialist surgical areas and minor oral surgery. The section on general surgical principles has been written mainly by general surgeons and provides core knowledge that informs the safe practice of surgery. It will be of practical help to those working as senior house officers in maxillofacial surgery wards. This section also considers cross-infection control and provides an overview of both general anaesthesia and conscious sedation.

The second section includes chapters on individual areas of specialist surgical practice of interest to oral and maxillofacial operators, written by experts. These are written to provide insight into these relevant areas of surgical practice so that the dentist can be confident in the information he or she provides to patients and can also make appropriate referrals. This section is not intended to inform practice in these areas and so it is short and readable.

The third section – oral surgery – is a practical guide to the practice of dentoalveolar surgery or surgical dentistry. It provides core information required to complete the undergraduate curriculum.

The integrated nature of this text, which includes general and oral surgery, is a companion to the *Textbook of General and Oral Medicine*, and is recommended for students studying human disease earlier in the undergraduate curriculum and, subsequently, oral surgery in the clinical years. Although intended primarily for undergraduate students, the book also provides a comprehensive range of information for those preparing for membership examinations and will be a useful bench book in a dental practice environment.

The authors have taken great pleasure and satisfaction in compiling this text, which is unique in bringing together succinct knowledge on the whole scope of surgical practice in dentistry. It is hoped that the reader will also be pleased and satisfied.

Finally, I would sincerely like to thank Dr Declan Millett, Senior Lecturer in Orthodontics, for providing his expertise in the areas where there is an interface with orthodontics. I would also like to record my thanks to Mrs Grace Dobson and Mrs Betty Bulloch for the manuscript, and to Mrs Kay Shepherd and Mrs Gail Drake of the Dental Illustration Department, in addition to those who have contributed to this text.

D Wray
Glasgow, 2003

Contributors

Professor Jeremy Bagg, PhD, BDS, FDS RCS(Ed), FDS RCPS(Glasg), FRC Path
Professor of Clinical Microbiology, University of Glasgow
Honorary Consultant Microbiologist, North Glasgow University Hospitals NHS Trust

Mr Philip Barlow, MPhil, BSc, MB ChB, FRCS(Ed)
Consultant Neurosurgeon, South Glasgow University Hospitals NHS Trust
Honorary Senior Lecturer, University of Glasgow

Dr Andrew J E Clark, BSc(Hons), MB ChB MRCS(Ed)
Clinical Research Fellow in General Surgery
Western General Hospital, Edinburgh

Mr Howard A Critchlow, BDS, FDS RCS(Eng), FDS RCPS(Glasg)
Consultant Oral Surgeon, South Glasgow University Hospitals NHS Trust
Honorary Senior Lecturer, University of Glasgow

Mr Hugh Harvie, BDS, FDS RCS(Ed), FDS RCPS(Glasg), Dip For Med
Head of Dental Division, Medical and Dental Defence Union of Scotland
Honorary Senior Lecturer, University of Glasgow

Dr James R I R Dougall, MB ChB, FFA RCSI
Consultant in Anaesthesia and Intensive Care, North Glasgow University Hospitals NHS Trust
Honorary Senior Lecturer, University of Glasgow

Mr W Stuart Hislop, BDS, MB ChB, FDS RCS(Ed), FRCS(Ed), FDS RCPS(Glasg)
Consultant Oral and Maxillofacial Surgeon, Ayrshire and Arran Acute Hospitals NHS Trust
Honorary Senior Lecturer, University of Glasgow

Mr David Lee, BSc, MB ChB, FRCS(Ed)
Consultant General and Endocrine Surgeon, Lothian University Hospitals NHS Trust,
Royal Infirmary, Edinburgh
Member of Council, Royal College of Surgeons of Edinburgh

Mr Jason A Leitch, BDS, FDS RCS(Eng)
Lecturer in Oral Surgery, University of Glasgow
Honorary Associate Specialist, North Glasgow University Hospitals NHS Trust

Mr Gerald W McGarry, MD, MB ChB, FRCS(Ed), FRCS(Glasg)
Consultant Otolaryngologist, North Glasgow University Hospitals NHS Trust
Honorary Senior Lecturer, University of Glasgow

Professor Khursheed F Moos, BDS, MB BS, FDS RCS(Eng), FDS RCS(Ed), FDS RCPS(Glasg), FRCS(Ed)
Honorary Professor, University of Glasgow
Honorary Consultant in Oral Surgery, North Glasgow University Hospitals NHS Trust

Mr Arup K Ray, MS, MB BS, FRCS(Ed), FRCS(Glasg)
Consultant Plastic and Reconstructive Surgeon, North Glasgow University Hospitals NHS Trust
Honorary Senior Lecturer, University of Glasgow

Mr R J Sanderson, MB ChB, FRCS(Eng), FRCS(Ed)
Consultant Otolaryngologist and Head and Neck Surgeon, West Lothian and Lothian University Hospitals NHS Trust

Mr David Soutar, ChM, MB ChB, FRCS RCPS(Glasg), FRCS(Ed)
Consultant Plastic Surgeon, North Glasgow University
Hospitals NHS Trust
Honorary Senior Lecturer, University of Glasgow

Mr David Stenhouse, DDS, BDS, FDS RCPS(Glasg)
Senior Lecturer in Oral Surgery, University of Glasgow
Honorary Consultant in Oral Surgery, North Glasgow
University Hospitals NHS Trust

Mr David Still, BDS, FDS RCPS(Glasg)
Lecturer in Oral Surgery
Honorary Consultant in Oral Surgery, North Glasgow
University Hospitals NHS Trust

Mr Graham A Wood, BDS, MB ChB, FDS RCPS(Glasg), FDS
RCS(Eng)
Consultant Oral and Maxillofacial Surgeon, South
Glasgow University Hospitals NHS Trust
Honorary Senior Lecturer, University of Glasgow

Professor David Wray, MD, FDS RCS(Ed), FDS RCPS(Glasg), F
Med Sci
Dean of the Dental School and Professor of Oral
Medicine, University of Glasgow
Honorary Consultant in Oral Medicine, North Glasgow
University Hospitals NHS Trust

Contents

CONTENTS

PART I
GENERAL SURGERY

Section A
Basic Principles

Introduction

If they are to achieve an acceptably high standard of clinical practice, it is essential that all surgeons – including dentists and oral surgeons – have a background knowledge of surgery in general. A specialised knowledge of oral and dental disorders and their management is not sufficient. An understanding of the basic principles of surgery is essential for all surgeons to be able to apply such knowledge to their specialty. Once they have acquired such knowledge, surgeons can use it to form the basis of their specialty knowledge and utilise it to achieve the standard required and desired.

Such a knowledge of 'surgery in general' is essential for dental/oral surgeons to ensure that they will be able to:

- recognise disease by detecting key abnormalities in the patient assessment
- recognise important disorders that might impinge on their practice
- assess and balance the needs for treatment against the risks of avoiding therapy in the patient with coincidental illness
- identify illness that needs to be treated
- refer patients with specific problems to appropriate specialists
- avoid operating on patients who have specific or relative contraindications to surgery
- understand the need to have the patient in optimal condition before surgery and how to achieve this
- treat and manage basic problems that might arise in the course of patient care
- afford a good level of patient care pre- and postoperatively
- understand the basic principles of surgical techniques
- be aware of potential problems, especially life-threatening complications, which may arise in the course of surgery and how to manage these

- understand the role of specialist colleagues in all aspects of patient care.

Part I of this book – 'General surgery' – affords a good basis, in simple text, to cover all aspects outlined above. This is subdivided into a section on 'Basic principles', which has been written by general surgeons, followed by a section on 'Specialist surgical principles', which has been written by surgeons who specialise in the field. This is followed by Part II – 'Oral surgery' – which is now able to develop the practice of oral surgery within the context of, and with the background knowledge of, surgery in general. The text is produced at a level that is suitable both for undergraduate and postgraduate students.

The chapters in the 'Basic principles' section have been selected carefully to cover those topics that are of immediate interest to oral and dental surgeons. These basic principles are detailed to allow clear understanding of the topic at undergraduate level. The detail is of more practical relevance to the postgraduate with patient-care responsibilities. A chapter on 'History taking' technique is followed by chapters highlighting:

- Wound healing, incisions and suturing to achieve the best surgical and cosmetic results.
- Complications of surgery and how to identify and manage these.
- Fluid balance, together with the potential problems and dangers of improper fluid and electrolyte balance, and how to avoid or deal with these.
- Blood disorders, which have a major impact on surgical practice. Many of the problems are avoidable and this chapter highlights relevant areas.
- Infections related to surgery, either as a presenting problem or as a consequence of surgery, which play a large part in patient management. Cross-infection can be a major problem and the principles of care and how to avoid the problems are highlighted. The role

of antibiotics, both prophylactic and therapeutic, is discussed.

- The basic principles of fracture management, which are very important to the oral surgeon; a full chapter covers this area.
- Anaesthesia and sedation, which form a major section of the care of the surgical patient and are discussed in detail.

The 'Specialist surgical principles' section provides a succinct overview of those specialist areas of surgical expertise that lie outside the remit of the dental surgeon, but a sound understanding of these areas is essential within the healthcare team to allow appropriate referral, provide appropriate information to the patient and to participate in the holistic care of the patient.

Part II – 'Oral surgery' – can then be studied based on a robust understanding of basic surgical principles.

As a final comment, it is good practice that all surgeons should document clearly each step of patient-care in writing, giving the reasoning behind each decision made. This is especially the case when making decisions that seem to lie outside the scope of normal practice. It is hoped that this book will afford a support for specialist oral or dental surgeons, to help them make accurate and calculated decisions that can be justified by the strength of a good background knowledge of basic surgical principles applied to good oral surgical practice.

2 History taking

Introduction

History taking is a most important process and must be rehearsed well. A patient who has not met the surgeon before is coming to explain about his or her problem and putting total trust in the surgeon's ability to sort this. The patient will be very apprehensive. No matter how efficient and skilled the surgeon is, he or she must make the patient feel confident. The surgeon's appearance and demeanor must exude professionalism. A hand-shake, a smile, a pleasant introduction and a caring gesture will make the remainder of contact with the patient much easier and more pleasant.

One's initial approach might have to be modified according to the patient, for example children, the very elderly and infirm, patients who are poor of hearing and patients who are mentally impaired all need different approaches. The surgeon must also take account of any accompanying relative or friend. It is very important, however, to ensure that the accompanying relative does not dominate the consultation.

The history should then be elicited in a rehearsed way as outlined in Table 2.1.

Part I of this text is concerned with basic principles, and so a detailed section on surgical history is not appropriate. Details relating to the specifics of history taking are given in Chapter 22. The sections below highlight certain basic points.

History of the presenting complaint

This is the patient's opportunity to tell the surgeon about the problem and it is important to avoid prompting with leading questions. Some patients will give a really good account of their problem but many will need guidance;

Table 2.1 History taking
History of present complaint
Relevant medical history
Family history
Social history
Drug and allergy history

many will also have difficulty in remembering the time-scale of the illness. A good initial beginning with history taking is to ask the patient to think back to the start of the problem to ensure that he or she gives an account in chronological order. It is also important, while the patient is giving the history, to ensure that he or she gives a clear account of what has happened, and does not discuss what he or she thinks is the cause of the problem.

Relevant medical history

This is the surgeon's chance to take a history from the patient. This part has two aspects: first, the opportunity to elaborate on any points in the history that the surgeon felt were unclear; second, to enquire from the patient any aspect of his or her health that might otherwise influence the treatment plan.

Family history

Two main items are worth enquiring regarding family history: (1) is there a genetic family problem, especially any blood-related problem such as haemophilia? (2) has any member of the family had any problem with anaesthetics, especially muscle relaxants? Prolonged action of depolarising agents such as suxamethonium runs in families and should be detected prior to any general anaesthetic.

Eliciting the significant diseases in family members or the cause of death of deceased members can give insight into disease susceptibility such as cancer or cardio-vascular disease.

Drug therapy

As outlined above, it is critical to know about certain drugs prior to performing any surgery. Dosage of corti-costeroids might need to be increased and anticoagulants need to be controlled and monitored carefully. Possible interactions between drugs need to be assessed.

Social history

The patient's occupation might be relevant to the complaint or to the opportunity for recovery. The patient's social circumstances and family support will also dictate opportunities for convalescence.

Knowledge of tobacco smoking and alcohol consumption will not only inform the surgeon of the potential risks for general anaesthesia and surgery but also the patient's likelihood of smoking- and alcohol-related diseases.

Allergies

A history of asthma and anaphylaxis is important. The surgeon must know about drug allergies and any idiosyncratic reaction that might have occurred at any time in the past, no matter how long ago.

Skin allergies, especially reaction to prepping agents such as iodine, must be discussed and these agents avoided.

3 Wound healing and suture materials

Introduction

The main goal when trying to get a wound to heal is to achieve anatomical integrity of the injured part and to restore full function. As a secondary consideration, this should be combined with an attempt to produce as perfect a cosmetic result as possible.

A sound knowledge of the principles of wound healing is necessary to achieve these aims and to allow appropriate planning of incisions and their closure. An understanding of the complications that can occur during wound healing is vital to try to avoid these or to treat them appropriately if they arise.

To achieve the best result during wound closure, every surgeon should be aware of the wide selection of suture materials available so as to be able to choose the most appropriate for each situation.

Classification of wound healing

A fundamental distinction in wound healing is between clean, incised wound edges that are closely apposed to each other, and wounds where the edges are separated. The former undergo healing by 'primary intention', the latter by 'secondary intention'.

Primary intention

Where the edges are clean and held together with ligatures, there is little gap to bridge. Healing, when uncomplicated, occurs quickly with rapid ingrowth of wound healing cells (macrophages, fibroblasts, etc.) and restoration of the gap by a small amount of scar tissue. Such wounds are soundly united within 2 weeks and dense scar tissue is laid down within 1 month.

Secondary intention

Wound healing by secondary intention occurs when the wound edges are separated and the gap between them cannot be bridged directly. This occurs when there has been extensive loss of epithelium, severe wound contamination or significant subepithelial tissue damage. Healing occurs slowly from the bottom of the wound towards the surface by the process of granulation. This larger defect results in a greater mass of scar tissue than healing by primary intention. In time, such scarring tends to shrink, resulting in wound contracture.

Normal sequence of wound healing

Despite the differences in time taken and amount of scar tissue produced, the sequence of events in wound healing by primary and secondary intention is similar:

- Skin trauma results in damage to superficial blood vessels and haemorrhage. Blood clotting results in fibrin clot formation, and this is stabilised by a number of factors, including fibronectin.
- Within 24 h neutrophils have migrated to the area, and epidermal cells have extended out in a single layer from the wound edges in an attempt to cover the defect.
- Between days 1 to 3 the neutrophils are replaced by macrophages, which clear debris and play a role in producing the environment that stimulates local and recruited fibroblasts to produce collagen. This milieu, along with new blood vessel formation (neovascularisation), constitutes 'granulation tissue'.
- Towards the end of the first week neovascularisation is at its peak. In healing by primary intention at this stage the incised gap is bridged by collagen. The full

thickness of epithelium is reconstituted, including surface keratinisation, a process that requires both epithelial cell migration and proliferation.
• During the second week there is increased fibroblast activity and collagen formation, with decreasing vascularity and cellularity in the wound.

With primary intention by 1 month there is a cellular connective tissue scar with normal overlying epidermis. By 2 months the wound has regained approximately 80% of its original strength. The redevelopment of strength in the wound involves remodelling and orientation of collagen fibres and continues for a number of months.

In healing by secondary intention there is more necrotic debris, exudate and fibrin, and a more intense inflammatory response results. There is a larger defect, therefore, with more granulation tissue and a greater mass of scar tissue. Wound coverage takes longer and wound contraction occurs caused by myofibroblasts.

Regulation of the complex interactions involved in wound healing is achieved by a number of local and systemic factors. These are produced both at distant sites (e.g. growth factor) and locally by the cells involved in the healing process. Many factors are involved, important examples including cytokines, platelet-derived growth factor and epidermal growth factor.

Factors affecting healing

A number of local and systemic factors affect wound healing (Table 3.1); these are discussed in turn.

Local factors

Wound sepsis

Removal of hair allows better visualisation of the wound. It also facilitates application of adhesive dressings and suture removal. However, evidence has shown that shaving of skin at an early stage preoperatively increases bacterial counts in the area, and shaving more than 12 h before incision can significantly increase the rate of wound infection. Hair removal should therefore be performed where necessary just prior to surgery (see Ch. 8).

Preparing the skin with antiseptic wash prior to surgery is vitally important. Preparation should be thorough. Chlorhexidine and povidone–iodine have been shown to reduce the skin bacterial flora by up to 95%. Most surgeons perform a double scrub of the area, preparing

Table 3.1   Factors affecting wound healing
Local
wound sepsis
poor blood supply
wound tension
foreign bodies
previous irradiation
poor technique
Systemic
nutritional deficiencies
systemic diseases
therapeutic agents
age

the skin well wide of the area of surgery. Careful hand wash by the surgeon using these antiseptics is also very important in reducing wound sepsis.

Poor blood supply

As described above, bleeding and neovascularisation play fundamental roles in wound healing. Areas with good vascularity, such as the scalp and face, heal well, whereas those with poor blood supply, such as pretibial skin, heal poorly. Surgical technique can also have a significant effect on the blood supply to the area. Care should be taken where possible to maintain the vascular supply to the incised area. For example, creation of a distally based skin flap is likely to disrupt the vessels to the skin of the flap, and impair wound healing. Appropriate planning of incisions minimises vascular damage.

Wound tension

Tension across a healing wound serves to separate the wound edges, impairs the blood supply to the area and predisposes to complications of wound healing. Care should be taken, therefore, when planning incisions to avoid creating tension if possible.

Where the gap between the wound edges is large, primary apposition of the edges might not be appropriate or even possible. Bridging of such a gap can be achieved by a number of plastic surgery techniques, including skin grafting or tissue flaps (see Ch. 15).

Better cosmetic results from surgery tend to be achieved if incisions are made along the lines of the collagen bundles of the skin (Langer's lines). These follow the natural skin creases on the face, transversely at the joints and longitudinally on the long parts of the limbs.

Foreign bodies

The presence of extraneous material within the wound predisposes to infection. It also results in a larger and more prolonged inflammatory reaction, which can predispose to excess scar tissue formation. Foreign material can enter a traumatic wound at the time of injury and should be removed at the onset of treatment with adequate debridement.

With surgical wounds, however, complications can result from endogenous material being inappropriately present within the wound, such as devascularised pieces of fat, necrotic tissue resulting from excess use of the diathermy, or the patient's hair. Thorough wound cleaning before closure helps to remove these materials.

Previous irradiation

Areas that have undergone preoperative radiotherapy suffer from a patchy vasculitis, impairing their blood supply and hence healing potential. Radiation also damages skin stem cells, resulting in poor re-epithelialisation.

Poor technique

Care should be taken when making an incision to create a clean precise cut. The incision should be made vertically through the skin. Gentle handling of tissues throughout the operation is important. Rough handling and damaging of tissues can result in tissue edge necrosis, predisposing to poor healing and infection. Careful haemostasis not only allows good visualisation during surgery but also reduces tissue bruising and haematoma formation.

Choice of appropriate suture material is important. Suture placement should be precise and suture tension sufficient to result in tissue apposition, but not too tight to cause tissue necrosis. Skin closure should include the strength-supplying dermis within the bite. Removal of sutures at the correct time (variable between sites) helps prevent scarring associated with the sutures themselves.

Systemic factors

Many systemic factors are necessary for wound healing and deficiency of these impairs the process. Certain diseases and therapies can also have detrimental effects on the wound.

Nutritional deficiencies

Vitamins important in the process of wound healing include A and C. Vitamin A is involved in epithelialisation and collagen production; vitamin C has an important role in the production and modification of collagen. This has been recognised for centuries by virtue of the disease scurvy caused by vitamin C deficiency.

Certain minerals are also essential in wound healing. Zinc acts as an enzyme cofactor and has a role in cell proliferation. It accelerates wound healing in experimental models. Deficiency may be encountered in patients on long-term total parenteral nutrition.

Protein is the main building block in wound healing. A malnourished, hypoproteinaemic patient has impaired inflammatory and immune responses, vital for normal wound healing and prevention of wound infection. Protein amino acids are essential for collagen production, which is itself a protein.

Systemic diseases

Several diseases are known to impair wound healing via a number of mechanisms. Important examples include diabetes, uraemia and jaundice.

Therapeutic agents

Immunosuppressive drugs dampen the inflammatory and immune responses, hence impairing wound healing. These include chemotherapeutic agents for malignancy and immunosuppressive and antiprostaglandin drugs used for inflammatory conditions such as rheumatoid disease. Probably the most important and widely used example is corticosteroid therapy. Steroids have the additional effect of increasing the fragility of small blood vessels.

Age

Prior to puberty, the rate of wound healing is increased compared to postpuberty.

Complications of wound healing

A number of complications of wound healing can occur; these are listed in Table 3.2.

Table 3.2	Complications of wound healing
Infection	
Dehiscence	
Incisional hernia	
Hypertrophic scarring	
Keloid scarring	
Contractures	

Infection

Wound infection is dealt with further in Chapter 8. As outlined in Table 8.2 (p. 54), several local and systemic factors predispose to wound sepsis.

Dehiscence

Total breakdown of all the layers of the surgical repair of a wound is called 'dehiscence'. The mortality of abdominal wound dehiscence is between 10 and 35%.

Dehiscence can be caused by a number of factors, including those that generally impair wound healing (Table 3.3). Incidence can be minimised by meticulous surgical technique to negate the technical factors that can cause dehiscence.

Suture breakage can result from poor suture selection. Knot slippage arises as a result of inadequate tying. 'Cutting out' of sutures can be due to failure to include layers with most strength within the bite of the suture. Excess tension on the suture line also impairs wound healing. Wounds should be sutured with only enough tension to close the defect.

Incisional hernia

Dehiscence of the deeper layers of a wound in which the skin layer remains intact will result in incisional hernia formation with protrusion of underlying structures through the deeper defect. This is of particular importance for abdominal wounds, where viscera such as small intestine can herniate, with the attendant risks of

Table 3.3	Factors causing wound dehiscence
Suture breakage	
Knot slippage	
'Cutting out' of sutures	
Excess tension on the suture line	

irreducibility, obstruction and strangulation. Incisional hernias in other areas can be unsightly and cause the patient discomfort (e.g. herniation of underlying muscle through a gap in fascia lata following hip replacement).

Hypertrophic scarring

Hypertrophic scarring is essentially excess collagen scar tissue formation – almost an overhealing of a wound. It is non-progressive after 6 months and does not extend beyond the edges of the wound. It occurs most frequently in specific areas, particularly around joints and where Langer's lines of tension are crossed by the incision. Poor skin suturing technique frequently results in hypertrophic scar formation, especially where the edges of the skin are overlapping instead of being accurately apposed.

Treatment is difficult and further surgery should not be attempted for at least 6 months. Excision of the scar and resuturing often has disappointing results, resulting in the same overhealing. Radiotherapy used to be used but has now been abandoned. Some improvement can be achieved with local injection of corticosteroids directly into the scar, a process that might need repeating several times.

Keloid scarring

Keloid scars are due to abnormal collagen metabolism. The excess scar tissue extends out beyond the wound edges and might continue to enlarge after 6 months. Prevalence is higher in patients with dark skin, especially those of African origin, in younger patients and in those with burn wounds.

Areas prone to this type of scarring are the face, dorsal surfaces of the body, sternum and deltopectoral region.

Excision generally results in a larger recurrence, although excision followed by compression bandaging can have slightly better results. Corticosteroid injections can give some improvement.

Contractures

Wound contractures can occur with any wounds but are more commonly associated with wounds that experience delayed healing (including infection), burns and those in which the incision crosses Langer's lines.

Contracture of a scar across a joint can result in marked limitation of movement. It is therefore essential to avoid vertical incisions across a joint if possible. At a joint, Langer's lines tend to run horizontally.

Surgical treatment of a scar contracture might be the only treatment available and can include skin grafting, local flaps or wound Z-plasty.

Suture materials

Classification

There is a wide variety of suture materials commercially available. Although the selection for a specific surgical repair will vary according to surgeon preference, financial considerations must be borne in mind.

Suture materials are classified as those that are absorbable and those that are non-absorbable (Table 3.4). Each of these categories is subdivided into sutures made from natural fibres, for example, silk, and those that are man made. In addition, sutures can be made from single strands (monofilament) or multiple strands (braided).

Most natural materials are now no longer used and catgut, for example, is no longer commercially available. These materials tended to have a variable suture strength, which was not entirely consistent through the length of the thread. Because of this, most surgeons now use synthetic materials.

Each suture type is available in a variety of widths, the larger the number, the finer the thread. For example, 1/0 suture is very thick whereas 6/0 suture is very fine.

Selection of materials

The first consideration when choosing a suture material is whether an absorbable or non-absorbable suture is required. Closing of the deep layers of a wound is usually performed with an absorbable suture, whereas vascular anastomoses are performed with fine-bore non-absorbable materials. Where an absorbable suture is required, a knowledge of the time taken for it to dissolve, and hence lose its strength, is necessary.

The strength of the suture also varies with the arrangement of fibres, such that braided sutures are stronger than monofilament sutures of the same material for the same thickness.

Different materials possess different handling properties, for example, Prolene has 'memory' (retains the bends in the suture that result from its packaging), and is more difficult to knot. With this in mind, the number of throws in a knot should be altered according to the suture material to prevent slippage and unravelling.

Tissue reactivity varies between sutures. Materials with high tissue reactivity, such as silk, cause inflammation at the site of the suture and are more likely to produce suture scarring. The different properties of various suture materials are listed in Table 3.5.

Needles

Sutures are supplied attached to a number of different needles and are swaged directly into the end of the needle rather than through the eye of a needle; this avoids having to pass a double thickness of suture.

Nowadays, most needles in common use are curved and are used mounted on a needle-holding forceps. Straight needles are available and used primarily for

---

Table 3.4   Classification of suture materials

Absorbable
  synthetic, e.g. polydioxanone (PDS) (monofilament), vicryl (braided)
  natural, e.g. catgut
Non-absorbable
  synthetic, e.g. Prolene (monofilament), nylon (monofilament)
  natural, e.g. silk (braided)

Table 3.5   Properties of different suture materials

	Absorbable or non-absorbable	Tissue reactivity	Duration of strength
Vicryl	Absorbable	Mild	60% at 2 weeks
Catgut	Absorbable	High	Lost in 7–10 days
Polydioxanone (PDS)	Absorbable	Mild	70% at 2 weeks
Silk	Non-absorbable	Moderate	20% at 6 months
Nylon	Non-absorbable	Low	Loses 20% per year
Polypropylene	Non-absorbable	Low	Indefinite

subcuticular skin closure, but are associated with a higher risk of needlestick injury to the surgeon. Other shapes are available for specific tasks, such as the J-shaped needle for femoral hernia repair.

Another variable is the shape of the needle in cross-section. Round-bodied needles are circular in cross-section and do not possess sharp edges. They are used for suturing delicate structures, such as bowel anastomosis, and are designed to push tissues to either side rather than cut through them.

Blunt needles are also available, and are most commonly used for closing the muscle layer of an abdominal wound or for suturing liver. They are intended to reduce the risk of needlestick injury to the operating staff and damaging adjacent structures.

For use on tough tissues, such as skin and fascia, there is a selection of needles with sharp edges at the tips. These are known as 'cutting' and 'reverse cutting', depending where the cutting edge of the tip is placed.

Nowadays, skin closure is commonly performed with the use of skin clips. These come in a disposable sterile stapler, are quick to use, cause minimal discomfort to the patient, and are easily removed.

Qualities of a good incision

An incision must give good access to the structures being explored. It should be positioned such that it can be extended to give greater access if necessary. It should be easy to perform and should be made with extreme care to avoid skin and tissue damage, which can affect subsequent healing. Consideration should be given to the final cosmetic result before deciding on the direction of the incision, for example, Langer's lines (see Ch. 15).

Surgery should be carried out with care to avoid tissue damage due to bad handling. Excess use of diathermy should be avoided, especially at the skin edge. Haemostasis should be meticulous and haematoma formation should be avoided.

For good wound closure, the correct suture materials and suture needles should be chosen. Where there is likely to be a high degree of tissue tension on the deeper layers of a wound, a strong suture is required and must be placed accurately to grip the strongest layer of the incision. Excess tension on this suture should be avoided to prevent wound-edge necrosis and wound dehiscence.

Skin closure should be meticulous. This is the surgeon's signature and poor suturing technique here can cause permanent disfigurement that could have been avoided. The skin edges should be apposed accurately with no overlapping. Where there is tension on the skin edges, for example, following excision of a skin lesion such as a mole, fine interrupted sutures or clips are ideal to support the skin tension until healing occurs. Where there is no skin tension, subcuticular suturing with either a braided absorbable suture such as Vicryl or a non-absorbable monofilament suture such as Prolene, which will be removed in a week, is ideal.

4 Complications of surgery

Introduction

All surgical procedures carry an innate degree of risk. The benefits of any procedure being performed need to be weighed against any potential complications so that the clinician and the patient can make a balanced and informed decision about whether the procedure should be performed. It is therefore fundamental to have a sound appreciation of adverse outcomes of surgery and to define the population of patients that is most likely to suffer from any such complications.

It is helpful to have a mental framework to categorise complications. One such framework that is in common use is temporal: early, intermediate and late. In addition, complications can be divided into those that are 'general' and could occur with any operation, and those that are 'local' or specific to a particular operation.

General complications

Surgery is a controlled insult to the patient, whose body responds with a number of well-defined physiological and pathophysiological responses that alter the body's homeostatic mechanisms.

In addition, outside influences are often therapeutically imposed, for example anaesthesia, intravenous fluids and immobility.

Table 4.1 Early-stage complications of surgery
Anaesthesia-related complications
Hypothermia
Nerve damage
Diathermy-related injuries
Hypotension
Metabolic complications
Pain

All of these factors have implications for the patient and for the outcome of surgery.

Early-stage complications

Early-stage complications (Table 4.1) will be considered in turn.

Anaesthesia-related complications

All but a few patients undergoing a surgical procedure require some form of anaesthetic, be this local, regional or general. The principles and adverse effects of general anaesthesia are described in detail in Chapter 10 and local anaesthetics are considered in Chapter 24. However, it is important to give some consideration to these because a significant proportion of complications from surgery are related to anaesthesia (Table 4.2). A patient's ability to withstand anaesthesia will often dictate his or her 'fitness' to undergo surgery or will have a bearing on the surgical approach.

Nausea and vomiting

Temporary nausea is common after general anaesthesia and might necessitate overnight admission for intended daycase patients. Administration of an antiemetic and a delay in restoration of oral intake usually suffice, although pathological causes should be borne in mind.

Table 4.2 Complications related to general anaesthesia
Nausea and vomiting
Sore throat
Muscle pain
Damage to teeth

Sore throat

The use of airway adjuncts during anaesthesia, such as an endotracheal tube or laryngeal mask, can cause mechanical irritation of the pharynx. The symptom resolves spontaneously and requires reassurance only.

Muscle pain

The use of depolarising muscle relaxants, such as suxamethonium, causes initial muscle contraction and might result in widespread postoperative muscle ache.

Damage to teeth

Teeth can be damaged during the process of intubation and the anaesthetist must be careful when using a laryngoscope.

Hypothermia

Surgical patients are relatively exposed to any drop in temperature during the course of surgery, especially if surgery is over a prolonged time period. Anaesthesia can alter the patient's ability to control body temperature, with many agents causing peripheral vasodilatation with the consequent danger of hypothermia. It is important, therefore, to maintain a suitable temperature and humidity within the operating theatre. The use of warming blankets and local hot-air circulating jackets can prevent a significant temperature drop.

Nerve damage

Care must be taken when positioning a patient, particularly when they are under general anaesthesia. Sufficient padding must be used, particularly over bony prominences. Pressure over peripheral nerves should be avoided where possible. Excessive movement of joints can also result in nerve damage. For example, the patient's arm should not be abducted more than 60 degrees (particularly in external rotation), to avoid brachial plexus damage.

Diathermy-related injuries

The high-frequency alternating current of diathermy is a versatile surgical tool used to produce haemostasis. The main risk from diathermy is of burns because of incorrect usage.

Diathermy can be monopolar or bipolar. The risk of burn is less with bipolar diathermy, where the tissue grasped between the forceps completes the circuit, with current flowing from one tip of the forceps through this tissue to the other limb of the forceps.

In monopolar diathermy the current travels in a circuit from the diathermy machine, via a cable, to the forceps that are holding the bleeding vessel, causing an electro-cautery of the vessel. The current then returns, via the path of least resistance, through the patient's tissues to the return plate (which is attached to a remote part of the body such as the thigh) and then to the diathermy machine. The plate must have a certain surface area such that the current is sufficiently dispersed so that the plate does not burn the skin it is attached to. If the plate is applied incorrectly, such that only part of it is touching the patient, the full power of the current might be too localised and a burn can occur in that area. Responsibility for diathermy, including the plate, rests ultimately with the surgeon. Metal objects touching other areas of the patient provide an alternative route for the current to flow and, again, burns will occur if there is a small surface area at the exit site, for example, when there is contact between skin and a drip stand.

The diathermy current can ignite flammable gases, including bowel gas, certain anaesthetic agents, and alcohol-based skin preparation solutions.

The presence of a cardiac pacemaker is not a contraindication to the use of diathermy. The return plate should be remote from the pacemaker and close to the operative site. Short bursts of current should be used. The anaesthetist should monitor pacemaker function by pulse measurement and cardiac monitoring.

Hypotension

Low blood pressure is a common complication in the postoperative period. The causes are numerous, of varying severity and can result in shock. Shock can be defined as inadequate tissue perfusion and tissue oxygenation, resulting in organ dysfunction. Postoperative hypotension is not always pathological. It might not require treatment and could even be the desired effect of therapy.

Therapeutic hypotension

Patients are often prescribed drugs that lower blood pressure, such as beta-blockers or ACE inhibitors, to reduce perioperative bleeding. For other medications, hypotension is a side-effect, an important example being morphine, which is often given postoperatively via infusion. However, it is dangerous to assume that post-operative hypotension is secondary to medication and a search for other causes should be performed.

Spinal/epidural anaesthesia

Local anaesthetic substances near the spinal nerves block not only the fibres carrying pain signals but also the sympathetic fibres that provide vasomotor tone to the lower limbs. Blockade of these fibres results in vaso-dilatation and hence hypotension. A degree of increased intravascular filling is required to compensate for this increased potential intravascular volume. However, it is important not to be overaggressive in fluid resuscitation in an attempt to restore a blood pressure. Clinical signs are the key and, if the patient is peripherally well perfused and there is evidence of normal end-organ function (e.g. good urine output), then the current status might be acceptable.

Again it is essential that hypotension is not attributed to regional anaesthesia until a search for other causes has proved negative, and it is important to recognise that the sympathetic blockade will decrease the patient's ability to compensate for fluid loss.

Clinical assessment and close monitoring of blood pressure should help to define the problem and its extent, and aid in prevention and treatment.

Shock

Shock is classified both in terms of cause and also in terms of severity. The types of shock are listed in Table 4.3.

Obstructive shock

The obstructive form is a rare type of shock, where venous return to the heart is impaired resulting in decreased atrial and ventricular filling and therefore decreased cardiac output. Important examples are massive pulmonary embolus, tension pneumothorax and cardiac tamponade.

Pneumothorax is the presence of air within the pleural space. Infrequently, the air can be trapped in this space by a 'flutter valve' effect from the lung, such that more air can get into the space but air cannot escape. This results in increased pressure within the pleural space with compression of thoracic and mediastinal structures including the lungs, the heart and great vessels.

Table 4.3	Types of shock
Obstructive shock	
Hypovolaemic shock	
Cardiogenic shock	
Septic shock	

Any pneumothorax has the potential to become a tension pneumothorax, especially under general anaesthesia where the patient is being ventilated under positive pressure. Urgent treatment is required.

Pneumothorax can be caused in the perioperative period as a complication of positive pressure ventilation or insertion of central venous access devices that inadvertently breach the pleura.

Hypovolaemic shock

The most common cause of postoperative hypotension is hypovolaemia, that is, insufficient intravascular volume.

Hypovolaemic shock is classified with regards to severity and the clinical signs that accompany it (Table 4.4). This classification is a broad outline and represents a spectrum rather than distinct clinical entities. There are also a number of situations where the clinical features are not reliable:

- Young children and fit young adults have a greater cardiovascular reserve, and might therefore be able to compensate for blood loss, maintaining their blood pressure until the blood loss is so large that they decompensate, resulting in a precipitous fall in blood pressure.
- Elderly patients have decreased cardiovascular reserve, such that relatively little blood loss can result in shock.
- Pharmacological agents designed to alter pulse rate and blood pressure naturally have an effect on the clinical signs, a common example being beta-blockers such as atenolol, which prevent a compensatory (and diagnostic) tachycardia. Where confusing variables are present, further monitoring modalities (e.g. such as central venous pressure recording) might be indicated to assess the patient's fluid status.

The causes of hypovolaemic shock are primary haemor-rhage, transcellular loss and insensible loss. Primary haemorrhage is defined as haemorrhage occurring within 24 h of surgery. It is generally due to inadequate

Table 4.4   Classification of hypovolaemic shock

	Class I	Class II	Class III	Class IV
Blood loss (mL)	<750	750–1500	1500–2000	>2000
Blood loss (%)	<15	15–30	30–40	>40
Pulse (beats per min)	<100	100–120	>120	>120, thready
Blood pressure	Normal	Normal	Decreased	Decreased
Pulse pressure	Normal	Narrow	Narrow	Narrow
Respiratory rate (breaths per min)	12–20	20–30	30–40	>40
Urine output(mL/h)	>30	20–30	10–20	Minimal
Colour	Normal	Pale	Pale	White
Mental state	Normal	Mildly anxious	Anxious, confused	Confused, drowsy

haemostasis at the time of operation. It can be clinically difficult to decide whether reoperation is required to halt the bleeding and when. Initial non-operative techniques can be tried (e.g. local pressure or reversal of coagulopathy). However, if there is evidence of ongoing bleeding causing shock, attempts should be made to arrest the bleeding.

A key clinical indicator of whether the blood loss is ongoing is the patient's response to fluid resuscitation. Before administering fluid resuscitation, it is important to consider cardiogenic causes of shock, which might be aggravated by further fluid load (see below). Monitoring of the response can be either by simple clinical means such as pulse and blood pressure recording, or by invasive monitoring techniques such as central venous pressure measurements. Three categories of response are classically described:

1. *Rapid response*: intravenous infusion of a fluid bolus, e.g. 2 L normal saline over 2 h, results in a fast, sustained improvement. This generally indicates a loss of less than 20% of circulating volume, without ongoing blood loss.
2. *Transient response*: Fluid bolus initially causes an improvement of clinical measures, although the improvement is not sustained. This indicates ongoing blood loss or inadequate resuscitation. Blood transfusion should be considered, as should measures to control haemorrhage.
3. *Minimal response*: Fluid bolus results in little or no clinical improvement. Blood loss is ongoing at a rate faster than the infusion of fluid. Blood transfusion and measures to arrest bleeding are urgently indicated.

Certain patients are more prone to haemorrhagic complications than others: patients with abnormalities of

blood clotting, such as those on the anticoagulant warfarin, and also those with fragile blood vessels, such as the elderly and patients on long-term corticosteroid therapy.

Transcellular loss can be considerable. An example is loss of fluid into the gastrointestinal tract in cases of bowel obstruction.

Insensible loss, such as fluid loss by sweating, can be greater than usual for patients in the perioperative period. Exposure of usually covered moist organs at surgery, for example, intra-abdominal viscera, can greatly increase fluid loss in this way. Postoperative pyrexia also increases insensible fluid loss.

These losses must be considered when evaluating the amount of fluid required to render the patient normovolaemic.

Cardiogenic shock

Cardiogenic shock occurs when the heart fails to produce sufficient cardiac output to maintain adequate tissue oxygenation, despite normovolaemia and sufficient venous return (Table 4.5).

Impaired contractile strength can be caused by myocardial infarction (MI) or left ventricular failure

Table 4.5   Causes of cardiogenic shock

Impaired contractile strength
  myocardial infarction
  left ventricular failure
Disordered contraction, arrhythmia
  atrial fibrillation
  other arrhythmias

(LVF). MI is the death of an area of cardiac muscle. It is differentiated from myocardial ischaemia in which there is a severe reduction in myocardial perfusion but not muscle death. Such ischaemia occurs, for example, when a patient suffers from angina.

Surgical patients with established ischaemic heart disease are at increased risk of undergoing perioperative MI. This is significantly greater in patients who have had an MI within the 6 months before surgery. As these patients have an increased risk of mortality, elective surgery is not recommended in this period if it can be delayed without undue risk to the patient. Diagnosis of perioperative MI can be difficult because pain is not always a feature, but monitoring during anaesthesia can detect changes in the electrocardiogram (ECG) pattern. Clinical features include the onset of arrhythmias and the symptoms and signs of heart failure.

Treatment of perioperative MI is a difficult clinical problem and specialist cardiology advice should be sought. Standard thrombolytic therapy is contraindicated in the postoperative period because of haemorrhagic problems.

Acute LVF can result from an acute MI or, more commonly, simply in patients with ischaemic heart disease. The diagnosis can be made clinically with breathlessness, elevated jugular venous pulse in the neck, and peripheral oedema. Simple investigations such as chest radiography should be performed. In severe cases, invasive monitoring techniques such as central venous pressure monitoring might be necessary.

Treatment of heart failure includes reduction of fluid load and administration of diuretics such as furosemide (frusemide) and digoxin.

Cardiology advice should be sought in patients who do not respond to standard therapy and further specialised tests might be performed, such as ECHO cardiography or cardiac catheterisation. Such patients probably require care in a high dependency unit. Fluid input and output charts should be kept, with the amount and rate of infusion of intravenous fluids being regulated carefully to prevent excess infusion and the development of cardiac failure.

To function as an efficient pump, the myocardium contracts in a synchronised order. Disorders of this rhythm – dysrhythmias – result in ineffective filling and emptying of the chambers of the heart and therefore in reduced cardiac output. A fundamental distinction in assessment of patients with dysrhythmias is whether there is associated cardiovascular compromise, such as hypotension and shock, or whether the patient is able to compensate and maintain blood pressure.

Atrial fibrillation (AF) is perhaps the most common perioperative dysrhythmia. The diagnosis of AF is divided into those with and without cardiovascular compromise. Most patients know if they have an irregular pulse but are asymptomatic. AF is often detected on admission to the unit when the pulse is noted to be irregular. Some patients, however, are symptomatic, possibly with palpitations, light headedness, syncope or cardiac failure. These patients usually have a rapid, irregular pulse with an uncontrolled ventricular response. As a result, the ventricles do not have time to fill adequately before contraction, causing decreased stroke volume and hence a drop in cardiac output. An ECG is diagnostic and can also show signs of myocardial ischaemia.

Urgency of treatment depends on the presence and degree of complications such as cardiac failure. In surgical wards, rate control is usually achieved by the use of drugs such as digoxin, which can be administered either orally or intravenously. Where digoxin fails to control the heart rate, a number of other antiarrhythmic drugs can be tried.

Many patients have chronic AF with a controlled ventricular rate. Research has demonstrated an outcome benefit of anticoagulation with warfarin for these patients, with a reduction in the incidence of embolic stroke. It is important in such patients to reduce or even stop the warfarin before surgery (Ch. 6).

Many other types of arrhythmia can occur in the postoperative period. Although a description of cardiac arrhythmias is beyond the scope of this chapter, it is important to note that many arrhythmias can result from or be exacerbated by electrolyte imbalance, particularly an abnormal potassium level. Electrolyte levels should be checked regularly and abnormalities corrected (see Ch. 5).

Septic shock

Septic shock is an intermediate-stage complication and is discussed below.

Metabolic complications

The insult of surgery causes an alteration in a number of metabolic processes (see Ch. 5). In particular, this can cause problems in diabetic patients. Requirements for insulin can change because patients have to fast. In

17

addition to this, however, the production of endogenous insulin and its effectiveness (end-organ resistance) are altered. As a result, blood glucose levels might be erratic. It is vital that this is controlled accurately. In this situation, for short-term control, diabetes is frequently regulated by the intravenous use of glucose, insulin and potassium.

Pain

One of the main reasons a patient might be reluctant to consider surgery is the thought of postoperative pain. The principles of pain control are dealt with in Chapter 23. However, it is worth considering briefly here, as there are some pathophysiological consequences of ineffective pain control.

Pain results in increased sympathetic activity, causing increased heart rate, vasoconstriction and hypertension. This produces an increased demand for cardiac work and the oxygen supply might not be sufficient to meet this demand. Pain can therefore reduce cardiovascular reserve and predispose to cardiovascular complications.

Intermediate-stage complications

Intermediate-stage complications are listed in Table 4.6 and are considered in turn.

Deep venous thrombosis (DVT)

Venous thromboembolism is a leading cause of preventable postoperative mortality. Clots form in the veins of the lower leg or in the pelvic veins during surgery.

Classically, the patient presents with symptoms of a deep vein thrombosis (DVT) between postoperative days 5 and 7, although it can occur at any stage. A number of factors predispose patients to DVT in the postoperative period (Table 4.7). The degree of risk varies between different operations, being very low in some but up to 40–50% in other operations, such as knee replacements.

Prophylaxis

Surgery predisposes patients to thromboembolism and prophylactic measures are essential. Most units will have a protocol indicating prophylactic measures to be employed for different operations. Patients will be categorised into low, intermediate and high risk; depending on the patient, the surgery and other factors as listed in Table 4.7. A suitable combination of measures will then be employed. Prophylactic measures are either mechanical or pharmacological.

Mechanical

Thromboembolic deterrent stockings (TEDS) provide graduated calf compression in an attempt to reduce venous stasis in the lower leg. TEDS can be either calf or full length.

AV boots are pneumatic devices attached to the patient's feet that intermittently dorsiflex and plantarflex, mimicking the venous pump action of the weight-bearing foot. These can be used postoperatively in high-risk patients.

Flotron boots are attached to the patient's calves intraoperatively. Inflation compresses the calf, producing

Table 4.6 Intermediate-stage complications of surgery
Deep venous thrombosis (DVT)
Pulmonary embolism
Secondary bleeding
Respiratory complications
Line infection
Urinary retention and urinary tract infection (UTI)
Sepsis
Systemic inflammatory response syndrome (SIRS)
Anaemia
Gastrointestinal ileus
Pressure sores

Table 4.7 Factors predisposing to deep venous thrombosis (DVT)
Immobility
Blood viscosity
Local trauma
Intraoperative blood stasis
Malignancy
Infection
Oral contraceptive pill
Pregnancy
Air travel
Thrombophilia
Previous DVT/pulmonary embolus
Cardiac failure
Inflammatory bowel disease

venous flow in the leg, similar to that induced by calf muscles in the process of walking.

Movement and early mobilisation are also important. All patients should be actively encouraged to move their feet and lower legs whilst still confined to bed. Mobilisation is important as soon as the underlying pathology and operation allow.

Pharmacological

Heparin is a mixture of polysaccharide substances with varying molecular weights that inhibits thrombosis by potentiating the action of antithrombin III. For DVT prophylaxis, low-dose subcutaneous heparin (e.g. 5000 international units (IU) twice a day) can be used. Monitoring of levels of anticoagulation is not necessary.

Low molecular weight heparin (LMWH) is thought to be more effective than standard heparin and is gradually replacing this. Standard heparin is enzymatically degraded into smaller molecules, which have a different anticoagulant effect. LMWH results in a reduced risk of bleeding complications. Also beneficial is the longer half-life, such that administration is only necessary once a day.

Aspirin has an antiplatelet action and therefore anti-thrombotic activity. However, its effects must be balanced against the adverse effects of gastrointestinal ulceration and precipitation of renal failure, particularly in elderly patients.

Clinical features

The majority of patients with DVT are asymptomatic and therefore might remain undiagnosed. Symptomatic DVT causes swelling and pain in the affected leg. This can be associated with engorged superficial veins and warmth with a tense and tender calf.

Irrespective of whether symptomatic or asymptomatic, a clot can be cast off from a DVT and float freely in the circulation until it lodges in the pulmonary vessels. This is known as a pulmonary embolus (PE) and can be the cause of sudden collapse and unexpected postoperative death.

Investigation

Clinical diagnosis is notoriously unreliable, with accuracy figures of around 50% even for experienced clinicians. Radiological imaging is essential to determine the extent of the clot and hence appropriate treatment. Venography is the gold standard, demonstrating all clots including those below the knee. However, this technique is very invasive and painful and there is evidence that it might potentiate further clotting. Doppler ultrasound scan is non-invasive and is good for detecting thigh thrombosis, which are arguably the clinically significant ones.

Treatment

Treatment is instituted to prevent propagation and embolism of the clot while the body's inherent thrombolytic mechanisms dissolve the clot that has already formed. The fact that DVTs situated solely below the knee are at low risk of embolisation very much influences the extent of treatment needed for these. In this situation, the need for anticoagulation is debatable.

Where anticoagulation is required (especially with thigh or pelvic vein thrombosis) this can be induced rapidly by intravenous heparin administered by a infusion pump. Longer-term anticoagulation is achieved by the use of the oral anticoagulant warfarin. How long therapy is continued depends on the patient's circumstances, but 3 months is a frequent length of time. Patients with recur-rent DVT/PE might require life long anticoagulation.

Pulmonary embolus (PE)

Aetiology

The majority of PE arise from thrombi in systemic veins as described above, emboli passing through the right heart chambers and lodging in the narrow calibre pulmonary arterioles or capillaries. Rarely the embolus can arise from the right chambers of the heart itself, for example, resulting from AF.

Pathophysiology

The effects of a PE depend entirely on the size of the clot. A large clot can block the total circulation from the heart causing cardiac arrest. Smaller emboli block blood flow to the alveoli of the affected part of the lung. This area of lung continues to be ventilated but is no longer perfused, resulting in a block of gas transfer to and from the bloodstream. With a larger embolus, blood pressure in the pulmonary circulation increases (increased resistance) and venous return to the left side of the heart is reduced with a consequent drop in cardiac output.

Clinical features

Clinical features are variable and relate to the amount and size of emboli. Small emboli can be asymptomatic, might cause a shortness of breath, or might induce a cardiac arrhythmia such as AF. Death of the affected area of lung tissue is known as infarction and is generally prevented in the case of small emboli by collateral supply from the bronchial blood vessels. Clinical signs are usually minimal.

However, moderate-sized emboli can cause lung infarction with the accompanying symptoms of pain, haemoptysis and more severe shortness of breath. Where infarction has occurred a pleural rub may be present on auscultation.

Large and massive PE constitutes a medical emergency and resuscitation might be required. Prevention of blood reaching alveoli results in profound hypoxaemia, and prevention of venous return to the left side of the heart can give a precipitous fall in cardiac output, shock and cardiac arrest. Signs are those suggesting outflow obstruction from the right side of the heart.

Investigation

Electrocardiogram (ECG)

ECG changes are not diagnostic. Most frequently there is sinus tachycardia. There might or might not be signs of right heart strain such as right bundle branch block.

Arterial blood gas analysis

Arterial blood gas analysis demonstrates hypoxaemia, often with hypocapnia, the result of increased respiratory drive 'blowing off' more carbon dioxide.

Radiology

A chest radiograph is rarely diagnostic. Most changes seen are non-specific with opacification secondary to atelectasis and possibly a pleural effusion. Larger emboli can result in a visible cut-off in the pulmonary artery, and lack of vascular pattern distal to this. Wedge-shaped pulmonary infarcts might be visible.

A ventilation/perfusion (V/Q) scan

Labelled isotopes are separately administered at the same time by inspiration and by intravenous injection. The perfusion (Q) and ventilation (V) of the lungs can then be compared, a PE producing a mismatch where an area is ventilated but not perfused. This picture is frequently obscured because, after a period of decreased blood supply, alveoli tend to collapse, resulting in reduced ventilation as well as perfusion. As a result, the results of V/Q scans can be indeterminate.

Angiography

Pulmonary artery angiography is the gold standard, directly visualising emboli. It is, however, technically difficult and invasive.

Computed tomographic (CT) pulmonary angiogram

The advent of spiral computerised tomography (CT), used in conjunction with intravenous contrast, has led to a widespread role for this non-invasive, sensitive test for PE.

Treatment

Prevention of further clot/emboli

The patient requires immediate anticoagulation with intravenous heparin. Low molecular weight heparin is now licensed for use in PE. However, conventional heparin infusion has some advantage in perioperative patients: namely (1) its effect is easily monitored using activated partial thromboplastin time (APTT); and (2) it can be reversed rapidly with protamine, should the patient develop life-threatening bleeding complications of surgery.

Oral anticoagulation with warfarin is indicated for a variable period. Patients who are unable to comply with or tolerate warfarin anticoagulation, or those who continue to have PEs despite a therapeutic dose of warfarin as monitored by the international normalized ratio (INR), might be suitable for a caval filter. This is a mechanical filter placed percutaneously through a neck vein into the inferior vena cava, which 'catches' emboli from the leg veins en route to the right side of the heart.

Removal of clot

Fibrinolytic therapy such as streptokinase (thrombolysis) might be indicated for patients with large PE. This is contraindicated in the postoperative period because of haemorrhagic complications. Surgical embolectomy is rarely required but is an alternative for life-threatening PE where thrombolysis is contraindicated.

Secondary bleeding

Secondary bleeding is defined as bleeding occurring more than 24 h after surgery. It has a number of causes, including dissolution of a clot sealing a blood vessel and erosion or unravelling of a haemostatic ligature. Secondary bleeding is rarely as significant as primary haemorrhage, but it can result in hypovolaemic shock and occasionally requires reoperation.

Respiratory complications

Respiratory complications are perhaps the most common postoperative complication. Their severity is a spectrum from an asymptomatic pyrexia to life-threatening pulmonary failure. The causes of respiratory complications are listed in Table 4.8.

A patient's risk of undergoing a respiratory complication depends on the underlying condition of his or her lungs and the circumstances they are exposed to. Smoking has a significant impact because smokers are predisposed to bronchitis and emphysema, ischaemic heart disease and heart failure. The normal action of the mucociliary apparatus in the tracheobronchial tree is to clear secretions and this is significantly affected in smokers.

Atelectasis

Atelectasis describes a degree of alveolar collapse that occurs after relative hypoventilation, inability to cough and suppressed ciliary action during general anaesthesia. Small mucus plugs block the alveoli causing them to collapse. Postoperatively, patients may develop a cough and a mild transient pyrexia. Deep breathing exercises, which might require supplementation with chest physio-therapy, clear the mucus plugs. It is important to do this because unresolved collapse and mucus clearance predispose to bacterial superinfection.

Lower respiratory tract infection (LRTI)

Microbial colonisation of the lung parenchyma causes inflammation, termed pneumonia or LRTI, where again a wide spectrum of severity is encountered.

By far the most common pathogens are bacteria, although other pathogens such as fungi can cause problems particularly in the severely ill patient requiring multiple system support. The bacteria implicated are numerous. Oropharyngeal and particularly tracheal instrumentation for anaesthesia introduce bacteria into the airways, which are normally relatively sterile. 'Community' and hospital acquired (nosocomial) bacteria can also be introduced to the patient's airways, where they colonise retained mucus. A full account of pneumonias is not in the scope of this chapter, but the principles of diagnosis and treatment are essential to any surgeon's practice. Pneumonia can be classified according to pathogen or anatomical site affected.

Clinical features

Patients develop a combination of symptoms of varying severity, including cough, production of discoloured sputum, pleuritic chest pain, shortness of breath, tachypnoea and pyrexia. Chest examination might reveal localised areas of decreased chest wall movement, dullness to percussion and auscultation reveals a combination of decreased air entry, crepitations and bronchial breathing.

Diagnosis

A radiograph can demonstrate areas of consolidation or associated features such as pleural effusion. Radiographic changes might take some weeks to clear after the pneumonia has clinically resolved.

Blood tests

The white cell count is usually raised, although there are exceptions, especially in elderly or immunosuppressed patients. Arterial blood gas analysis reveals abnormalities, particularly of partial pressure of oxygen, which will help direct supportive therapy.

Table 4.8 Causes of respiratory complications of surgery
Atelectasis
Lower respiratory tract infections
Aspiration
Adult respiratory distress syndrome (ARDS)
Pulmonary embolus
Pneumothorax

Sputum culture

It is fundamental to try to isolate the infecting organism, so that appropriate antibiotics can be given. This is not always possible, and repeated cultures and multiple changes in antibiotic treatment might be required.

Treatment

General supportive treatment should be instituted quickly. Oxygen should be administered at a concentration guided by blood gas analysis. Saline nebulisers and aggressive chest physiotherapy help to clear the consolidation. The patient should be sat up in bed to improve ventilation/perfusion matching. Bronchodilators may be indicated where there is evidence of some reversible airway narrowing such as a wheeze.

Antibiotic best-guess therapy should be started at the time of diagnosis. At this stage, culture results are not available and therapy should be directed at organisms that are most likely to be involved. This might involve the use of more than one antibiotic, and the combined therapy has a broader spectrum of activity than a single drug. Targeted therapy should be tailored accordingly when results of sensitivities from sputum culture are available. Where severe chest infection occurs, or in cases that are failing to resolve, the input of chest physicians is invaluable.

Aspiration

The protective airway reflexes that prevent inhalation of substances from the gastrointestinal tract in the fully conscious patient are depressed by general anaesthesia. Inhalation of regurgitated gastric contents is known as aspiration and results in a potentially virulent form of pneumonia. Appropriate antibiotics should be given to cover gastrointestinal bacteria. The acid and digestive juices from the stomach also contribute in causing a severe chemical pneumonitis.

Adult respiratory distress syndrome (ARDS)

ARDS is a syndrome resulting in lung failure. It is characterised by respiratory distress, hypoxaemia that is difficult to treat, decreased lung compliance and diffuse pulmonary infiltrates. Its precise aetiology is not clear, but is probably involved in a systemic inflammatory response syndrome (SIRS). As such, it essentially constitutes 'lung failure' and frequently precedes or is part of a multiorgan failure syndrome (MOFS)

There are many known precipitants of ARDS, and effective treatment of these in an attempt to prevent ARDS occurring, is the best form of management. Treatment other than that of the underlying cause is supportive, with the administration of oxygen often requiring mechanical ventilation, careful fluid balance and monitoring of cardiovascular parameters to minimise pulmonary oedema. The prognosis for established ARDS is poor, with figures quoted of around 50% mortality.

Pulmonary embolus and pneumothorax

These conditions have been discussed above.

Line infection

Surgical patients tend to have numerous lines inserted perioperatively. Intravascular lines that are inserted percutaneously have an inherent risk of becoming infected, predominantly with skin flora. Certain bacteria have an affinity for sticking to the synthetic material of the cannulae. It is important that all lines are inserted with an aseptic technique and adequately prepared skin. Lines should be inspected regularly for signs of infection and replaced where necessary. Lines should be removed as soon as they are no longer required. Blood cultures, taken from a line that is suspected as a source of sepsis and also from a peripheral vein, can help elucidate if the line is the cause.

Urinary retention and urinary tract infection (UTI)

Both men and women are at increased risk of UTI postoperatively, predominantly due to urinary tract instrumentation. Males who have any prostatic symptoms preoperatively are at risk of developing postoperative urinary retention; preoperative bladder catheterisation should be considered. Urinary catheters are commonly inserted before major surgery to ensure accurate measurement of postoperative urine output. This aids the monitoring of fluid balance and makes nursing care of the patient easier. Catheters should be inserted under an aseptic technique.

Patients with catheters in situ are at risk of urinary infections but might be asymptomatic because of the catheter. Pyrexia and cloudy urine should alert the clinician. A specimen of urine should be sent for culture and sensitivity and an appropriate antibiotic started while awaiting the results. Where metal implants have been used, as in total hip replacement, prophylactic antibiotics are commonly used while the patient has a urinary catheter in situ, or, alternatively, individual doses are given at insertion and removal of the catheter. This is in an attempt to prevent blood-borne spread of the urinary tract pathogens to the prosthesis, with potential implant failure.

Sepsis

Sources of postoperative infection are multiple, the most common ones having been dealt with above, and are discussed in detail in Chapter 8. Other causes are specific to particular operations or types of surgery, such as intra-abdominal sepsis due to a leaking intestinal anastomosis, meningitis after breach of the meninges and deep-seated prosthetic infection in arthroplasty surgery. Often, the only overt symptom is pyrexia and a thorough, systematic search for the cause is needed, bearing in mind that it may not be infective (e.g. DVT). Failure to identify a cause should be met by starting the process again, reculturing specimens and widening the search to more obscure causes. Early diagnosis and treatment of infective complications is necessary to prevent progression to septicaemia and septic shock. Pathogens spread from the site of initial infection to the bloodstream, where they multiply, resulting in septicaemia and spread to any part of the body.

Septic shock

The presence of bacteria in the bloodstream, particularly those that possess endotoxin (Gram-negative bacteria), has a profound effect on the cardiovascular system and can induce septic shock. There is a complex interaction between the pathogen and host via multiple mediator systems. By a complex process, endotoxin induces increased permeability and reduced vascular tone in blood vessels by direct damage to the endothelial lining. This results in a profound decrease in peripheral vascular resistance, and hence hypotension. A greatly increased cardiac output is required to maintain adequate tissue oxygenation, and might not be achieved, causing shock.

Classically, therefore, the patient has warm peripheries and a large cardiac output. This, however, assumes adequate intravascular volume and fluid resuscitation is often necessary before these features are seen.

Septic shock has a high mortality rate (up to 50%) and often requires the support afforded in an intensive care unit. Septic shock often precedes, and can even be the cause of, multiorgan failure, which in part explains its high mortality.

Systemic inflammatory response syndrome (SIRS)

The term SIRS has been coined to describe this common pathophysiological state and its clinical features. The complex mixture of chemicals produced by the host in response to severe sepsis has been implicated as the pathophysiological cause of septic shock and its complications. Similar host responses might occur as a result of other, non-infective, insults to the patient such as major trauma, burns and pancreatitis. Multiorgan failure can be precipitated, with a high mortality.

Anaemia

Blood loss at operation results in a fall in haemoglobin concentration. Unless the haemoglobin is replaced, the blood has a decreased oxygen carrying capacity with wide-ranging effects including decreased cardiovascular reserve and impaired wound healing. Oral iron therapy is given for mild to moderate postoperative anaemia. Lower levels of haemoglobin, or cases where oxygen delivery must be maximised (coexisting disease, or concurrent complication), should be restored with blood transfusion.

Gastrointestinal ileus

The insult of abdominal surgery can result in temporary intestinal dysfunction and lack of contraction and peristalsis. Although this is particularly the case for intra-abdominal surgery, it can occur in any severely ill patient especially those with deranged blood electrolytes. When this occurs, nutrition might need to be given by an alternative route, and this is discussed in Chapter 5.

Pressure sores

Breakdown of the skin over an area where pressure has been applied too long is a common postoperative problem. Pressure sores can become infected and cause sepsis, or grow to involve a significant area of skin. Prevention is the key, as these lesions are notoriously difficult to treat once established. Expert nursing care is required from an early stage.

Patients with increased risk of pressure sores are those with severe immobility, altered skin sensation, such as those with spinal cord lesions, and those with poor skin quality such as the elderly and those on corticosteroid therapy.

Late-stage complications

The main aim of surgery is to return the patient to his or her previous good state of health. For numerous reasons this might never be achieved. Apart from a failure to 'cure' a patient's illness, other patient factors can play a role in the development of long-term disability

Psychological

A minority of patients has difficulty adjusting to illness and the fact they have had to have an operation. Naturally, this depends on the extent of surgery and the disease process that has necessitated it. In extreme cases, this attitude can result in adoption of the 'sick role', with abnormal conceptions of health and healthcare-seeking behaviour. Support groups and psychiatric services can be beneficial.

Pain

Chronic pain syndromes can occur postoperatively for complex reasons. Where simple measures are unsuccessful, referral to a pain team might be indicated.

Specific complications

Operation-specific complications are generally considered when discussing that operation. It is helpful to maintain a framework into which specific complications can fit. These are listed in Table 4.9.

Local complications

Local complications related to the wound are listed in Table 4.10 and are discussed in detail in Chapter 3. The temporal classification of local complications of surgery is also listed in Table 4.10.

Table 4.9   Specific complications of surgical operations
Approach used
Surrounding structures might be damaged accidentally or sacrificed by necessity
Hazards of repairs made, including complications of wound closure
Risks associated with materials implanted
Effect of removal of diseased tissue

Table 4.10   Local complications of surgery
Early
damage to surrounding structures
haematoma/bruising
Intermediate
wound infection
wound dehiscence
wound seroma
breakdown of repair
failure of implant
Late
abnormal wound healing
loss of function
psychological

Early complications

Damage to surrounding structures

A detailed knowledge of anatomy is necessary to avoid unnecessary damage to nearby structures and plan suitable surgical approaches. Patients should be warned of the side-effects of damage to structures liable to be affected such as scrotal paraesthesia following damage to the ilioinguinal nerve in revision inguinal herniorrhaphy.

Haematoma/bruising

Patients can be alarmed by bruising around the wound. Bruising and haematoma formation cause pain and predispose to wound complications including infection.

Intermediate complications

Complications relating to the surgical wound itself are discussed in Chapter 3. Other complications are discussed below.

Surgical repairs made during the operation can fail for a number of reasons, including patient factors (poor healing), inadequate surgical technique and failure of materials used to carry out the repair. The expected results of repair breakdown should be considered and the patient observed closely for these, followed by appropriate investigations. The action required once repair failure has been ascertained varies widely between types of repair and the extent of failure.

An enormous range of surgical implants is available, all with their own idiosyncrasies. However, they can fail for a number of common reasons, for example, incorrect application results in forces being applied that the implant is unable to cope with. Material defects occur occasionally and design faults can take up to several years to become apparent and be corrected. Synthetic materials are prone to infection, which often leads to failure, and prophylaxis might be required.

Late complications

Abnormal wound healing

Hypertrophic and keloid scarring are discussed in Chapter 3.

Loss of function

Where diseased tissue has been removed, the previous function of that area is either compensated for by another area, or the patient suffers effects of loss of function. This is an expected side-effect of surgery, rather than a complication *per se*, but often requires symptomatic treatment.

Psychological complications

Psychological problems often relate to loss of function and any disability that arises from this. Obviously, this varies enormously between operations and should be borne in mind preoperatively, especially for high-risk operations such as limb amputations. The patient should be directed to suitable support groups.

5 Fluid balance, metabolism and nutrition

Fluid and electrolyte balance

The fluid in the body is separated into different 'compartments' – the intracellular compartment (within the cells) and the extracellular compartment, which is further subdivided into interstitial (between the cells) and intravascular (in the blood vessels) – and in each of these areas the concentration of salts, or electrolytes, differs. These variations are subject to highly complex control mechanisms and this degree of tight control is essential to maintain efficient cell function. Abnormalities of fluid and electrolyte concentrations can induce life-threatening cellular dysfunction, e.g. cardiac arrhythmias.

The body normally maintains excellent electrolyte balance, better than any doctor could hope to achieve by careful fluid and electrolyte infusions, and in this regard the kidneys play a vital role. However, as with any body system, diseases occur that prevent normal homeostasis. In addition, during the perioperative period, patients are subjected to a number of exogenous influences, for example, fasting and intravenous fluid administration, which can outstrip the body's normal homeostatic capabilities. As a result, great care needs to be taken at this time with regard to fluid and electrolyte administration, and careful monitoring of electrolyte levels in the body is needed.

A consideration of the principles of electrolytes balance will be followed by a discussion of normal homeostatic mechanisms, abnormalities of body water and electrolytes and finally, a further discussion of fluid replacement and acid–base balance as listed in Table 5.1.

Principles of electrolyte balance

Some common principles apply when considering homeostasis of any electrolyte. These are based on a number of factors:

Table 5.1   Fluid and electrolyte balance
Principles of electrolyte balance
Normal homeostasis
fluid compartments
barriers between compartments
homeostatic mechanisms
Abnormalities of body water
dehydration
fluid overload
Abnormalities of electrolytes
sodium
potassium
Fluid replacement
Acid–base balance
abnormalities
compensation

- *Distribution and barriers*: it is important to know the normal concentration of an electrolyte in any given fluid compartment. Fundamental to this is an appreciation of how a concentration gradient between compartments is maintained and can be manipulated.
- *Output*: it is necessary to know the amount of the electrolyte that is consumed each day through normal cellular and systemic functions, and also how much is lost normally by excretion.
- *Intake*: the amount of the electrolyte that needs to be acquired to maintain normal concentrations of the electrolyte in the body should be balanced with the amounts actually taken in. Any inefficiency in uptake, either lack or excess from the method of administration, needs to be noted and corrected.

Normal homeostasis

Fluid compartments

A patient's body water content depends on the constitution of that person's body. This varies according to

Table 5.2 Fluid compartments (70-kg man)	
Intracellular fluid (ICF)	28 L
Extracellular fluid (ECF)	14 L
interstitial fluid	10.5 L
intravascular fluid	3.5 L

age, sex and percentage of body fat, and can range from 50 to 75% of body weight. For simplicity an account of an average 70 kg man is given.

A 70 kg man is 60% water, and therefore contains 70 kg × 0.6 = 42 L water (1 L weighs 1 kg). This is distributed between the two main compartments as shown in Table 5.2.

There are a number of other small extracellular compartments, which are of less clinical relevance with regards to salt and water homeostasis, namely transcellular water (e.g. cerebrospinal fluid) and water associated with bone and dense connective tissue.

Barriers between compartments, osmolality and electrolyte concentrations

Osmolality (measured in milliOsmoles; mOsm) is defined as the strength of a solution. It is derived from the amount of active ions in that solution. Cations are positively charged ions and anions are negatively charged. In each body compartment, there is normally a balance between cations and anions. The main extracellular cation is sodium (Na^{2+}) and the main intracellular cation is potassium (K^+). The osmolality of plasma is derived from the equation:

$$2 \times sodium\ (Na) + urea + glucose$$

The normal range is 280–290 mOsm/L. This value allows the clinician to estimate whether the patient has a relative excess or lack of water in the body and can be measured easily clinically.

The above equation is an approximation only because, although sodium is the main extracellular cation, various factors can affect plasma osmolality, causing inaccuracies that must be noted clinically. The presence of an exogenous, osmotically active molecule such as alcohol in the blood is a good example, and the body will try to maintain the correct osmolality of plasma by recruitment of water from the intracellular compartment.

The intracellular and extracellular fluid are separated by the cell membrane. This acts as a semipermeable membrane, allowing free passage of water but not electrolytes. Because of the difference in concentration of electrolytes between the two compartments, water will move from the compartment with lower osmolality to that with higher osmolality, therefore diluting it. This is known as an osmolality gradient

To maintain the differences in ions between intracellular and extracellular fluids, sodium ions are constantly driven from the intracellular compartment by a pump mechanism, which actively drives them out in exchange for potassium ions. The enzyme involved in this active pumping mechanism is ATPase, and thus this process is known as the ATPase exchange pump. As a result sodium is the major extracellular cation and potassium is the major intracellular cation. To maintain the balance of electrical charge, chloride (Cl^-) is associated with sodium ions outside the cell and potassium is balanced mainly by the anion phosphate (PO_4^{2-}) and anionic protein inside the cell.

In the extracellular compartment, intravascular and interstitial fluid are separated by the endothelium or blood vessel membrane, which, at capillary level, is one cell thick. Fluid balance between these two compartments is determined by hydrostatic or blood pressure forcing fluid out from the intravascular area, and oncotic pressure sucking fluid in. The endothelium is freely permeable to small molecules such as sodium and potassium ions, and relatively impermeable to the larger protein molecules in the plasma. As a result, there is a protein concentration gradient across the endothelium, caused mainly by the plasma protein albumin, which has an appreciable effect on water movement between the compartments. Again, fluid moves towards the area of highest concentration and this is called oncotic or colloid osmotic pressure.

Homeostatic mechanisms

Sodium regulation

The volume of extracellular fluid (ECF) relates directly to the total amount of sodium in the body, the vast majority of which is extracellular. The concentration of sodium is maintained between narrow limits by free transfer of water between the ECF and the intracellular fluid (ICF). Hence, a large amount of total sodium, held in the extracellular compartment, recruits water from the ICF, increasing the volume of the ECF and diluting the sodium such that it is maintained at a normal concentration.

Control of total body sodium therefore relates directly to control of ECF volume. This is subject to homeostatic mechanisms that are both renal and extrarenal in origin, but ultimately alter sodium excretion by the kidney.

Sodium is ultrafiltrated by the glomerulus of the kidney; the rate of this process (the glomerular filtration rate; GFR) relates directly to renal plasma flow (RPF) or renal blood flow. Renal blood flow, like the flow of blood to the brain, is autoregulated such that this is constant within a range of systemic blood pressures. The majority of the filtered sodium is resorbed in the renal tubules, mainly in the proximal tubule with fine tuning occurring in the distal tubule.

Renal mechanisms can involve blood flow or sodium concentration. Changes in renal blood flow alter GFR and hence the amount of sodium that is filtered.

Blood flow to the glomeruli of the kidney is monitored via receptors in the afferent arterioles. Changes in perfusion activate messenger systems in the arterioles, which alter the renal vascular tone and correct the abnormality in blood flow. This process is known as 'autoregulation' and attempts to maintain the glomerular perfusion as a constant.

One of the factors involved in autoregulation is local production of prostaglandins, which alter arteriole wall tone. This is an important precipitant of renal failure, particularly in elderly surgical patients with decreased renal reserve. The administration of non-steroidal anti-inflammatory drugs (NSAIDs) impairs the patient's ability to produce prostaglandins and hence regulate renal blood flow.

Changes in renal blood flow also result in modulation of the renin–angiotensin–aldosterone system. Renin is produced in the juxtaglomerular apparatus in the kidney. A drop in renal perfusion pressure results in release of renin into the systemic circulation. This in turn results in conversion of angiotensinogen to angiotensin I and then to angiotensin II, which in turn results in release of aldosterone by the adrenal glands.

Aldosterone causes increased permeability of the distal renal tubules to sodium and, as a result, more sodium is reabsorbed, with resultant increased loss of potassium. The sodium pulls water with it back into the circulation, causing salt and water retention and a consequent rise in blood pressure.

Extrarenal mechanisms can also occur via the mechanisms of autoregulation of blood flow as described above; the renal circulation is relatively detached from the general vascular tone. However, volume receptors present in the great vessels in the chest have an effect on renal perfusion via the sympathetic nervous system. Additionally, activation of stretch receptors in the right atrium causes release of a hormone called atrial natriuretic factor. This peptide causes increased sodium excretion by reducing sodium resorption in the distal tubule. Hence, sodium and accompanying water is excreted, resulting in a fall in the ECF volume.

Potassium regulation

Potassium excretion and secretion by the kidney is intimately associated with sodium reabsorption. Nearly all the potassium that is filtered in the glomerulus is reabsorbed in conjunction with sodium (cotransporter) in the proximal nephron. In the distal tubule the reabsorption of sodium causes an electrochemical gradient, resulting in secretion of potassium (and hydrogen ions). Therefore, the more sodium that is reabsorbed, under the action of aldosterone, the more potassium is excreted.

Water regulation

As described above the main determinate of water reabsorption is the osmotic drive associated with sodium reabsorption. There is capacity for fine-tuning of water reabsorption, independent of sodium, which occurs in the most distal part of the nephron, called the collecting duct. The hormone antidiuretic hormone (ADH) is produced by the posterior part of the pituitary gland. Its release is influenced by numerous factors including plasma osmolality, stress, surgery and thirst. ADH increases the permeability of the collecting duct to water, increasing its reabsorption. This results in water conservation by the body and is the basis of the ability to concentrate urine. The stress of surgery results in increased ADH release, causing a degree of water retention.

Normal daily water losses in a healthy 70-kg man are listed in Table 5.3. These losses are balanced by an intake

Table 5.3 Normal daily water losses (70-kg man)	
Gastrointestinal (faeces)	100 mL
Respiration	500 mL
Insensible (latent evaporation from skin)	700 mL
Urine	1700 mL (variable, depending on fluid status)
Total	3000 mL

Table 5.4 Normal daily water intake sources	
Ingested fluids	1750 mL
Food	900 mL
Metabolism	350 mL
Total	3000 mL

Table 5.5   Causes of dehydration
Insufficient fluid intake
Excess loss of fluid
Haemorrhage
Diarrhoea, bowel obstruction, bowel preparation
Vomiting
Fistulae
Diuresis
Insensible losses
Respiratory

of about 3 L water per day from the sources in Table 5.4. These amounts can be drastically different in the conditions described below, where the correct amount of fluid to be administered is guided by monitoring fluid output and electrolyte concentrations in the blood.

Abnormalities of body water

Dehydration

In the case of water or electrolyte deficiency the kidney is acted upon by numerous systems (as discussed briefly above) to prevent further excess loss while maintaining adequate waste product excretion. However, in extreme circumstances these compensatory mechanisms are outstripped, causing shrinkage of the body fluid compartments. Insufficient fluid in the interstitial space results in loss of skin turgor. Shrinkage of the intravascular volume causes circulatory changes, which, in extreme cases, can result in shock. Relative hypovolaemia can occur in conditions affecting vascular tone, such as septic shock (see Ch. 4).

Monitoring of the intravascular fluid is achieved by clinical examination and particularly by measurement of heart rate and blood pressure. Invasive monitoring of the central venous pressure is helpful in severe cases or those with confounding variables. The causes of dehydration are listed in Table 5.5 and are now discussed in turn.

Insufficient intake

Failure to match fluid output with sufficient intake results in dehydration. This is a common danger in surgical practice, with patients undergoing periods of starvation due to disease processes, preoperative preparation and postoperative recovery. Examples are found in all branches of surgery and include inability to swallow (coma, oral disease) and enforced starvation (prior to anaesthesia, postoperative resting of the gastrointestinal tract). Adequate input is maintained with intravenous fluids, guided by output monitoring and electrolyte measurement, bearing in mind that a pre-existing deficit must be compensated for.

Excess loss

Common surgical procedures, diseases and complications cause an abnormally high fluid loss. The principles for management of these are the same. Treatment should be directed at the underlying cause, in an attempt to decrease future losses. Supportive replacement therapy is determined by measuring the amount and type of fluid loss, with special note being made of its electrolyte concentration so that appropriate loss can be corrected. Direct analysis of the electrolyte concentration of the fluid lost (by laboratory testing) can be helpful.

Haemorrhage

Bleeding can lead to a fluid deficit that requires replacement, the principles of which are considered in the section on shock (see Ch. 4).

Diarrhoea, bowel obstruction and bowel preparation

Gastrointestinal secretions are rich in solutes and the increased losses occurring in the above conditions can need aggressive replacement. When the bowel is obstructed, the fluids do not leave the body but accumulate in the gut lumen, outside the extracellular fluid compartment. This is known as a third-space loss.

Vomiting

Vomitus is also solute rich. In addition, it is highly acidic and the loss of hydrogen ions has an important effect on acid–base balance in the body.

Fistulae

Gastrointestinal fistulae bypass the capability of fluid reabsorption further down the gastrointestinal tract.

Losses therefore, particularly from high fistulae and particularly to the skin, can be large and solute rich.

Diuresis: drugs and renal disease

Diuretic drugs used for the treatment of fluid overload (see below) can be overeffective and result in dehydration by losses into the urine. Similarly, a number of renal diseases, including common disorders such as diabetic nephropathy, result in production of excess amounts of urine.

Insensible losses

Losses through the skin can be significant. A common example is pyrexia, whereby water evaporates from the surface using latent heat of evaporation.

Massive amounts of plasma are lost from the surface of burns, and one of the mainstays of burns management is fluid resuscitation.

Respiratory losses

The tachypnoea and pyrexia of respiratory complications of surgery can result in appreciable fluid loss.

Fluid overload and oedema

Excess body water occurs in several disease processes. The symptoms depend on the cause and the compartment in which the excess fluid is distributed (Table 5.6).

Excess intake

By far the most common cause of fluid overload in surgical practice is excessive intravenous administration. This is more likely to occur in patients with pre-existing renal and cardiovascular disease, and such patients therefore require careful thought about their fluid regime and may need close monitoring modalities. Maintenance of accurate fluid balance charts is essential. In such

Table 5.6   Causes of fluid overload
Excess intake
Decreased loss
Renal disease
Liver disease

patients, generalised oedema and acute heart failure can be easily precipitated.

Decreased loss

Several medical conditions result in pathophysiological salt and water retention. They are of relevance to surgical practice as these patients might require surgical intervention, where inappropriate fluid management can exacerbate their condition. The altered cardiovascular dynamics of cardiac failure results in pathophysiological alterations in the renin–angiotensin–aldosterone axis, causing salt and water retention and further increases in venous pressure.

A low plasma albumin concentration – hypoalbuminaemia – results in a decreased colloid osmotic pressure of the blood. This results in more fluid shifting into the interstitial space, causing peripheral oedema. This fluid is lost from the intravascular space and results in activation of mechanisms effecting salt and water retention.

Renal disease

Diseases that reduce the glomerular filtration rate result in an impaired ability to excrete sodium. Complex interactions are seen in many renal diseases that alter tubular reabsorption of sodium and lead to retention of sodium and its accompanying water.

Liver disease

Patients with cirrhosis have raised portal venous pressure, causing similar changes to those seen in cardiac failure and hence salt and water retention. Many of these conditions require tight fluid restriction. In those patients who become overloaded with fluid, reduction in body water is achieved predominantly with diuretic drugs, of which there are several different classes with different mechanisms of action.

A commonly used class of drugs is loop diuretics, e.g. furosemide (frusemide), the main effect of which is to block the sodium–chloride cotransporter in the loop of Henle. This results in an increased sodium load in the distal tubules. The tubule attempts to reabsorb this extra sodium, at the expense of excreting potassium and hydrogen ions, but its capacity is not sufficient and more salt and water is lost to the urine. As a result, the major side-effects of furosemide (frusemide) therapy are hypokalaemia, metabolic alkalosis and the effects of overaction (i.e. salt and water depletion).

Abnormalities of electrolytes

Sodium

As discussed above, sodium and water homeostasis are intimately related. The classic abnormalities described below relate to plasma sodium concentrations. These can occur in the presence of low, normal or high levels of total body sodium. Daily requirements of sodium in a normal patient are around 120–140 mmol per day (i.e. 1 L of 'normal' saline).

Hypernatraemia

Raised concentration of sodium in the plasma most often results from water deficiency. The raised plasma osmolality results in activation of mechanisms to conserve water and increase intake (e.g. stimulating thirst).

There are many causes of hypernatraemia and only those of surgical relevance are given here:

- Insufficient intake of water, e.g. perioperative fasting.
- Excessive insensible and respiratory water loss, e.g. pyrexia, tachypnoea secondary to respiratory complications.
- Administration of excess sodium, either with intravenous sodium solutions or medications containing large amounts of sodium.
- Diabetes insipidus (DI), which is either a failure of production (pituitary DI) or lack of response to ADH (nephrogenic DI).

Generally, these causes are easily prevented by consideration and monitoring the patient's fluid balance. Correction of the water deficiency is effected with administration of appropriate intravenous fluids. Sodium concentration should be corrected gradually to minimise the risk of inducing cerebral oedema (as water shifts from the newly hypotonic or isotonic plasma). Treatment of DI depends on the underlying cause.

Hyponatraemia

Low serum concentrations of sodium can occur in the presence of high, normal or low total body sodium levels. The clinical picture seen and treatment required depends on which of these is present.

Most commonly seen in surgical practice is combined salt and water depletion. The disease processes are the same as those causing dehydration from excess fluid losses (see above), particularly where the losses are solute rich. The decreased extracellular fluid stimulates water reabsorption under the influence of ADH. More water is therefore preserved relative to sodium, diluting sodium in the ECF, and hence resulting in hyponatraemia. The clinical signs are as for dehydration. Treatment is by restoration of salt and water by intravenous administration of normal saline.

The processes involved in fluid overload can also result in hyponatraemia, with more water being retained relative to sodium. The total body sodium is therefore increased, but not as much as the total body water, causing dilution and hyponatraemia. Treatment is as described for fluid overload above.

Potassium

Daily requirements of potassium are between 60 and 140 mmol per day. This is dependent on the rate of excretion and also the rate of liberation from the intracellular fluid compartment (see below).

Hyperkalaemia

A significantly raised serum potassium concentration (>7.0 mmol/L) can cause life-threatening cardiac arrhythmias and urgent treatment is required to prevent these. Symptoms are rare until complications have occurred, so awareness and prevention are essential. Treatment is resuscitative, performing life support manoeuvres where required. If complications have not yet occurred, treatment is directed at preventing complications and reducing serum potassium levels. Calcium gluconate (10 mL of 10%) protects the heart from arrhythmias.

Insulin drives potassium into the intracellular fluid. There is some debate as to whether glucose should be given simultaneously to prevent a fall in blood glucose concentration. Treatment is then directed at the underlying cause, e.g. renal support may be required. Causes include either increased release or administration, or decreased excretion.

The vast majority of body potassium is intracellular. Cell lysis, or inefficient functioning of the sodium–potassium exchange pump in the cell membrane, results in liberation of potassium into the circulation. As a result, processes that cause cellular damage or cellular dysfunction (e.g. surgery, trauma, acidosis) can increase serum potassium levels.

Excessive administration of potassium is most frequently iatrogenic. Patients receiving supplementation should receive this slowly, and close monitoring of blood levels is required.

Renal insufficiency results in impairment of potassium excretion and acute renal failure can result in a precipitous rise in serum potassium levels. Severe chronic renal failure can have a similar effect, particularly where tubular function is affected.

Drugs that affect distal tubular function can cause inefficient potassium excretion. An example is the class of diuretics that antagonises the action of aldosterone (e.g. spironolactone, which prevents the reabsorption of sodium at the expense of potassium). Similarly, drugs and diseases that affect the rennin–angiotensin–aldosterone axis result in hyperkalaemia (e.g. ACE inhibitors, Addison's disease).

Hypokalaemia

Low serum potassium levels result from insufficient intake or excess loss of potassium. Again, symptoms are rare, but the deficit is rarely life-threatening, unlike hyperkalaemia. An exception is concomitant treatment with digoxin, where hypokalaemia causes a dangerous potentiation of the drug's action and can result in cardiac arrhythmias. Treatment of hypokalaemia is based on replacing the deficit either orally or in dilute intravenous fluids (never as a potassium salt bolus), and treatment of the underlying cause.

There are very many causes of hypokalaemia and descriptions of all of these are beyond the scope of this chapter. Examples of those most commonly encountered in surgical practice are given in Table 5.7.

Fluid replacement

There is a long-standing debate over the relative value of fluid replacement with crystalloid and colloid solutions,

there being some evidence that use of colloids in critically ill patients actually increases mortality. However, the fundamentals of fluid replacement remain unchanged and a knowledge of the constituents of the infused fluid and its pattern of distribution within fluid compartments, is important. Solutions available for fluid replacement are listed in Table 5.8.

Crystalloid

Crystalloid solutions are those with dissolved solutes. They are cheap, natural and safe when given appropriately. Potassium can be added to bags to maintain plasma potassium levels.

Dextrose

Glucose solution is isotonic at 5%, and this is the standard fluid infused. It is transferred freely between all fluid compartments so that only 8% remains in the intravascular space. Its energy content is negligible, the glucose in each 500 mL bag producing only 100 calories of energy.

Saline

Isotonic saline is 0.9%, and is called 'normal saline'. Each 500 mL bag contains 75 mmol of sodium, balanced with 75 mmol of chloride. Following intravenous infusion, it is distributed freely within the ECF, with 25% remaining intravascular.

Colloid

Colloid solutions contain large-molecular-weight substances that are designed not to cross the vascular

Table 5.7 Common causes of hypokalaemia
Insufficient intake: inadequate intravenous replacement
Excess gastrointestinal losses: diarrhoea, fistulae, villous adenomas
Excess renal losses: diuretic therapy

Table 5.8 Solutions for fluid replacement
Crystalloid
dextrose
saline
Ringer's lactate
Colloid
gelatines
dextrans
heta starch
human albumin solution
Blood

endothelium and thus remain within the intravascular space. They are used to increase the colloid osmotic pressure causing retention of fluid in the circulation. However, some molecules do cross to the interstitial space, and this proportion can be increased in disease processes where vascular permeability is affected.

Blood

Where fluid loss is by way of significant haemorrhage, replacement with blood is appropriate. The principles of blood transfusion are discussed in Chapter 6.

Acid–base balance

For efficient cellular function to occur, the cellular and plasma pH, or hydrogen ion concentration, must be maintained between narrow limits (pH 7.36–7.44). Values outside these parameters result in cellular and system dysfunction, which become profound and can ultimately result in cell death and system failure.

Hydrogen ions are generated by several metabolic processes, and by equilibration of carbon dioxide (CO_2) in solution. Maintenance of normal pH is achieved through a number of different systems: namely, buffering, respiration and renal excretion of hydrogen ions and bicarbonate.

The main determinant of pH is the equilibration of CO_2 in solution. CO_2 is generated as a waste product in normal aerobic respiration. It is excreted by the lungs during respiration. Transport of CO_2 from the tissues to the lungs is performed by the blood, with the CO_2 being dissolved in solution. The enzyme carbonic anhydrase forms carbonic acid according to the Henderson–Hasselbach equation:

$$CO_2 + H_2O \longleftrightarrow H_2CO_3 \longleftrightarrow H^+ + HCO_3^-$$

This equation has to remain in equilibrium, and is therefore dependent on CO_2 excretion by the lungs and the bicarbonate (HCO_3^-) concentration in plasma. Bicarbonate concentration is controlled by renal excretion.

Other forms of acid are produced by tissues, e.g. lactic acid from anaerobic metabolism. These are buffered in plasma by bicarbonate, phosphate, haemoglobin and other plasma proteins. Renal excretion of hydrogen ions is important in their elimination.

An important effect of the interaction between hydrogen ions and haemoglobin (Hb) is the reduction in the affinity of Hb for oxygen. As a result, when oxy-haemoglobin reaches the tissues, where there is a higher concentration of carbonic and other acids, it more readily releases the oxygen it is carrying for use in that tissue.

Abnormalities of acid–base balance

The hydrogen ion concentration can either be increased (acidosis) or decreased (alkalosis). This can be caused by imbalance at any point of the Henderson–Hasselbach equation as a result of either respiratory or renal changes in acid–base management.

Respiratory acidosis

Decreased CO_2 excretion by the lungs results in increased plasma carbonic acid and hence hydrogen ion concentration. Causes include decreased respiratory drive (e.g. opiate overdose) and diseases of lung parenchyma that result in inefficient gas transfer.

Respiratory alkalosis

Overventilation increases CO_2 excretion, decreasing plasma carbonic acid and hence hydrogen ion concentration. Hyperventilation can be psychological, pathological (e.g. tachypnoea of respiratory tract infection) or iatrogenic (e.g. overventilation of mechanically ventilated patients).

Metabolic acidosis

Metabolic acidosis is an increase in plasma hydrogen ion concentration derived from another source than CO_2. Examples include lactic acidosis and diabetic ketoacidosis.

Metabolic alkalosis

This is a fall in plasma hydrogen ion concentration not related to carbon dioxide. It can result from many processes that cause either increased renal H^+ excretion or from excess plasma bicarbonate (e.g. iatrogenic administration, renal conservation of bicarbonate).

Compensation

The clear-cut abnormalities described above are rarely seen because the system not affected by the abnormal process will act to compensate for the problem. Thus, in respiratory acidosis the kidney will retain bicarbonate and excrete H^+. This in effect causes a partial metabolic alkalosis and combats the fall in pH driven by CO_2 retention. Similarly, in metabolic acidosis, respiration is increased, blowing-off more CO_2, causing a compensatory partial respiratory alkalosis.

Metabolic response to surgery

The insult of trauma, including surgery, results in a number of metabolic changes directed at containing and repairing the damage. This response is complex and involves many metabolic processes and body systems. The effects are mediated by the sympathetic nervous system, endocrine, inflammatory and endothelial responses. Not only has the response been implicated in healing but, more recently, has been suggested to play an important pathophysiological role in the complications of trauma, such as systemic inflammatory response syndrome (SIRS) and multiorgan failure (MOF). A full description of the changes observed is excessive for the purpose of this chapter, but it is worth highlighting a number of points that have bearing on everyday clinical practice.

Sympathetic activity causes a rise in heart rate and blood pressure, increasing cardiac work. Mobilisation of energy stores occurs shortly after injury, causing relative hyperglycaemia and insulin resistance. ADH secretion is increased resulting in water retention and a fall in urine output. Vascular permeability is increased, predisposing to oedema formation. Inflammatory mediators (e.g. prostaglandins and leucotrienes) are produced, causing systemic effects such as pyrexia; they might also be implicated in trauma pathophysiology. The immune system is impaired, predisposing to infective complications. After the initial brief mobilisation of energy stores (catabolic state) the body enters a more prolonged reparative anabolic state with increased energy and nitrogen demands. Activation of platelets leads to a hypercoagulable state.

Postoperative feeding

For effective healing to occur after trauma or surgery, the body must be supplied with the correct substrates in sufficient amounts. Whereas these are normally supplied via the gastrointestinal tract by a balanced diet, demand for, and the ability to attain, the substrates can be dramatically altered perioperatively.

Patients' ability to ingest, digest, absorb and utilise substrates is affected by any number of disease processes. In cases where the effects of these processes are expected to be prolonged, or are superimposed on a background of malnutrition, nutritional support may be indicated. This support can be provided either to the gastrointestinal tract (enteral) or intravenously (parenteral).

Trauma and major surgery induce metabolic changes such that energy and nitrogen demands are increased, and this should be taken into account when deciding on a feeding regime. Reasonable figures for normal daily requirements of energy and nitrogen are 2000–2500 kcal and 14–16 g, respectively.

Enteral feeding

Where possible, enteral dietary supplementation is preferable. Stimulation of the gut mucosa with food has been implicated in reducing sepsis in critically ill patients. It is thought that continued mucosal activity maintains a barrier to bacteria in the gut lumen, preventing them from translocating into the circulation, where they are thought to play an important role in the pathophysiology of multiorgan failure.

Enteral nutritional support can be given as oral supplements, or where appropriate by intubation of the gastrointestinal tract (e.g. nasogastric, feeding jejunostomy). The feed needs to contain each food group – carbohydrate, fat and protein. These can be given in several different proportions and forms, particularly relating to protein and its degree of predigestion prior to administration. Disease-specific diets are also available. Trace elements are also added (e.g. zinc and magnesium). Enteral feeding is appropriate in patients who are comatose, those with oropharyngeal diseases that prevent ingestion, mastication and swallowing, and some patients with certain diseases further down the gastrointestinal tract.

In the presence of a poorly functioning gastrointestinal tract, enteral feeding can lead to further complications, including diarrhoea, vomiting and aspiration. Complications relating to method of administration are not uncommon, including incorrect positioning of the feeding tube and bacterial growth in the excellent medium that the feed provides.

Parenteral feeding

When patients with a non-functioning gastrointestinal tract require nutritional support, and when it is not practical to gain access for enteral feeding, feeding can be given intravenously. The feed is designed to meet all the body's requirements and is termed 'total parenteral nutrition' or TPN.

Constituents

To meet the body's needs, TPN solutions contain fat, amino acids and carbohydrate (mainly glucose). The composition of a feed varies, is prepared for individual patients and is tailored to their needs. There are a number of standard feeds with different amounts of nitrogen, and the majority of energy supplied by carbohydrates or fats. These are further manipulated, for example, with the addition of potassium, as guided by monitoring of serum levels and markers of metabolic state.

Complications

The constituents of TPN solutions render them hyperosmolar, and hence irritant, and when given through peripheral veins cause thrombophlebitis. They are therefore administered via a large-bore central venous cannula. There is, however, an increasing role for peripherally sited 'long' feeding lines.

The hyperosmolality of TPN solutions can also cause metabolic complications, most commonly hyperglycaemia. If this occurs, insulin might be required and, in future feeds, more of the energy should be supplied as fat. Rebound hypoglycaemia can occur on cessation of feeding.

Patients on TPN are more prone to hepatobiliary disease.

Trace element and vitamin deficiencies can occur, more commonly in prolonged TPN administration, and these should be replaced accordingly.

However, the majority of complications of TPN relate to the feeding line. The majority of these lines are sited centrally, and so are subject to the risks of central line insertion (e.g. pneumothorax or arterial puncture). Infection is a common problem, as is secondary line thrombosis and failure. Patients requiring long-term TPN can benefit from the placement of a buried subcutaneous feeding line to minimise these risks. All TPN should be administered through a lumen dedicated solely to it and not used for other purposes such as intravenous antibiotic administration or blood transfusion.

6

Blood disorders and their management in surgical practice

Introduction

Poor haemostasis (control of bleeding) is one of the most common surgical complications and can range from catastrophic blood loss causing hypovolaemia and shock to small wound haematomas that provide an excellent growth medium for microorganisms. By virtue of the coagulation or clotting cascade, blood and blood vessels are a self-sealing system, and therefore have an inherent ability to provide haemostasis. However, there is no substitute for careful technique and meticulous surgical haemostasis.

This chapter describes, under the headings shown in Table 6.1 the normal sequence of events involved in blood clotting and also those mechanisms that prevent clotting in normal, undamaged vessels. Also described are conditions where abnormalities in clotting occur, their recognition and treatment. The implications of anaemia in surgery are considered, the principles of blood transfusion are described and a guideline for the recognition and care of a patient with potential bleeding problems is provided. The specific management of a dental post-extraction haemorrhage is considered in Chapter 26.

Normal clotting

The whole process of blood clotting, limitation of propagation of clot and ultimate dissolution of clot is a complex interactive system interdependent on, and subject to, numerous feedback controls. Blood clotting will be considered under the headings listed in Table 6.2.

The immediate response to vessel damage is vasoconstriction, which reduces blood flow in the area thereby reducing blood loss and preventing the fledgling blood clot from being washed away. This is mediated both as a local reflex and by a number of mediators that are released mainly from activated platelets, such as thromboxane

Table 6.1   Blood disorders and their management
Normal clotting
Abnormal clotting
increased bleeding tendency
increased clotting tendency
Patients with anaemia
Transfusion
Summary and guidelines

Table 6.2   Normal blood clotting
Initiation of clotting
platelet adhesion
platelet activation
platelet aggregation
Stabilisation
coagulation
intrinsic pathway
extrinsic pathway
common pathway
Limitation of clotting
Dissolution of clot
Prevention of inappropriate clotting
structural
chemical mediators

(TxA_2). Thus, although coagulation, as measured by clotting time, takes around 8 min to occur, haemorrhage is reduced and arrested much sooner.

Initiation of clotting

Circulating platelets play a central role in the initiation of blood clotting by three main mechanisms:

1. *Platelet adhesion*: platelets possess membrane receptors to many proteins not encountered in normal blood

or endothelium. Disruption of endothelium exposes platelets to 'foreign' proteins, for example, different types of collagen, to which they have receptors and to which they therefore stick.

2. *Platelet activation*: platelet adherence results in a change in the shape of platelets. Within seconds, by way of complex intracellular messaging, the platelet becomes 'activated'. This results in synthesis and release of mediators such as histamine and TxA_2 from intracellular stores (lysosomes).

3. *Platelet aggregation*: the conformational changes in the platelets and the milieu of mediators released attract other platelets and allow them to stick to one another. This is known as aggregation.

Platelet adhesion, activation and aggregation result in the formation of a platelet plug, which is an attempt to cover the breach in the endothelium and acts as the starting point from which the rest of the process of coagulation occurs.

Stabilisation

Coagulation

A mature blood clot is a combination of cross-linked fibrin admixed with blood cells and plasma. Platelet events described above stimulate a stepwise pathway that results in the formation of cross-linked fibrin. This system is known as the 'coagulation cascade', which consists of two routes that run in parallel – the intrinsic pathway and the extrinsic pathway. Current thinking in coagulation research is that this might be oversimplified and there are now thought to be multiple interactions between the pathways, resulting in a more integrated system. However, the sequences described here are accurate and provide a good framework for understanding the process of coagulation.

Ionised calcium is a crucial cofactor for many of the clotting factors, and deficiency has an important effect on coagulation.

Intrinsic pathway

This is the more intricate portion of the coagulation cascade, and there is debate over the relevance of different aspects seen in vivo compared to results seen in vitro experiments. Essentially, contact with injured tissue results in activation of factor XII, which in turn activates factor XI, which in turn cascades to the common pathway as shown in Fig. 6.1.

Extrinsic pathway

This is coagulation initiated by tissue factor. Tissue factor (TF) is expressed on the surface of the subendothelial tissue that is exposed when endothelium is damaged. Tissue factor activates factor VII, which, in turn, activates factor X, the beginning of the common pathway.

Common pathway

This is the common endpoint of the intrinsic and extrinsic pathways. It begins with activation of factor X and, via the steps in Fig. 6.1, results in the formation of cross-linked fibrin.

Limitation of clotting

It is vital that clotting is limited to the local area of damage to prevent propagation of clot throughout the vascular system. Activated clotting factors are removed from the propagating clot by blood flow. There is also a form of negative feedback on clotting by naturally occurring substances that inhibit coagulation, some of which are activated by products of the coagulation cascade itself. Examples of these are proteins C and S and antithrombin III. Abnormalities of these factors can cause disease (antithrombin III deficiency, see below) and knowledge about these can be utilised for therapy (e.g. heparin potentiates antithrombin III).

Dissolution of clot (fibrinolysis)

Ultimately, when the damaged vessel has healed and re-endothelialised, the adherent clot will be removed. This is known as fibrinolysis. In this process, tissue plasminogen activator (TPA), produced by vascular endothelium in the presence of thrombin, acts on circulating plasminogen to form plasmin; this action is dependent on the presence of fibrin. Plasmin now acts in turn on fibrin, which is degraded to soluble fibrin degradation products (FDPs).

Fibrinolysis maintains vessel patency and helps to prevent overpropagation of clot. Not surprisingly, there are also inhibitors of plasmin and plasminogen activators.

Levels of fibrinogen and FDPs can be measured and provide helpful diagnostic clues, for example elevated D-dimer FDP levels are indicative of the presence of blood clot and can be used in the diagnosis of suspected deep venous thrombosis (DVT).

This very intricate system of control prevents excessive bleeding while at the same time preventing

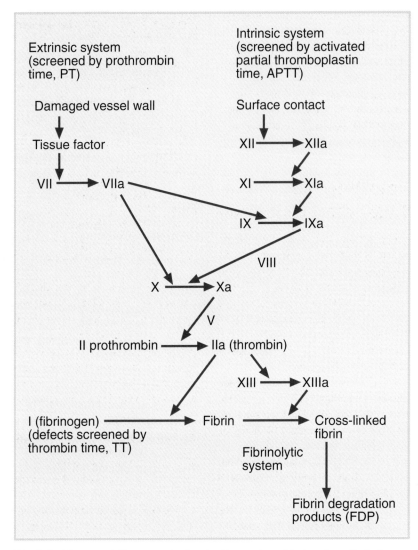

Fig. 6.1 The coagulation cascade showing the numbered factors (a, activated form). The factors involved in the intrinsic system, beginning with the activation of factor XII and ending with the activation of factor X are all present in the circulating plasma: the extrinsic system consists of tissue thomboplastin and includes factor VII, not involved in the intrinsic system. Activated factor X, along with factor V, initiates the final steps, culminating in the conversion of fibrinogen to fibrin by thrombin.

excess intravascular coagulation once clotting has been initiated: the body has developed a very finely balanced feedback system.

Prevention of inappropriate clotting

To prevent inappropriate clotting in normal blood vessels, physiological systems act to counteract those that stimulate blood clotting. Interference with these systems stimulate the initiation of blood clotting, as described below. The mechanisms that prevent blood from clotting in normal blood vessels can be divided into structural and chemical:

• *Structural prevention mechanisms*: the smooth lining of the blood vessel provided by endothelium does not express surface proteins that stimulate platelet adhesion as has been described above. Rough or damaged endothelium (e.g. atherosclerotic plaques) not only allows platelets to come into contact with proteins that they adhere to but also results in turbulent blood flow, which also predisposes to blood clotting.

- *Chemical mediators*: normal vascular endothelium produces the prostaglandin, prostacyclin (PGI_2). This opposes the actions of TxA_2, causing vasodilatation and opposing platelet activation and aggregation.

Abnormal clotting – increased bleeding tendency

Careful history taking is fundamental in the diagnosis of bleeding disorders and is essential before surgery. In patients who express a past history of bleeding problems, the site and type of bleeding (e.g. spontaneous Vs induced by trauma) needs to be determined accurately. This can give clues to the type of bleeding disorder. A history of excess bleeding at the time of previous surgery is very important to note. A detailed family history can suggest if such a disorder is inherited or acquired.

Full physical examination can show further evidence of a bleeding disorder, including bruising, petechiae (subcutaneous red spots that do not blanch on pressure and which represent areas of small capillary bleeding) or previous bleeding into joints.

However, despite a careful history and examination, excessive bleeding at the time of surgery might be a patient's first presentation of a bleeding disorder, and it is therefore important for a surgeon to be aware of the concepts and how to control bleeding in this situation should it occur. Close liaison with a haematologist will be necessary at this time. The causes of an increased bleeding tendency are listed in Table 6.3.

Platelets disorders

These can be either quantitative (number) or qualitative (function). Disorders of platelets can result in bleeding from small vessels in mucous membranes such as nose bleeds (epistaxis), or in skin causing bruising or petechiae.

Decreased numbers

This is known as thrombocytopenia. Platelet count is measured routinely as part of a full blood count. A normal

Table 6.3 Causes of increased bleeding tendency
Platelet disorders
decreased numbers
idiopathic thrombocytopenic purpura (ITP)
hypersplenism
disseminated intravascular coagulation (DIC)
decreased function
Vessel disorders
Coagulation disorders
inherited
haemophilia A
haemophilia B
von Willebrand's disease
Acquired
liver and biliary disease
DIC
massive blood transfusion

value is $150–400 \times 10^9$ per litre. Bleeding is rarely a problem when the platelet count is above 50. Severe or spontaneous bleeding occurs with values below 20.

There are multiple causes of thrombocytopenia, which can be broadly divided into those with excessive loss or consumption of platelets and those with impaired production. Either form can be congenital or acquired. Important examples are discussed below.

Idiopathic thrombocytopenic purpura (ITP)

This condition is also known as autoimmune thrombocytopenic purpura and the platelet count might be undetectable.

Treatment of thrombocytopenia is directed at the underlying cause (e.g. ITP might respond to steroid therapy or splenectomy). During surgery, if a patient is actively bleeding with a low platelet count, platelet transfusion can provide a temporary solution. However, these transfusions are prone to the same fate as the patient's endogenous platelets (e.g. rapid consumption).

Hypersplenism

This occurs where platelets are sequestered in an enlarged spleen.

Disseminated intravascular coagulation (DIC)

This occurs where platelets and coagulation factors are consumed in widespread inappropriate coagulation within normal blood vessels (see below).

Decreased function

These disorders can also be congenital or acquired. Assessment of platelet function is difficult and reliance is initially on the bleeding time, which is the time taken for bleeding to stop under standard test conditions. However. this is a difficult test to standardise and has a wide normal range between 2 and 10 min.

An important acquired cause of decreased platelet function is medication, the most common of which is aspirin. This is now widely used in prophylaxis and treatment of vascular disease because of its effect on platelet function and its effects can last up to 10 days. Aspirin should therefore be withheld for 10 days prior to major procedures associated with a potential high risk of bleeding complications.

Vessel disorders

These form a generally rare, heterogeneous group with a clinical presentation similar to that of platelet disorders, but where investigations of platelet number and function are normal. Essentially, the capillaries are fragile and bleeding occurs more easily. Again, there are congenital and acquired forms. Corticosteroid therapy is a common example of an acquired cause.

One of the interesting congenital causes is hereditary haemorrhagic telangiectasia, characterised by recurrent bleeds from mucous membranes. The lesions look like small blood blisters and occur particularly on the face, lips, tongue and hands. They bleed freely if traumatised. Control of bleeding is very difficult and this condition should be identified before surgery. This is of particular relevance to dentists.

Coagulation disorders

Disorders of coagulation factors are characterised by a more generalised bleeding tendency than platelet and vascular disorders, including spontaneous bleeding from larger vessels and into joints. The vast majority of coagulation factor defects encountered in surgical practice are acquired. The most common cause is iatrogenic, related to treatment with warfarin. Inherited disorders are uncommon but require special consideration.

A number of laboratory investigations can help elucidate the type of a coagulation defect. Although some of these are specialised, an appreciation of standard clotting tests is essential for surgeons:

- *Prothrombin time (PT)*: this gives an indication of the extrinsic and common pathways of the coagulation cascade. Abnormalities in these portions of the cascade result in a prolonged time. Times are related to an international standardised sample designated international normalised ratio (INR). An INR of 1.0 is normal, whereas an INR of 2.0 denotes that the patient's blood takes twice as long as 'normal' to clot under test conditions.
- *Activated partial thromboplastin time (APTT)*: this measures the efficiency of the intrinsic and common pathways.

If abnormalities of INR or APTT are discovered then normal plasma is added to the sample in the laboratory. If this corrects the abnormality, then the problem must relate to a factor deficiency or dysfunction (because the factors present in the normal added plasma corrected the problem). If the abnormality is not corrected then it is likely to be due to the presence of a substance that inhibits coagulation. This procedure is known as 'correction testing'.

Inherited coagulation disorders:

Inherited defects are specific genetic abnormalities that generally affect only one clotting factor.

Haemophilia A

This is an X-linked recessive disorder that therefore affects only males but which is transmitted by females. The prevalence is about 1:10 000. Statistically, all the daughters of haemophiliacs will carry the gene and none of the sons will inherit the disease or transmit it. However, in the second generation, only 50% of the sons of female carriers will inherit the disorder and only 50% of their daughters will inherit the gene.

Haemophilia A can be caused by a number of genetic abnormalities, all of which result in decreased or absent factor VIII:C. Deficiency of factor VIII:vWF results in the closely related von Willebrand's disease (see below).

Different affected individuals have a different level of VIII in the blood and there is therefore a spectrum of disease. Factor VIII levels can be measured in the patient's plasma and are expressed as a percentage of normal.

Bleeding into joints causing arthritis is common and produces clinically obvious joint deformities in many cases. Bleeding can also occur into body cavities and intracranially.

Preoperative transfusion of factor VIII concentrate is aimed at raising factor VIII levels to nearer normal, for example, 60% for dental extraction, and as near 100% as possible for major surgery. These levels need to be maintained postoperatively.

Tragically, many haemophiliacs who received blood transfusions prior to HIV blood donor screening introduction in the UK contracted HIV, and in these patients high-risk precautions are indicated perioperatively.

Haemophilia B

This is also known as Christmas disease. It is similar to haemophilia A but the disorder is related to deficiency of factor IX. The incidence is less common, with a prevalence of around 1:100 000 and the defect can be corrected by the transfusion of fresh-frozen plasma (FFP).

von Willebrand's disease

von Willebrand's disease is not sex-linked and can occur via a number of genetic abnormalities. It is usually due to autosomal dominant inheritance.

Surgery – elective or emergency – on any of the above patients should only be performed in close consultation with a haematologist (preferably the patient's own).

Acquired coagulation disorders

Bile salts are produced by the liver and enter the duodenum via the common bile duct to aid the absorption of fats and fat-soluble vitamins such as vitamin K. The presence of vitamin K is essential for the synthesis of coagulation factors II, VII, IX and X (and also proteins C and S). Disorders of bile production and of biliary drainage will affect coagulation.

It should be noted that the majority of clotting factors are produced by hepatocytes. Remembering this physiology is helpful in understanding acquired coagulation defects, of which there are many causes.

Liver and biliary disease

There are many causes of liver dysfunction and a description of each of these is beyond the scope of this chapter; one common cause is alcohol-related cirrhosis.

The coagulopathy that results from diffuse liver dysfunction is complex. The damaged liver produces too few clotting factors. Bile salt synthesis, needed for vitamin K absorption, is also impaired. Portal hypertension can result in hypersplenism, and therefore thrombocytopenia.

Surgical jaundice secondary to obstruction of the common bile duct due to gallstones or malignancy of the pancreas prevents bile salts reaching the duodenal lumen. Vitamin K malabsorption results, followed by deficiencies of factors II, VII, IX and X. Other causes of vitamin K deficiency, such as dietary deficiency, have the same result. However, the effect of 'back pressure' on hepatocyte function also plays a role in the coagulopathy of biliary obstruction.

Vitamin K deficiency can be corrected by parenteral injection of a water-soluble vitamin K analogue before elective surgery, but this will not be immediately effective. It will be several days before the liver can synthesise sufficient factors to correct the bleeding tendency. Urgent or emergency surgery might therefore require infusion with solutions containing the deficient factors. The INR should be checked immediately before surgery, with the aim of reducing it to 1.

Warfarin therapy

Warfarin, a coumarin drug, is a vitamin K antagonist (it prevents conversion of vitamin K to an active form). Warfarin therapy is indicated in a number of common conditions including atrial fibrillation, pulmonary embolus and prosthetic heart valve replacement. Normal medical practice for most conditions dictates that warfarin therapy should be administered to achieve an INR of around 3. Excessive bleeding will occur where the INR is greater than 2.

The effects of warfarin are slow to reverse because, again, even if vitamin K is administered, the clotting factors still have to be synthesised. When emergency surgery is needed, vitamin-K-dependent factor concentrates can be administered intravenously, reducing the INR quickly, as noted above in obstructive jaundice. This must always be done with care. A balance needs to be achieved between maintaining an acceptable level of anticoagulation (e.g. to prevent thrombosis of a prosthetic heart valve) and not exposing the patient to the risk of haemorrhage during surgery. It is vital, therefore, that the administration of these concentrates is done in consultation with a haematologist, and that the INR is maintained well above 1. It is recommended that patients undergoing elective surgical should have their warfarin stopped for 2–3 days before surgery and, depending on the procedure to be performed, are perhaps switched perioperatively onto faster and more malleable anticoagulation therapy with heparin. Coagulation tests should always be performed on the morning before operation. In most cases, an INR of 2 is acceptable. In dental procedures, an INR of less than 4 is acceptable because local haemostatic measures can be used as an adjunct (see Ch. 26).

Disseminated intravascular coagulation (DIC)

DIC is a major complication seen in seriously ill or injured patients. The triggers to DIC are multiple and include infections, malignancy and trauma. Inappropriate extensive coagulation occurs, often in fundamentally normal blood vessels. This process uses up clotting factors, fibrinogen and platelets, resulting in an increased bleeding tendency.

Clinical features are paradoxically of both bleeding and organ dysfunction from ischaemic damage caused by microthrombi. Investigations show consumption of fibrinogen and platelets, an increase in FDPs and deranged clotting studies. Treatment is based on the underlying cause, along with supportive therapy and transfusion of clotting factors and platelets that have been consumed. As can be appreciated, this is an extremely serious condition.

Massive blood transfusions

Stored blood has relatively low concentrations of platelets and clotting factors, particularly factors V and VIII. This is not only because of the short lifespan of these substances but also because platelets and clotting factors are often removed from fresh blood for specific infusions as described above. In addition to this, stored blood must contain an anticoagulant to prevent it clotting while in storage. Citrate, which binds ionised calcium, is used for this purpose. As outlined above, calcium is an important cofactor in the coagulation cascade. Although this effect of citrate is essential for storage, it means that transfused blood has poor clotting ability. This is not usually a problem clinically, unless the patient has received a 'massive transfusion' (defined as receiving a transfusion volume greater than the patient's normal blood volume, i.e. 4–5 L). If this happens, the recipient is reliant on transfused factors, of which there are not enough in stored blood. The recipient will therefore require simultaneous transfusion with platelets and

clotting factors along with calcium. The management of such patients is again done in close collaboration with a haematologist.

Abnormal clotting – increased clotting tendency

This group of diseases is actually more prevalent than diseases with increased bleeding tendency. Their relevance to surgical practice relates to an increased risk of deep venous thrombosis (DVT). Thrombosis can be recurrent or atypical, as in spontaneous axillary vein thrombosis.

Patients with suggestive features require referral to haematology for further investigation before surgery. Patients already diagnosed with an increased clotting tendency require prophylactic measures against DVT no matter how minor the procedure (Ch. 4). Patients who have previously been diagnosed with such a problem might already be receiving treatment with warfarin, which will alter operative preparation (see above).

Patients with anaemia

There are many different forms of anaemia, and multiple causes for each type. A description of these is beyond the scope of this chapter. However, the existence of anaemia in surgical patients has implications that are worth brief consideration.

Anaemia is defined as a haemoglobin concentration below an arbitrary designated level, which is generally accepted as 13 g/dL for men and 12 g/dL for women. Anaemia has a number of pathophysiological consequences of surgical relevance (Table 6.4) as a consequence of the decreased oxygen-carrying capacity of the blood.

Cardiorespiratory problems

The reduced oxygen-carrying capacity of the blood results in an impaired ability to cope with the stresses of

Table 6.4 Consequences of anaemia
Cardiorespiratory problems
Impaired wound healing
Precipitation of haemolysis

anaesthesia and surgery. For example, myocardial ischaemia is more easily induced and might result in an increased incidence of myocardial infarction (MI). Postoperative respiratory complications are less well tolerated.

Wound healing

Relative hypoxia impairs tissue healing, and increases the risk of infection (Chs 3 and 8).

Precipitation of haemolysis

The hypoxia of anaesthesia can induce haemolytic crises in certain hereditary haemolytic anaemias such as sickle-cell disease. Preoperative planning, with or without transfusion, and careful anaesthesia aim to prevent this.

Operating on a background of anaemia will result in the patient having fewer reserves to compensate for operative blood loss. There might be associated depletion of other blood cells, including white blood cells (which increases susceptibility to infection) and platelets (which increases the bleeding tendency).

As a result, the haemoglobin concentration should be returned to near normal preoperatively, for example, with iron therapy in elective patients (failure to respond could indicate an alternative cause of anaemia), or transfusion for emergency operations.

The oxygen-carrying capacity of transfused blood is lowered by the presence of high concentrations of 2,3 diphosphoglycerate (DPG) and hydrogen ions, which shift the oxygen–haemoglobin dissociation curve to the right (this is known as the Bohr effect).

Replacement of blood loss: transfusion

Whole blood is rarely given because the scarce resources of donated blood are used more efficiently when given in constituent parts. Blood is commonly fractionated into its constituent parts, which are used for specific indications. This ensures more efficient use of each unit of donated blood.

It is essential that each patient is cross-matched correctly before transfusion. Patients are grouped according to antigens expressed on their red blood cells as A, B, AB and O. Each group contains antibodies against foreign antigen, for example, group A blood possesses anti-B antibody. AB possesses no antibodies and is therefore the 'universal recipient'; group O individuals possess antibodies to both A and B.

The other major blood grouping is Rhesus factor, and patients are either positive or negative.

Patients that are group O rhesus negative have no A or B antigens and no rhesus factor, and can therefore be transfused to other groups with minimal risk of reaction ('universal donors').

Blood products

The range of blood products available is listed in Table 6.5 and are discussed below.

Red cell concentrate (RCC)

Red cells are extracted and suspended in a near optimum solution containing glucose, adenine, mannitol, sodium chloride and citrate (the last prevents clotting). Cell lysis during storage means that each unit contains a high concentration of extracellular potassium. RCC has a haematocrit of 65–70% and hence has poor flow characteristics. Simultaneous crystalloid infusion reduces the haematocrit and provides volume repletion.

RCC is used for transfusion in patients with anaemia and in those suffering acute blood loss, but it has a reduced oxygen-carrying capacity (see above). It must be blood group ABO- and Rhesus-factor-compatible (see below).

One unit of RCC is derived from one donation. The shelf-life is 35 days at 4°C. The volume varies by unit, but is approximately 400 mL.

Platelets

Infused platelets are suspended in plasma (and therefore infusions contain some clotting factors). Full cross-match is not necessary before transfusion.

Table 6.5   Blood products
Red cell concentrate
Platelets
Fresh-frozen plasma
Cryoprecipitate
Factor concentrates
Albumin solution
Other

43

One unit is obtained from 4–6 blood donations. The shelf-life is 5 days at room temperature and the volume is 300 mL. No viral inactivation procedures are used in processing. Platelets are used perioperatively in patients with thrombocytopenia.

Fresh-frozen plasma (FFP)

This is pure plasma that is separated and frozen shortly after donation. It contains all the plasma-derived clotting factors, but has relatively low levels of factor VIII and fibrinogen. The shelf-life is 1 year at –30°C and its volume is 150–300 mL per unit. FFP is used for correcting factor deficiencies.

Cryoprecipitate

Contains high levels of factor VIII and fibrinogen. Again, the shelf-life is 1 year at –30°C. Each unit is approximately 10–20 mL and the standard dose is 10 units.

Factor concentrates

Multiples are available and are either derived from plasma or are manufactured using recombinant DNA technology.

Albumin solution

This is derived from whole blood after removal of cells and factors. Shelf-life is 3–5 years. It is used to expand intravascular volume, although it has now been largely superseded by synthetic gelatin solutions such as gelofusin and haemacel. It is also used for fluid replacement after burns and during plasmapheresis

Other

There are multiple other blood products available for treatment of more unusual conditions, including specific immunoglobulins.

Complications

The complications of blood transfusion can be immunological, infective or due to miscellaneous causes (Table 6.6).

Table 6.6 Complications of blood transfusion
Immunological
immediate haemolytic
non-haemolytic
delayed haemolytic
Infective
Miscellaneous
fluid overload
hyperkalaemia
coagulation disorder
haemosiderosis
hypothermia

Immunological complications

Immediate haemolytic complications

This can result from mismatched blood-cell antigens between donor and recipient. The most important antigens are those of the ABO system. These reactions are severe and sudden and most often result from human error, for example if the wrong unit of blood is given to the wrong patient because of a labelling, handling or patient identification error. Activation of the complement system occurs when the recipient possesses antibodies to an antigen on the donated red blood cells, and haemolysis (breakdown of the red blood cells) ensues.

Clinically, the patient rapidly becomes unwell with fever, hypotension and difficulty breathing. Activation of coagulation can occur, leading to DIC. The haemoglobin released from the haemolysis, along with hypotension, can cause acute renal failure.

Treatment involves preventing further reaction by stopping the transfusion immediately. The patient might require life-saving resuscitation, including measures to maintain oxygenation and blood pressure. Intensive care might be appropriate.

Where a reaction occurs, the unit of blood must be returned to the laboratory, along with a cross-match sample from the patient.

Non-haemolytic complications

Febrile, allergic and anaphylactic reactions can occur and will necessitate immediate cessation of the transfusion and possibly medical resuscitation, depending on the severity. Allergic and anaphylactic reactions might require immediate treatment with adrenaline (epinephrine), antihistamine or corticosteroids.

Delayed haemolytic complications

These result from incompatibility of blood with regards to less important antigens. They occur in patients who have previously been sensitised to the antigens. Examples include Rhesus antibodies and rarer antibodies to minor antigens such as Kell and Duffy. Haemolysis occurs several days after the transfusion. The patient is not generally acutely unwell and might develop jaundice and anaemia several days after the transfusion.

Infective complications

Blood that is donated in the UK is routinely screened for HIV, syphilis, hepatitis B and hepatitis C. However, a number of these diseases have a latent period before their detection is possible and so transmission of infection can still occur. Before screening for certain diseases was introduced, many blood recipients were infected with hepatitis C and people with haemophilia contracted HIV.

The risk of transmission of infection is related to how many donors the blood product was derived from and to the pretransfusion treatment the product has received (see above).

Miscellaneous complications

Fluid overload

The volume load of the transfusion might precipitate heart failure in the elderly or those with a history of heart disease, particularly as a unit of blood has to be transfused in less than 4 h. Prophylactic diuretic therapy is often given with a transfusion to prevent this. Central venous pressure monitoring, in a surgical high dependency or intensive care unit, can help to prevent this.

Hyperkalaemia

As mentioned above, stored blood has a high concentration of potassium and when multiple units are given the recipient's serum potassium level can rise to dangerous levels. Electrolyte levels must therefore be monitored.

Coagulation disorder

This was considered under massive transfusion, above.

Haemosiderosis

Patients who receive regular or multiple blood transfusions can suffer from iron overload. Excess iron is deposited in vital organs such as the pancreas, myocardium or liver, causing them to dysfunction. This is reduced by using an iron chelator such as desferrioxamine.

Hypothermia

Blood is stored cooled to 4°C. If large volumes of unwarmed blood are transfused the patient will suffer hypothermia. The role of blood warmers is particularly important in trauma cases.

Summary and guidelines

Bleeding is a potentially serious surgical complication and a knowledge of the principles of coagulation and of the disorders that can precipitate bleeding is essential for all surgeons. Recognition and prevention of a problem is obviously preferable to having to deal with a haemorrhaging patient, particularly if the problem could have been recognised and avoided.

A careful history is essential. This should include a history of any previous bleeding problem, especially if related to surgery, a family history of any bleeding problem and a drug history, especially to note if the patient is on anticoagulants, aspirin or corticosteroids.

Examination should look for abnormal bruising or petechiae, and telangiectasis around the mouth.

If there is any doubt, the advice of a physician or haematologist should be sought before embarking on even the most minor surgery.

Where a significant bleeding problem is encountered at surgery, immediate control by compression should be followed by urgent admission to hospital for investigation and correction of any coagulopathy.

Cross-infection

Introduction

To a large extent, the heightened professional and public awareness of the potential for cross-infection in surgical and other medical settings has followed the discovery of human immunodeficiency virus (HIV) as the cause of AIDS. However, although transmission of blood-borne viruses, especially hepatitis B, has been documented in surgical practice, many other microorganisms also pose a significant threat and most of them are far more infectious than HIV. In surgery, bacteria are the major cause of postoperative sepsis (see Ch. 8). These can be acquired from a number of sources, including the patient's own bacterial flora and by cross-infection from other contacts including – importantly – healthcare workers such as doctors and nurses.

The extent of the problem and other aspects important in cross-infection will be considered as described in Table 7.1.

The extent of the problem

Surgical-site infections account for 14–16% of all nosocomial infections and are the third most frequently reported nosocomial infection. A UK study published in 1993 of the excess costs attributable to nosocomial infection in surgical patients reported a mean extra cost per patient of £1041 and an increased length of hospital stay of 8.2 days. A more recent study has calculated that hospital-acquired infections (HAI) cost the NHS in England £1000 million per annum, and it is believed that 5000 patients die of HAI in the UK every year. Similarly large figures are available from the USA where, in 1992, the cost of treating nosocomial infections was estimated at $4.5 billion, of which $1.6 billion was allotted to surgical-site infections (SSI). These data highlight the enormous problem posed by infection for the health services and indicate the importance of measures to improve infection control.

Routes of transmission

The possible routes for cross-infection in surgery are summarised in Fig. 7.1. Direct contact is an important mechanism of transmission for hospital-acquired infections, particularly in surgical units. The best example is the fundamental role played by hands as vectors for spread of microorganisms. Many infections acquired in hospitals are transmitted on the hands of healthcare workers and it is known that regular hand-washing between the examination or treatment of individual patients results in a significant reduction in the carriage of potential pathogens on the hands. Hand-washing has, therefore, been stressed as a simple, cheap and highly effective infection control intervention. Unfortunately, both European and US studies have shown repeatedly that handwashing compliance rates in hospitals are lower than 50%. The use of alcoholic hand rubs, rather than handwashing, is now recommended by some authorities as a convenient means of improving compliance with hand hygiene protocols.

It has been recognised for many years that healthcare workers can acquire occupational infections, for example hepatitis B, from patients they are treating. Transmission

Table 7.1 Aspects of infection control
Extent of the problem
Routes of transmission
Universal infection control
Occupationally acquired infection
Healthcare workers infected with blood-borne viruses
Antimicrobial prophylaxis in surgery
Creutzfeldt–Jakob disease

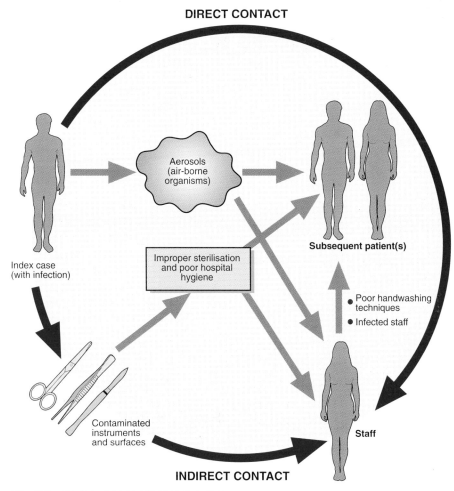

DIRECT CONTACT

Aerosols
(air-borne
organisms)

Index case
(with infection)

Improper sterilisation
and poor hospital
hygiene

Subsequent patient(s)

● Poor handwashing
techniques
● Infected staff

Contaminated
instruments
and surfaces

Staff

INDIRECT CONTACT

Fig. 7.1 Routes of cross-infection in surgery.

of these infections can occur by direct contact with the patient or indirectly through contact with contaminated instruments or surfaces. More recently, there has been considerable professional and media interest in the possible risk of patients becoming infected from healthcare workers who are themselves carriers of blood-borne viruses (see below).

Some microorganisms are transmitted by droplet spread and aerosols are, therefore, another important potential mode of spread of infection in surgery. Airborne spread of infection is a major hazard, for example, in total joint replacement surgery, and use of 'hypersterile' (laminar airflow) operating theatres can play an important role in preventing infection.

Finally, there is a risk that patients might become infected from instruments or other items contaminated during treatment of a previous patient. Effective sterilisation of instruments, which is central to all infection control policies, will prevent this route of transmission. The importance of thorough decontamination and sterilisation of used surgical instruments cannot be overstressed. However, the emergence of prion diseases, in particular variant Creutzfeldt–Jakob disease (vCJD), is now proving a major challenge, because these agents are resistant to standard sterilisation procedures (see below).

Universal infection control

In the light of the multiple routes of transmission noted above, the key principles that underpin modern infection control procedures are shown in Table 7.2. These apply in all healthcare settings, including dental surgery.

Table 7.2 Principles of universal infection control
Many different pathogenic microorganisms pose a problem
There are many sources of infection
Any patient might be a carrier of pathogenic microorganisms
Routine procedures must be effective in preventing cross-infection
All blood, regardless of source, is potentially infectious
The same cross-infection control procedures must be used for all patients

Table 7.3 Key elements of universal infection control
Medical history
Cleaning instruments
Sterilising instruments
Use of disposables
Decontamination of operatory surfaces
Protective workwear
Avoiding needlestick injuries
Immunising staff
Safe waste disposal
Effective training of staff

First, although there is widespread concern about blood-borne viruses such as HIV, a wide range of pathogenic microorganisms is encountered in clinical practice. Thus, attention must be given to preventing the spread of all infections, both rare and common.

Second, there are many potential sources of infection, most of them unrecognised. For example, carriers of hepatitis B virus frequently appear clinically well and are unaware of their carrier status. Similarly, patients could be colonised by antibiotic resistant bacteria, such as methicillin resistant *Staphylococcus aureus* (MRSA), with no outward clinical signs or symptoms. Thus any patient, regardless of background or medical history, must be considered to pose an infection risk.

The logical conclusion to these concepts is the adoption of universal infection control, whereby every patient is treated as a potential carrier. The infection control protocol adopted must be sufficiently stringent to reduce the risk of contamination of patients or staff to a level that is highly unlikely to cause infection. It also follows that patients who are known carriers of pathogens, including blood-borne viruses, will pose no additional risk and can be treated safely under the same operating conditions.

Key elements of universal infection control

The key elements of universal infection control are listed in Table 7.3 and will be discussed in turn.

Medical history

The collection of an accurate medical history is part of good clinical practice and is helpful in the identification of immunocompromised patients. However, although a medical history can provide useful information in respect of previous infectious diseases the clinician must be aware that it does not allow for the categorisation of patients into 'high risk' and 'low risk' from the point of view of infectivity to staff and other patients. One current exception to this concept relates to patients who fall into the risk groups for CJD (see below).

Cleaning instruments

The cleaning of used surgical instruments to remove visible deposits is an essential step prior to their sterilisation. In hospitals, both the cleaning and the subsequent sterilisation procedures are usually performed in a Central Sterile Supply Unit (CSSU). However, increasing amounts of minor surgery are performed in primary care and, under these circumstances, the decontamination of used instruments might be performed in a medical or dental practice. In such cases, instrument cleaning may be achieved by hand scrubbing in soap or detergent, but ultrasonic baths and washer disinfectors are very useful and more effective for many items. Heavy-duty protective gloves should be worn during instrument cleaning, and care taken to avoid sharps injuries.

Sterilising instruments

After clinical use, all surgical instruments must be sterilised before they are used to treat a subsequent patient. The sterilisation method of choice for heat-stable instruments is the autoclave. It is critical that the steam makes physical contact with the surfaces of all the instruments and care must be therefore be taken not to overload the autoclave and impede steam penetration. Effective monitoring of autoclave efficacy is important. Physical, chemical and biological tests of efficacy are available; for example, a chemical indicator strip can be placed in the centre of the load as a check on the effectiveness of each cycle of a bench-top autoclave.

Hot air ovens are microbiologically acceptable as a sterilisation measure and are used for specific purposes, such as the sterilisation of greases. However, the higher temperature and longer cycle time (160°C for 60 min) make them more damaging to instruments and they are not ideal for routine sterilisation procedures.

Chemical agents such as aldehydes are not appropriate for routine sterilisation of surgical items and equipment. They are unreliable and some are toxic or corrosive. However, for certain expensive, heat-sensitive items such as endoscopes, high level disinfection with chemicals, under strictly controlled conditions, is employed.

In the light of concerns over the resitance of prions to sterilisation procedures, there are now calls for the 'tagging' (e.g. by bar coding) of all individual surgical instruments. This would permit the recording, in a patient's notes, of exactly which instruments were used and so introduce 'traceability' of instruments into the recycling process. It would, however, be a massive logistical exercise with major cost implications.

Use of disposables

Disposable items are generally recommended, although there is a cost implication. Disposable items must always be used once only and then discarded. The routine use of disposable instruments for surgery involving tissues that pose a risk from vCJD, for example tonsillectomies, has been recommended in the UK.

As needles cannot be reliably cleaned and sterilised, they must always be discarded into a sharps bin after use on a single patient. Similarly, a local anaesthetic cartridge must never be used for the treatment of more than one patient.

Decontamination of operatory surfaces

Good hygiene in healthcare facilities is an important and underrated element of infection control, with particular relevance to surgical sepsis. In addition to general environmental contamination, surfaces in clinical areas can become contaminated with microorganisms following contact with tissues and body fluids of patients. Regular cleaning of surfaces with detergent, together with application of disinfectants in appropriate sites, are essential. Other 'surfaces' can also pose a problem, for example the pens used by healthcare workers, many of which have been shown to be contaminated with pathogens such as MRSA.

In the event of an overt spillage of blood or other body fluid, it should be soaked into an absorbent cloth and a disinfectant such as hypochlorite (10 000 ppm available chlorine) applied. Alternatively, commercially available spillage granules could be used.

Protective workwear

All staff should wear protective coats on wards to protect their outdoor clothing from contamination. However, white coats themselves become contaminated with microorganisms, especially at points of frequent contact, such as the sleeve and pocket. Indeed, the uniforms worn by healthcare workers have been shown to play a role in transmitting bacteria in the hospital setting and the importance of hygiene, with regular laundering of uniforms, should again be stressed. Appropriate theatre dress, including operating gown, gloves and eye protection must be worn routinely when undertaking surgical procedures, together with a well-fitting surgical facemask.

Avoiding needlestick injuries

Sharps injuries are common among staff performing surgical procedures and many go unreported to occupational health departments and so are not followed up. However, occupationally acquired infections with hepatitis B and C viruses, and with HIV, have been recorded following needlestick injuries and related sharps accidents. It is, therefore, essential that healthcare workers are encouraged to seek appropriate management following such incidents. The principles of management of needlestick and related injuries are discussed below. Although some of these injuries are unavoidable, many are essentially preventable and great care must be taken when handling and disposing of all sharps.

Needles should never be resheathed after use, unless a safe resheathing device is used. Care must also be taken not to injure other staff, for example when sharp instruments are being passed between surgeons and nurses. Unsheathed needles must never be left exposed where others might injure themselves. All contaminated sharp items must be discarded into a sharps box (see below) and staff must never put their hands into the opening of the box.

Immunising staff

Vaccination against hepatitis B virus is now a requirement in the UK for all healthcare workers undertaking exposure-prone procedures. This vaccine, which contains hepatitis B surface antigen (HBsAg), provides protection from one of the most important and serious occupational infections of healthcare workers. The course of three doses of vaccine must be followed by a blood test to ensure that the recipient has developed a protective level of antibody.

For healthcare workers who are non-responders to the vaccine, further serological tests are required to ensure that they are not high-risk carriers of hepatitis B. High-risk carriers are those who are HBeAg positive or who are HBeAg negative but with a viral load exceeding 10^3 genome equivalents per mL. Such individuals pose a potential risk of infection to patients and would not be permitted to undertake exposure-prone procedures, which clearly include all forms of surgical practice.

Immunisation against other infectious diseases such as tuberculosis (in the UK), tetanus and poliomyelitis is also recommended and non-pregnant female personnel of child-bearing age should be protected against rubella.

Safe waste disposal

Hospitals have a responsibility to ensure the safe disposal of all contaminated waste generated during surgery. Arrangements must be made with a local authority or private contractor for final collection and disposal. Regulated waste includes contaminated sharps, liquid blood and other body fluids, tissues, and non-sharp solid waste that is saturated or caked with body fluid.

All sharp items must be consigned to rigid, puncture-resistant containers, which should never be filled to more than two-thirds of their capacity. The containers should be securely closed and fastened before uplift for incineration. Soft waste contaminated with blood must be placed into sturdy, impervious, sealed bags and clearly labelled as infective waste.

Effective training for staff

Good training of all staff engaged in patient care is an important element of infection control. Good infection control procedures should become an automatic part of clinical practice for all healthcare workers but, unfortunately, they are often not afforded the priority

they deserve. A written infection control policy must be available in all healthcare facilities and procedures reviewed on a regular basis. The overseeing of all aspects of infection control in hospitals, including training, is the responsibility of the Infection Control Committee, which is usually chaired by a Consultant Medical Microbiologist. This committee will also include one or more specially trained Infection Control Nurses, who play an important role in dealing with day-to-day cross-infection issues in hospitals.

Occupationally acquired infections

The main concern of healthcare workers relates to the risk of infection with blood-borne viruses, notably HIV. Hepatitis B remains the major infectious occupational hazard for surgeons and other healthcare workers who, prior to the availability of a vaccine, were up to ten times more likely to become infected than members of the general population. Table 7.4 summarises the relative risks of infection with HIV and hepatitis B virus. Hepatitis B virus is far more infectious than HIV and it is fortunate that most healthcare workers respond to the hepatitis B vaccine, thereby gaining protection.

According to the most recent figures available, the totals of 'definite' and 'possible' occupationally acquired HIV infections have amounted to 319 cases worldwide. These have comprised 102 definite (5 in UK) and 217 possible (8 in UK), most of which followed sharps accidents with large-bore needles.

The occupational risk of infection with hepatitis C virus is not yet clear but several recent studies suggest that the overall risk is low. However, well-documented

Table 7.4 The relative risks of occupational infection with HIV and hepatitis B virus (HBV)		
	HIV	*HBV*
Minimum volume of blood to transmit infection	0.1 mL	0.00004 mL
Risk of infection following needlestick injury from a seropositive patient	0.3%	7–30%*
*The risk of infection with hepatitis B virus depends on whether the source patient is a high-risk carrier		

seroconversions following needlestick accidents have been reported and emphasise the importance of avoiding such injuries.

Other infections can be occupationally acquired by surgeons: there is a documented occupational risk for healthcare workers of infection with *Mycobacterium tuberculosis*. There is no evidence of an occupational risk for healthcare workers from prion diseases such as CJD.

Management of sharps injuries

Prevention of sharps injuries is extremely important but it is recognised that, within healthcare facilities, and particularly during surgical procedures, such incidents are still fairly common. A significant proportion are essentially preventable if staff follow guidelines on handling sharps and, in addition, many commercial companies are now developing new 'needle-less' devices. However, it is impossible to eliminate the risks completely. The effective management of sharps injuries is, therefore, an important issue in the prevention of occupationally acquired infections with blood-borne viruses; it also has medicolegal implications.

Every hospital should have a policy and procedure for managing sharps injuries, and this should be well publicised and readily available to all staff. The principles of management are summarised in Fig. 7.2. All such events should be officially recorded in an accident book. Immediate first aid involves cleaning the wound under running water, without scrubbing or manipulation, and the application of a waterproof dressing. Expert medical advice should then be sought.

Ideally, blood should be taken at the time of the accident from the healthcare worker and the titre of anti-HBs antibody measured. Residual serum is stored so that it is available in the future for HIV and hepatitis C virus antibody testing, if necessary.

Although the concept of approaching the source patient is controversial, ideally blood should also be collected from this individual. Appropriate discussion and counselling are obviously essential but, if consent is given, the blood can be screened for hepatitis markers and HIV antibody, which in most cases will be negative. Such information can be very reassuring to a healthcare worker who has sustained an injury, but no pressure should be exerted on the source patient to donate the appropriate sample.

Immediate treatment for the healthcare worker might include passive immunisation for a hepatitis B vaccine

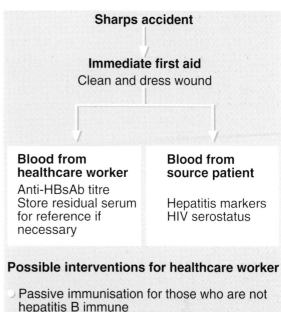

Fig. 7.2   Management of sharps injuries.

non-responder, or a vaccine booster for those whose anti-HBs antibody titre has waned. The administration of prophylactic azidothymidine (AZT) for those who have sustained an injury from a known HIV-positive patient has been controversial but recent evidence suggests that, in combination with other antiretroviral drugs, it can further reduce the risk of infection. Such prophylaxis is now officially recommended for significant injuries and should be administered promptly, ideally within 1 h of the injury. However, the treatment is not without side-effects and the risk assessment of the injury should be made in conjunction with a physician who is experienced in this area.

Healthcare workers infected with blood-borne viruses

There is strong epidemiological evidence that healthcare workers who are high-risk carriers of hepatitis B virus, as defined earlier, can transmit hepatitis B to patients if they undertake exposure-prone procedures. Exposure-prone procedures are those in which there is a risk that injury to the worker could result in the exposure of the patient's open tissues to the blood of the healthcare worker. Those who are HBsAg positive but not HBeAg positive, and whose viral load does not exceed 10^3 genome equivalents per mL, are permitted to continue with exposure-prone procedures, providing they have not been associated with spread of infection to patients.

Apart from the case in which a Florida dentist with AIDS apparently transmitted HIV to several patients, there is only one other report of an HIV-infected healthcare worker transmitting the virus to a patient. This involved an HIV-seropositive orthopaedic surgeon in France, who apparently transmitted HIV to a patient during hip surgery in 1992. At the time, the surgeon was asymptomatic and unaware of his infection. Thus, currently available data suggest that the risk of transmission of HIV to patients from HIV-infected healthcare workers is extremely low. Nevertheless, healthcare workers who are known to be HIV seropositive are not permitted to undertake exposure-prone procedures in the UK.

There is increasing epidemiological evidence that hepatitis C virus can be transmitted from seropositive healthcare workers to patients during exposure-prone procedures. UK guidelines published in 2002 place restrictions on the clinical activities of healthcare workers who are infected with hepatitis C (HCV RNA positive).

Antimicrobial prophylaxis during surgery

A number of factors can increase the risk of surgical site infection and these are considered in detail in Chapter 8; they can be patient-related or procedure-related (see Table 8.2). The risk of surgical site infection also depends on whether the surgical procedure is a clean, clean-contaminated, contaminated, or dirty-infected procedure (see Table 8.3).

Improvements in operating room ventilation, sterilisation methods, barriers and surgical techniques have all helped to reduce the incidence of surgical site infections, but the use of topical, oral and intravenous antimicrobial prophylaxis has also played an important role. However, in the current climate of increasing antimicrobial resistance, it is important that prophylaxis is not overused but is reserved for well-defined indications.

Table 7.5 Goals of surgical prophylaxis
Prevent postoperative infection of the surgical site
Prevent postoperative infectious morbidity and mortality
Reduce the duration and cost of health care
Produce no adverse effects
Have no adverse effects for the microbial flora of the patient or hospital

Perioperative antimicrobial surgical prophylaxis is recommended for operative procedures that have a high rate of postoperative wound infection, when foreign materials are to be implanted, or when the wound infection rate is low but the development of a wound infection results in a disastrous event. It is beyond the scope of this chapter to provide details of all those surgical procedures for which prophylaxis is indicated but examples include colorectal surgery and joint replacement surgery. The goals of an anti-infective drug used for surgical prophylaxis are summarised in Table 7.5. To achieve these goals, an ideal prophylactic antimicrobial agent should be bactericidal, non-toxic, inexpensive and have in vitro activity against the common organisms that cause postoperative wound infection after a specific surgical procedure.

There is no benefit in commencing intravenous antimicrobial therapy before the perioperative period. Normally, prophylactic antimicrobial agents should be administered no more than 30–60 min before surgery. A common practice is to administer the intravenous prophylactic agent at the time of induction of anaesthesia. Therapeutic concentrations of antimicrobial agents in tissues should be present throughout the period that the wound is open. For prolonged procedures, or antimicrobial agents with short half-lives, an additional dose may need to be administered intraoperatively. The duration of antimicrobial prophylaxis for most procedures is controversial, but expert opinion recommends at most one or two postoperative doses. Prolonged prophylaxis should be discouraged because of the possibility of added antimicrobial toxicity, selection of resistant organisms and unnecessary expense.

Creutzfeldt–Jakob disease

The transmissible, spongiform encephalopathies (TSEs) comprise a group of neurodegenerative disorders caused by infection with agents called prions. This group of diseases includes sporadic, familial and iatrogenic forms of Creutzfeldt–Jakob disease (CJD). The description of a new form of CJD, now called variant CJD (vCJD), together with evidence that it is caused by the same agent as bovine spongiform encephalopathy (BSE), has significantly raised the profile of the TSEs.

The relevance of TSEs to this chapter is that these diseases are causing serious concerns in relation to infection control procedures. Prion proteins are remarkably stable and resistant to most conventional sterilisation measures. Iatrogenic transmission of human prion diseases via neurosurgical instruments has been reported and there is some evidence that transmission via other surgical procedures can also occur. For the sporadic, familial and iatrogenic forms of CJD, the tissues in which there is a high level of infectivity are the brain, spinal cord and eye. However, the position is further complicated because vCJD differs from the sporadic, iatrogenic and familial forms in that the lymphoreticular tissues of vCJD cases are also consistently infected with prion proteins.

Current guidelines are that all the instruments used in a surgical procedure on a patient suffering from a TSE must be disposable and destroyed by incineration. In addition, current recommendations from the Spongiform Encephalopathy Advisory Committee suggest using the medical history form to identify patients who may be at risk of (although not clinically suffering from) iatrogenic or familial forms of CJD. Questions enquire about previous brain surgery (to identify possible recipients of dura mater grafts), growth hormone use before the mid-1980s (after which artificially synthesised growth hormone came into use), and close family members who might have had CJD (to identify those at risk of familial CJD). For patients who are identified as being at risk, any surgery involving the brain, spinal cord or eye should be undertaken using disposable instruments that are subsequently incinerated. Surgery involving other tissues in such patients is ideally also undertaken with disposable instruments and, if non-disposable instruments are used, they must pass through a stringent decontamination process, separately from other instruments. This involves two washing cycles and a total of 18 min in a porous load (vacuum) autoclave.

However, no questions in the medical history will identify those patients at risk of sporadic or vCJD. The latter is a major concern because of the infectivity in lymphoreticular tissues. The number of cases of vCJD in the UK is still low (122 confirmed cases to 3 February 2003), and a preliminary screening study of vCJD reactivity in approximately 3000 archived tonsils and appendix specimens revealed no positive results. However, there is still concern among many experts that an epidemic, linked to consumption of meat from BSE-infected herds, could develop. The routine use of disposable instruments for all patients undergoing certain surgical procedures that involve high-risk tissues is now being given serious consideration and, where practicable, implemented.

8 Surgical sepsis

Introduction

The principles of the control of cross-infection were discussed in Chapter 7. Sepsis as a specific complication of surgery is considered in this chapter (Table 8.1).

The body possesses a complex system of mechanisms to protect itself from infection. These include:

- methods to prevent entry of bacteria into the body, such as skin and mucous membranes, which act as a barrier to penetration by organisms
- the mucociliary apparatus in the respiratory tract, which washes bacteria from the respiratory tract
- methods to deal locally with organisms if they manage to invade the body tissues, for example, the local inflammatory reaction resulting in cellulitis and abscess formation
- methods to deal with organisms if they start to invade tissues, including lymph node reaction and systemic lymphocyte response.

Surgery predisposes to infection by affecting the body defences at all levels. It also causes a breach in the protective barrier, allowing organisms a portal of entry. However, tissue damage will also inhibit the inflammatory response locally by causing tissue ischaemia or by formation of haematoma. Surgery also affects the systemic response of the body to trauma.

Thus, postoperative sepsis may be local – affecting the wound itself – or sepsis may occur at a remote site. Chest sepsis is the most common remote site infection but other sites may be involved. For example, patients may be predisposed to chest sepsis if they have a pre-existing upper respiratory tract infection, if they smoke or if they have chronic lung disease such as asthma or bronchiectasis. An example of sepsis at another site is urinary tract infection resulting from a poor catherisation technique. Factors that may increase the risk of wound

Table 8.1   Wound infection following surgery
Classification of wounds
Infecting organisms
Prevention of wound infections
Clinical features of wound sepsis
Diagnosis of wound sepsis
Treatment

Table 8.2   Factors that may increase the risk of surgical site infection
Patient-related
age
nutritional status
diabetes mellitus
cancer
uraemia
jaundice
smoking status
obesity
coexisting infection at a remote site
colonisation with microorganisms
altered immune response, e.g. HIV
drugs, e.g. corticosteroids, anti-inflammatories, chemotherapy
length of preoperative stay
Procedure-related
duration of surgical scrub
skin antisepsis
preoperative shaving
duration of operation
operating room ventilation
inadequate sterilisation of instruments
foreign material at the surgical site
surgical drains
surgical technique
haematoma
poor blood supply

sepsis are listed in Table 8.2. These may be patient-related or they may be local, procedure-related factors. This chapter will concentrate primarily on wound sepsis.

Wound infection is defined as a collection of pus in a wound. In the initial phase of bacterial penetration of the tissues, the body will host an inflammatory response against the invading organisms to try to contain them in the area and to destroy them. This inflammation will be apparent clinically as cellulitis, which is a tender redness of the tissues. However, a similar response may result from inflammation from other causes (e.g. haematoma, excess tissue handling or trauma during surgery). Because of this, the presence of cellulitis alone may not always indicate infection.

One can only be sure that a wound is infected when pus forms, hence the above definition. Studies comparing methods to control wound infection only discuss wounds where pus is confirmed to be present.

For a wound infection to occur, there must be a sufficient number of organisms inoculated into the wound ($>10^7$ viable cocci must be injected into a wound in a normal person to cause an abscess) and conditions within the wound area must be suitable for growth of the organisms. The presence of necrotic tissue, haematoma, seroma and foreign bodies all predispose to sepsis.

Classification of wounds

Certain wounds are more prone to infection than others. Surgeons therefore divide wounds into different types according to the level of risk of sepsis (Table 8.3).

Clean wounds

These are wounds in which no viscus has been entered, no septic area has been encountered and there has been no break in aseptic technique. Such wounds should never become infected; infection rates with such wounds should be less than 3%.

Clean contaminated wounds

In this situation, the operation enters a non-infected area but may encounter bacteria. Careful control of the area should result in minimal spillage of organisms. Examples of this include surgery on the upper gastrointestinal tract, biliary tree or respiratory tract. Infection rates for this type of surgery should be less than 10%.

Table 8.3 Classification of wounds
Clean wounds
Clean contaminated wounds
Contaminated wounds
Dirty wounds

Contaminated wounds

This is surgery where there is gross spillage of organisms, where there is infection already present but without pus formation, where there is a major break in aseptic technique or where there is an open wound that has been exposed for less than 4 h (e.g. following major trauma). In this type of wound, sepsis frequently exceeds 30%.

Dirty wounds

This is an operation through an infected area (e.g. perforated viscus, abscess or traumatic wound) that has been exposed for over 4 h. By definition, all these wounds are infected.

This classification of wounds allows comparative studies to be conducted between centres and of varying techniques to try to control wound sepsis. It also allows surgeons to monitor their own data to ensure that they are achieving acceptable standards of surgery with regard to sepsis.

Infecting organisms

Infecting organisms can be subdivided into two types.

Exogenous organisms

Exogenous organisms are organisms introduced into a wound from an external source. The two main exogenous organisms responsible for wound sepsis are *Staphylococcus aureus* and *Streptococcus pyogenes*. These are encountered much less frequently than they used to be, with the exception of patients with trauma and/or burns, in whom they are as prevalent as ever. When wound sepsis occurs with these bacteria, it usually indicates a breakdown of sterile surgical technique. The longer an operative procedure, the more likely the procedure is to become infected by an exogenous organism.

Endogenous organisms

Endogenous organisms are bacteria that are usually present in the body but are non-infective under normal circumstances. Such organisms are known as commensals. These organisms are encountered in clean-contaminated, contaminated and dirty wounds. Such organisms are common in gastrointestinal surgery, for example, *Escherichia coli*, enteroccocci and *Bacteroides* species. In clean-contaminated and contaminated wounds, where it is expected that a significant number of organisms may be encountered, the use of prophylactic antibiotics given from the time of surgery has been shown in many cases to significantly reduce the risk of wound infection. Such use of antibiotics, however, must not be seen to be an alternative to meticulous and careful atraumatic surgical technique.

Excessive use of prophylactic antibiotics is not without problems, for example, allergic side-effects to the drug, development of bacterial resistance to specific antibiotics and cross-transfer of these resistant strains within the hospital environment (see Ch. 7).

Prevention of wound infections

'Clean wounds' lend themselves to studies of techniques of control of infection. When the wound sepsis rate of clean wounds is unacceptably high, it suggests that a problem within the unit is allowing the introduction of large numbers of exogenous organisms into the operation field.

The infection rate due to exogenous organisms has reduced dramatically because of aseptic techniques. It is impossible to sterilise the atmosphere in an operating theatre, to sterilise the skin of a patient completely and to avoid the carrying of microorganisms into the operating area by theatre personnel. However, equipment and drapes can be sterilised and much can be done to reduce

Table 8.4 Prevention of wound infection
Environment
Theatre personnel
Patient preparation
Operating technique
Prophylactic antibiotics

the transport of organisms to the patient's wound. Key elements of universal infection control were discussed in detail in Chapter 7 but factors relating specifically to prevention of wound infection (Table 8.4) are discussed here.

Environment

The design of a modern operating theatre with laminar air-flow and air-filtering systems has significantly reduced the number of organisms in the atmosphere. In recent years, however, further advances have made little effect on wound sepsis rates because most infections are now endogenous in nature.

The longer the duration of surgery and the greater the number of personnel in theatre, the higher the wound sepsis rate.

Theatre personnel

Contamination of a wound occurs easily from theatre staff.

The surgeon, theatre assistant(s) and nursing staff should wash/scrub their hands and forearms with an antimicrobial agent such as chlorhexidine or povidone–iodine to reduce bacterial load on the skin. The initial scrub of the day is the most important and should include a careful nail scrub and a wash lasting at least 5 min. Thereafter, scrubbing for further operations requires only a 1 min careful wash and nail scrubbing is no longer necessary. This reduces the numbers of skin organisms but, after 30 min, the bacterial count on the skin starts to rise again and may exceed the prescrub levels after 2 h. Staff in intimate contact with an operation should therefore wear suitable sterile protective clothing with sterile gowns and gloves. As there can be a glove puncture rate of up to 10% by the end of an operation, many surgeons now double-glove. This may also protect the surgeon from organisms that might be acquired from a patient.

The use of theatre masks is controversial, with evidence to suggest that they are ineffective within a relatively short period of time.

The number of personnel in theatre should be reduced to the minimum, with little movement of staff through theatre while surgery is being undertaken.

Staff with a severe upper respiratory infection or sore throat should be excluded from the theatre area.

Patient preparation

Patients who have been inpatients in hospital for a significant period prior to surgery tend to develop a skin contamination of 'hospital-acquired' organisms. These bacteria tend to be highly resistant to commonly used antibiotics. In such patients, bacterial scrub the night before surgery may be beneficial, although this is unproven.

Any patient harbouring an infection at a site distant to the operation wound has a significantly increased risk of wound sepsis, perhaps doubling the incidence. Therefore any patient with an infected lesion should have this treated before surgery is contemplated.

Shaving the skin in the area of the operation on the night before surgery has now been shown to increase wound sepsis rates. Tiny nicks in the skin acquire bacterial contamination, which is at a much higher level than in the unshaven skin. Hair removal by clipper is advised, or it should not be done at all. Certainly, if shaving is to be performed, this should be done in the anaesthetic area immediately before surgery is about to take place.

Various skin preparation agents for 'sterilising' the skin in the operation field are available, the most commonly used being chlorhexidine and povidone–iodine. A double wash is traditionally performed and the operation area is covered with sterile drapes leaving only a window for surgery. However, it is not possible to sterilise skin completely by the use of such agents.

Operating technique

Surgical technique is most important in control of wound sepsis. Wound sepsis rates vary between surgeons and are almost certainly related to individual technique such as careful handling of tissues, removal of all foreign bodies or dead tissue, avoiding the use of excess diathermy and sutures, avoiding excessive suture tension, accurate placement of sutures, and avoiding the formation of haematoma. Monofilament sutures are probably associated with less wound sepsis than braided suture materials.

A careful audit comparing one surgeon's infection rates with those of another surgeon usually results in a steady reduction in infection, and this is certainly related to increased careful technique. Surgeons should therefore keep a close audit of their own sepsis rates and, if they are unacceptably high compared with other surgeons, must address the reasons for this.

Prophylactic antibiotics

As discussed in Chapter 7, antibiotics have been shown to reduce wound sepsis in clean/contaminated and contaminated wounds only. The use of antibiotics in clean wounds is of no value in reducing wound sepsis but they should always be given if there is insertion of foreign material or if the patient has cardiac valvular disease. This is especially important during dental procedures.

Clinical features of wound sepsis

Classically, wound sepsis produces a tachycardia and pyrexia approximately 2–4 days postsurgery. The patient usually complains of increasing pain in the wound, perhaps exceeding that noted immediately after surgery.

The features of an infected wound usually develop very rapidly. The wound develops a cellulitis, perhaps with some purulent material oozing from the surface of the incision or from the suture sites. The wound then becomes oedematous and bronzed in appearance with marked swelling. Attempted palpation reveals a marked local increase in temperature and exquisite tenderness.

At this point, removal of some or all of the sutures results in release of pus and the wound margins will then be noted to be lined with slough.

In severe cases, haemorrhagic vesicles may appear, with areas of frank necrosis of tissue.

Especially after bowel surgery, the surgeon should always be aware of the fact that the sepsis may be arising from the peritoneal cavity and not just be superficial under the skin. Severe wound sepsis may result in complete breakdown or dehiscence of the wound, necessitating wound resuture.

Diagnosis of wound sepsis

This is usually made on clinical grounds alone. Bacteriology culture swabs may allow confirmation of the infecting organism(s) and their antibiotic sensitivity. This is especially useful if the patient does not seem to be responding satisfactorily to apparently adequate therapy and knowledge of the infecting organisms now obtained by such swabs will allow a more accurate choice of antibiotic to be made.

Treatment

Initial treatment of a suspected wound infection is usually by antibiotics. The choice depends on the type of wound and the nature of the surgery. In contaminated and clean/contaminated wounds, antibiotic therapy may merely consist of continuing the prophylactic antibiotic originally used. Certainly, if there is severe or spreading cellulitis, antibiotic usage is essential and may be more effective if given intravenously.

Where there is obvious pus formation, sutures should be removed from the skin and the wound allowed to gape or, if necessary, probed. Any pus obtained should be forwarded to the bacteriologist for culture. If there is no significant cellulitis, lymphangitis or lymphadenopathy, simple release of pus may be all that is indicated and antibiotics may not be necessary.

After release of pus, the wound should be left open. It may be filled with antiseptic packs. There are many different techniques and agents available for dressing such wounds and each unit tends to have its own preferences. Normally, an infected wound is left to heal by granulation from below, with the packs being changed regularly to keep the wound as clean as possible and to allow the granulation to fill the cavity. When the wound is clean and granulating, if it is large, it may be secondarily resutured. In many instances, however, these wounds reheal rapidly without the need for resuturing and, as soon as the wound has healed by granulation, it will rapidly re-epithelialise.

Abdominal wounds that have been badly infected and allowed to heal by this method are commonly weakened, with the subsequent formation of incisional hernia.

9 Fractures

Introduction

A fracture is a break in the continuity of bone; it can be complete or incomplete. Fractures are the cause of a considerable degree of morbidity and even mortality across all age groups. Patients suffer both in the short term from pain and in the long term from disability and deformity. These effects are, in the main, largely preventable. A sound appreciation of the principles of fractures and their management has a profound effect on patients' quality of life, not only in orthopaedics but in many other specialties including maxillofacial and oral surgery, neurosurgery and accident and emergency surgery.

A discussion of the aetiology of fractures is followed by their diagnosis and classification. The process of fracture healing will also be discussed, followed by consideration of the management of fractures and the complications that can occur (Table 9.1).

This chapter deals with the general principles of fracture management and gives specific examples as appropriate. The detailed management of maxillofacial fractures and its variance from general principles is considered in Chapter 12.

Aetiology of fractures

Fractures can be caused by a number of different mechanisms (Table 9.2) and this leads to a variation in the pattern of fractures. The vast majority of fractures are caused by an excessive force applied to that bone, causing it to break. Biomechanics are the key in relation to bony injury, both in terms of the injury sustained and its appropriate management. A direct force applied to a bone will cause a fracture at the site of impact. Indirect forces cause fractures distant to where the force is applied, such as spiral long-bone fractures.

Table 9.1 Important considerations in the management of fractures
Aetiology of fractures
Diagnosis of fractures
Classification of fractures
Fracture healing
Principles of management
treatment of closed fractures
treatment of open fractures
Complications

Table 9.2 Mechanisms of bony fracture
Direct force
Indirect force
Stress fractures
Pathological fractures

The pattern of fractures also differs with age, relating to the nature of the patient's skeleton and bone stock. Different types of bone tend to show different types of fracture. For example, cancellous bone, when put under sufficient stress, generally undergoes crush fracture, which can be comminuted.

The history will indicate which injuries are likely to be present and will help to direct investigation. For example, in the driver of car involved in a road traffic accident, the presence of a broken windscreen will alert to the probability of head and facial injuries.

Stress fractures are caused by repeated relatively minor injury. Their exact aetiology is not known but again, a detailed history alerts to their possibility as, for example, in a runner with painful metatarsals.

Pathological fractures occur in abnormal bone. The force applied would not normally be enough to cause a break if the bone was normal. The weakness of the bone can be caused by very many disease processes. The most common underlying pathologies for pathological fractures include osteoporosis and malignant infiltration of the bone, either secondaries or rarely primaries. Naturally, the diagnosis of a pathological fracture, and the underlying pathology, have a bearing on appropriate subsequent management.

Diagnosis of fractures

Clinical examination

Injuries to bone are often present in combination with other injuries, and initial consideration should be directed to the patient as a whole and particularly if there is need for resuscitation.

The fundamentals for diagnosis are based on history and examination. History has been alluded to above. A detailed clinical examination, with emphasis directed by the history not only indicates which investigations are required for definitive diagnosis but also alerts to injury of underlying or surrounding structures.

Look, feel, move is a good way to approach the examination of bony injury:

- *Look*: for signs of injury; swelling is often the most useful sign. Fractures are associated with a greater degree of swelling than soft tissue injuries. The distribution of the swelling can also be enlightening. For example, if confined to the joint, swelling can indicate excess fluid or blood in that joint. Deformity generally leaves little doubt about the existence of underlying bony injury. Bruising might be present if there is delay in presentation. It is important to look for and document the integrity of the skin overlying the injury, as this will allow classification into open (compound) or closed fractures, and will affect management. Colour – particularly distal to the injury – will give clues to vascular status.
- *Feel*: palpation needs to be done carefully, but sufficiently firmly to give the answers. Often large areas around the site of injury are tender, but it is important to elicit the area or areas of maximum tenderness to direct subsequent investigations, and focus analysis of those investigations. Temperature of the injured area should be noted and may indicate infection, for example, if presentation is delayed.
- *Move*: initially, patients should be asked to perform relevant movements themselves. If there is significant

injury minimal movement is possible. Often patients feel that they are unable to move any of the joints in a large surrounding area such as a whole limb. Careful 'passive' movements can be carried out, always gently and never forcing the movement.

Other tests

The important structures most commonly affected by limb fractures are either blood vessels or nerves and it is essential to document neurovascular status around, and particularly distal to, all fractures. Vascular compromise in particular will alter immediate management, in an attempt to restore blood flow.

Vascular

Pulses and capillary refill distal to the site of injury should be assessed. Although this is performed at this stage in a systematic examination, an early assessment of vascular status should be carried out, for example during preliminary history taking.

Neurological

Sensory and motor function should be tested in the distribution of nerves that may have been affected by the injury.

Other

Surrounding structures can be affected and are often fracture specific. Tendons might be disrupted by the sharp edges of the fracture, for example in the hand. Any structure lying in proximity to the fracture is at risk and careful examination should be carried to assess for damage to underlying structure, such as orbital blow-out fractures (where the inferior rectus can be tethered) or pelvic fractures (where there might be urethral injury); rib fractures can cause lung injury or pneumothorax.

Radiographic examination

There is no place for blanket radiographs. Clinical suspicion is of paramount importance. Radiographs are sometimes indicated where bony tenderness cannot be excluded. For example, unconscious trauma patients must have cervical spine films.

Radiographs of at least two views at 90° to each other are essential. A fracture cannot be excluded without these views and accurate classification and description of an obvious fracture cannot be complete without them.

Obvious signs of bony injury show as disruption of the cortex. However, cortical breaks can be difficult to see and clinicians should develop a systematic routine for reviewing radiographs that involves tracing around the cortical lines. It is useful to stand back from the radiograph to assess if its overall appearance is normal, and also whether the general state of the bone looks normal.

Once a fracture is seen, it is important to look for other fractures associated with it. Rings of bone rarely break in only one place and a second fracture should be suspected, for example, in the pelvis or mandible. It might be necessary at this stage to obtain further radiographs (e.g. of the joint above and below the fracture).

It is sometimes necessary to rely on more subtle evidence that is visible radiographically. The only clue to a bony injury might be surrounding soft tissue swelling or blood visible within usually empty spaces, such as in maxillary sinuses.

Further imaging

When used appropriately, plain radiographs have both high sensitivity and specificity. However, they can be fallible and, in the presence of a negative radiograph, reliance is on clinical suspicion. If either the mechanism of injury or the clinical examination suggests a particular injury then further imaging is necessary.

Further plain radiographs might be indicated, either different views or films taken with a joint in a particular position or under stress (for example, flexion/extension views).

More sophisticated forms of imaging might be necessary and computerised tomography (CT) scanning is particularly good at showing bony detail. Magnetic resonance imaging (MRI) is excellent at showing soft tissue detail. Radioisotope-uptake bone scans also have a role in advanced investigation.

Classification of fractures

Fractures are classified in many different ways, and often the same fracture is classified simultaneously a number of different ways. For example, a single fracture can be open, pathological, displaced, oblique, intra-articular and unstable.

Table 9.3 Classification of fractures
Site
Extent
Configuration
Overlying skin integrity
Pathological
Displacement
Angulation, rotation, impaction and distraction
Joint involvement
Stability

The following classifications are the most common and most helpful with regards to treatment and referring the patient to a surgeon who will undertake treatment (Table 9.3).

Site

The most important consideration is which bone is fractured and which part of that bone is fractured, clearly documenting the side, for example, fractured right distal third of radius.

Extent

This differentiates between a complete disruption of cortex and a partial disruption of cortex or a crack. Incomplete fractures are more common in children and are known as greenstick fractures.

Configuration

This is essentially the shape or direction of the fracture line. Transverse fractures extend at right-angles to the cortical surface. Oblique fractures are as their name suggests, as are compression fractures. Spiral fractures tend to occur in long bones and are the result of twisting forces applied distant to the fracture site. 'Comminuted' means that there are a number of bone fragments.

Overlying skin integrity

A breach in the skin over a fracture makes the fracture open or compound and changes the subsequent management required, the principles of which are considered later in this chapter.

Open fractures can be further classified with regards to how 'open' they are (the Gustillo and Anderson

Table 9.4 Classification of open fractures
Grade I : less than 1 cm wound
Grade II : greater than 1 cm wound
Grade III: extensive skin and soft tissue damage
IIIA: wound can be covered with remaining soft tissue
IIIB: wound cannot be covered with soft tissue, periosteal stripping
IIIC: associated arterial injury

classification), which has bearing on how likely it is that the wound will become infected (Table 9.4).

Pathological fractures

Pathological fractures were considered on page 59, under the heading 'Aetiology of fractures'.

Displacement (apposition)

A fracture is displaced if the two ends are not in exact anatomical apposition. This is caused by the force of the injury and/or the action of muscles around the fracture site. The degree of displacement or shift is often described subjectively (e.g. 'moderately' displaced). However, perhaps a more useful description is a measurement of the displacement, for example with respect to the width of the fractured bone. Correcting displacement has an important impact on fracture healing, deformity and function.

Angulation, rotation, impaction and distraction

These are other forms of deformity relating the fracture ends to each other. Angulation can be thought of as tilt between the ends, and rotation is the degree of twist. Impaction is where the ends are forced into each other and distraction where there is a gap between the ends in the axis of the fractured bone. All of these can also result in healing and functional problems and they might require close clinical and radiological examination to detect them.

Joint involvement

If the fracture line extends into the joint it disrupts the articular surface and can be regarded as intra-articular. This predisposes to long-term sequelae, mainly osteo-arthritis. This type of fracture therefore requires an accurate degree of reduction.

Stability

Unstable fractures are those whose positions are prone to change. This is often the case even after initial reduction. These injuries therefore require more immobilisation, for example, with internal fixation. Unstable fractures of the mandible are specifically discussed in Chapter 12.

Fracture healing

The process of fracture healing can be conveniently divided into stages (Table 9.5). It is important to realise that these stages are not discrete entities, but rather overlap and blend into one another. Mediators and factors affecting fracture healing are broadly similar to those involved in wound healing (described above).

Inflammatory phase

- *Bleeding and clot formation*: bleeding occurs from the fracture ends, predominantly from periosteal and endosteal vessels. A clot forms between the ends of the fracture.
- *Acute inflammatory reaction and swelling*: an inflammatory infiltrate of white blood cells invades the clot and fracture site. Resultant swelling causes loosening of the periosteum.
- *Bone necrosis*: blood vessel disruption deprives osteocytes at the fracture end of oxygen and they undergo necrosis.
- *Macrophage infiltration*: macrophages and osteoclasts are recruited to the area and remove dead material including bone.

Table 9.5 Stages of fracture healing
Inflammatory phase
bleeding and clot formation
acute inflammatory reaction
bone necrosis
granulation tissue
Reparative phase
provisional callus
healing across fracture gap
Remodelling phase

- *Granulation tissue*: the blood clot is organised by around day 3–4 and osteoblasts are generated within it. Simultaneously, locally released factors stimulate angiogenesis, revascularising the area.

Reparative phase

- *Provisional callus*: the organised clot contains fibroblasts producing collagen, chondroblasts and osteoblasts laying down matrix. The initial result is a mixture of cartilage and connective tissue called fibrocartilage. This material matures, over the course of 2–6 weeks, into bone, and is described as callus.
- *Healing across fracture gap*: ossification begins at the fracture ends, starting subperiosteally. Initially relatively immature and less stable woven bone is produced. Over 6–12 weeks, ossification occurs throughout the provisional callus, bridging the fracture gap. At the same time, maturation to more structurally robust lamellar bone occurs and the fracture is united.

Remodelling phase

The healing fracture site continues to adapt to its environment and particularly the forces applied to it for up to 2 years. Different bones have different capacities to remodel and children have a marked ability to remodel compared to adults, particularly the elderly.

Principles of management

The patient must be considered as a whole, not as isolated injured parts. As always, the priority is to treat life-threatening injuries by way of resuscitation. Bony injury can indeed be life threatening in itself and hence require early treatment, as in the case of maxillofacial fractures such as Le Fort III, which can displace and obstruct the patient's airway, and pelvic fractures, blood loss from which can cause haemorrhagic shock.

With regards to orthopaedic injuries the priority is to treat limb-threatening injuries such as displaced fractures causing vascular compromise.

Analgesia is an important early consideration for the obvious reason of patient comfort but also to combat the pathophysiological effects of pain and distress.

Definitive fracture management is determined by the type of fracture. A fundamental distinction is manage-ment of open compared to closed fractures.

Table 9.6   Treatment of closed fractures
Reduction
Immobilisation
plaster
traction
external fixation
internal fixation
Stress and movement

Treatment of closed fractures

The treatment of closed fractures is outlined in Table 9.6.

Reduction

Reduction should be carried out without any delay if vascular compromise is present, and should take precedence over investigation including radiographs. Provided the blood supply is unaffected reduction can be carried out under more considered circumstances.

Reduction is often not required. This is the case with minimally displaced fractures where the process of remodelling will compensate in the long term.

Where reduction *is* required, it is ideally effected by closed manipulation, thereby minimising the risk of introducing infection to the fracture site. It is important to provide adequate analgesia for reduction and this can involve regional or general anaesthesia, with their attendant risks. These risks of reduction might outweigh the benefits where the displacement or deformity will result in no loss of function.

Different fractures require differing accuracy of reduction. In general, alignment is more important than apposition, which the process of fracture healing is good at compensating.

Intra-articular fractures are a group that require reduction to as close to the anatomical normal as possible. This is mainly due to the risk of osteoarthritis. Often, this can be achieved by closed manipulation. More precise reduction can be achieved by operative open reduction, and this is indicated when closed reduction has not produced a satisfactory result including if there are soft tissues interposed between fracture ends. This is also the case for extra-articular fractures. Fractures that require internal fixation are reduced operatively to the position that they are to be held in, during the same operation.

Open reduction requires a form of anaesthesia and – importantly – breaches the protection against infection that the skin provides.

Immobilisation

A degree of movement at the fracture site is beneficial for fracture healing, by providing a stimulus to callus formation.

Splintage can be thought of as artificial callus put in place early on. It prevents excessive movement at the fracture site, relieving pain and keeping the fracture ends in close proximity to undergo healing and union, and therefore also minimising deformity.

There are several methods available for providing immobilisation; the indications, risks and benefits are described below.

Plaster

Plaster casts are easy, cheap and safe. Modern plaster materials are light, waterproof and easy for the patient to manage. They allow patients to mobilise and go home early and maintain the fracture in good position. However, they allow little movement, particularly of the joints surrounding the fracture, and therefore predispose to stiffness.

Plaster casts are most suitable for fractures that are minimally displaced, or those that have been adequately reduced and whose new position is stable.

The main dangers of casts are if they are applied incorrectly. A tight cast can act as a constraint and hence cause a kind of iatrogenic compartment syndrome. This is particularly the case shortly after injury, or manipulation, and often a 'backslab' (i.e. a plaster that does not go around the whole circumference of the injured part) is applied.

Pressure sores can occur within the plaster and skin breaks can be induced by the patient trying to relieve the itch in the plaster, for example with a knitting needle. These predispose to infection.

Traction

This is used to immobilise some long bone fractures. Force is applied along the long axis of the fractured bone, distracting the fracture ends and keeping them aligned. Traction devices can be attached to bone, skin or bandaging on the injured body part.

External fixation

Pins or screws are inserted proximal and distal to the fracture site, and these 'anchors' are attached to a rigid external device. This allows unique manipulation and can also act as a form of localised traction device, or even provide a force compressing the fracture ends together, helping to bridge a fracture gap. Wounds can be left open to drain and to be easily inspected with external fixation, and skin reconstruction can be carried out around it.

The types of fractures best treated by external fixation are those that would benefit from the above features, particularly fractures at risk of infection or with significant soft tissue damage, such as open fractures. External fixators are unsightly but, more important, they prevent normal force loading of the fractured bone, slowing healing. Although the force applied through the device might be excessive, for example resulting in over distraction of the fracture ends, the same device can be manipulated to compensate this. However, external fixators are not devoid of the risk of infection and pin-track infection is a considerable problem that can result in chronic osteomyelitis.

Internal fixation

This form of immobilisation is achieved by open, operative reduction of the fracture, which is then held in place by any number of devices, most of which are metal, that are left in place and the wound closed over them. The variety of products available is enormous and includes pins, plates and screws, the particular indications for which are generally fracture specific. These are considered further in Chapter 12.

The main advantage of this form of treatment is the accuracy of reduction that can be achieved and indeed maintained by the firm immobilisation provided.

This high degree of rigidity at the fracture site is not completely beneficial, however, as it does not induce callus, as previously mentioned. However, the main disadvantage of internal fixation is the higher risk of infection. Not only is the skin's barrier to infection breached at operation but microorganisms also tend to stick to prosthetic materials, including metal. Infection on metal implants is hard to clear, as little systemic antibiotic gets to the site, as do few of the body's natural defences. Other complications include fracture of the internal fixation device, particularly if it takes too great a proportion of the load rather than the healing bone.

Stress and movement

Physiological loading of the fracture site not only allows early return of function but also aids healing in the short term by stimulating callus formation, and in the long term by providing the basis of remodelling. Early movement and physiotherapy of areas and joints around the fracture site help prevent stiffness and deformity in the longer term.

The caveat is inducing excessive movement at the fracture site, which can also delay healing. This is a delicate balance and the degree and duration of immobilisation is fracture specific, and often even patient specific. Therefore regular clinical review is essential, as is close communication with paramedical specialties such as physiotherapy.

Treatment of open fractures

The main risk of an open fracture *per se* is that of infection. This risk is the result of breach of the barrier provided by skin, the presence of foreign material and dead tissue in the wound, and impaired blood supply preventing the body's innate defences getting to the area as normal.

One of the main principles of treatment is therefore prevention of infection. This cannot be instituted too early and the wound should be covered with a non-adherent sterile dressing as part of first aid management. Ideally, this dressing should be left in place. Antibiotic prophylaxis should be given early, as there is inevitably some delay in definitive management. Intravenous broad-spectrum antibiotics are indicated to cover Gram-negative, Gram-positive and anaerobic organisms. Tetanus immunisation status should be considered early and a booster given if indicated. Operative treatment is based on the principles of debridement and fixation.

Current thinking is to aggressive debridement, removing all foreign material and dead tissue. Thorough washing of the wound should be followed by excision of appropriate tissue. Several visits to theatre might be required as it becomes apparent postoperatively that further tissue is not viable. Although this can result in a significant defect, a clean wound is amenable to later closure and reconstruction, whereas an infected wound is ultimately likely to produce more of a defect. A common dilemma at initial operation is whether to close the wound. In general, only small, clean wounds with minimal soft tissue damage should be closed at the initial operation. The fracture ends need to be washed and reduced to an acceptable position. Holding the fracture in the reduced position is most often achieved with external fixation, which allows best drainage of the wound. Occasionally,

fixation is achieved with plaster or traction. Internal fixation is relatively rare because of the risk of infection of the implants; however, in experienced hands, and in particular fractures, it can produce the best results (see Ch. 12).

A postoperative course of antibiotics should be continued irrespective of the method of fixation.

Complications of fractures and fracture healing

As discussed in Chapter 4 'Complications of surgery', it is helpful to divide complications into general and specific (or local), and to subdivide with regards the timeframe they occur in – early, intermediate and late (see Table 4.10).

General

Early

As alluded to earlier, attention must be paid initially to associated injuries, most often to other systems, that might require life-saving resuscitation treatment.

Injuries to bones, particularly the pelvis and long bones, can result in significant blood loss into the pelvic cavity or soft tissues that can cause shock in their own right, or exacerbate shock of other causes.

Intermediate

Some patients require treatment in hospital and are subjected to a degree of immobility. This predisposes them to a number of conditions, perhaps most importantly deep venous thrombosis (DVT) and pulmonary embolism (PE). Prophylaxis for DVT is an important consideration in inpatients with bony injury, and most centres will have a form of protocol for this. Other risks of immobility include pneumonia, constipation and pressure sores, for which careful nursing prevention is the best form of treatment. Patients requiring operative treatment are exposed to the general risk of anaesthetic, as discussed in Chapter 10.

Fat embolism syndrome is a phenomenon seen 3 to 10 days postinjury, and is most often seen following long bone or pelvic fractures. Clinically, it is characterised by an unwell patient with respiratory distress, who might have visible petechial haemorrhages, particularly on the trunk. Other clinical indicators are tachycardia and pyrexia. Treatment is supportive. Crush syndrome is the consequence of major trauma whereby muscle crushing causes significant muscle destruction, with release of proteins from the damaged muscle. These substances prevent normal renal tubular function, and acute renal failure and shock supervene. Treatment is again largely supportive, with careful fluid and protein balance. Prevention is also important and includes radical measures including removal of severally damaged tissues, e.g. amputation.

Late

Patients might be left with disability, deformity and handicap. These factors can result in significant social, occupational and psychological sequelae.

Local

Early

The important local early complications have already been dealt with, being injuries to surrounding structures including blood vessels and nerves.

Intermediate

Local problems occurring at an intermediate stage are listed in Table 9.7.

Compartment syndrome

This phenomenon generally occurs within hours of injury and is associated with injuries in certain areas. Whereas compartment syndrome is most commonly associated with fractures, this is not always the case, as it relates to soft tissue swelling. Swelling within a relatively fixed compartment (e.g. enclosed by bone and non-compliant fascia) results in compression of the soft structures within that compartment. Both blood vessels and nerves are squashed, reducing their blood supply and impairing their function. Tissue ischaemia results in tissue damage and oedema, and therefore further swelling, causing a vicious circle. This pathophysiology explains the symptoms, signs, sequelae and treatment of compartment syndrome.

The earliest symptom is of pain in the injured area. This might not seem terribly helpful but the pain of compartment syndrome is disproportionately great compared to the underlying injury and has a less-than-expected response to analgesics.

The area is exquisitely tender and pain is experienced on stretching (passively) any muscles that are also being squashed within the compartment, or whose blood supply is impaired. From these early features there is a spectrum to the late features of compartment syndrome that should not be seen (as treatment will have been instituted). The late features are classically described as the five Ps (Table 9.8).

A high level of suspicion allows monitoring and prevents occurrence. If compartment syndrome is developing, constricting dressings and traction should be removed and the area elevated to try to reduce oedema. If unresolving, it might be necessary to surgically decompress the compartment, for example by fasciotomy.

Infection

Infection can seriously impair the physiological process of fracture healing described above, and is one of the more common causes of malunion and non-union described below. Infection is much more common in open fractures and this is one of the main reasons they are treated differently.

Another risk factor for the development of infection is the insertion of foreign bodies. This is particularly important when considering the insertion of metal such as plates and screws.

Table 9.7   Local intermediate problems complicating fractures
Compartment syndrome
Infection
Delayed union
Non-union

Table 9.8   The five Ps of compartment syndrome
Pale
Pulseless
Paraesthesia
Painful
Paralysed

Delayed union

In delayed union, fracture healing takes longer than expected. This is predominantly a clinical diagnosis with persistent pain and excessive mobility at the fracture site. Even under normal circumstances, radiological union takes longer than clinical union.

There are numerous causes of delayed union and it is less common in cancellous bone than cortical bone. Infection is a common cause and the presence or absence of infection has an influence on management. Other important causes include poor alignment of the fracture (inadequate reduction), poor blood supply to the fracture site and excessive mobility at the fracture site.

Non-union

Causes are similar to those of delayed union, with the addition of interposition of soft tissues. A gap remains between the ends of the fracture, which is radiographically visible, and it might also be possible to see that the medullary cavities have sealed off. Clinically, the patient has persistent pain and mobility, with or without crepitus, on stressing the fracture site. The diagnosis is therefore both clinical and radiological.

Treatment of abnormal fracture union depends on whether there is infection present. Healing in the presence of pus and dead bone (sequestrum) is unlikely, and surgical debridement with antibiotic therapy is often required.

Delayed union is classified into fractures with hypertrophic callus and hypotrophic callus. Where there is excess callus, normal healing is the rule with a prolonged period of immobilisation. Where there is minimal or no callus, healing is likely to remain inadequate and operative treatment, for example with bone grafting may be indicated.

Late

The late local complications are listed in Table 9.9.

Table 9.9 Late local complications of fractures

Loss of function
Osteoarthritis
Post-traumatic ossification
Nerve tendon and muscle complications
Avascular necrosis
Suedeck's atrophy

Loss of function

Uncorrected deformity can result in loss of function, as relationships are no longer anatomical. Similarly, prolonged immobilisation can result in soft tissue fibrosis, resulting in contractures, for example, fixed flexion deformity. Other causes of dysfunction include muscle weakness and loose ligament complexes.

Osteoarthritis

Intra-articular fractures that are not correctly aligned result in abnormal wear of the articular surface, osteoarthritis. Altered biomechanics from a fracture, for example, gait, can result in abnormal loads through joints not involved in the original injury, also leading to premature wear and tear.

Post-traumatic ossification

This is the laying down of bony elements within soft tissues around the site of injury. Its aetiology is not known. Clinically patients have pain and may have a tender palpable mass. Treatment is with rest, and can be followed up by elective excision of the affected tissues.

Nerve, tendon and muscle complications

Callus or irregularly healed fracture edges can impinge on adjacent tendons or nerves, with either rupture or dysfunction ensuing. These features are often fracture specific, and seen in classic patterns. Muscles that have been involved in compartment syndrome die and contract, producing so-called Volkmann's contractures.

Avascular necrosis

Where the fracture disrupts the blood supply to a piece of bone, it can undergo necrosis. An example is the femoral head that derives some of its blood supply through the femoral neck. The head of femur can undergo late death (avascular necrosis) following a fractured neck of femur, particularly if the fracture is displaced.

Suedeck's atrophy

This is a phenomenon of unknown aetiology, often precipitated by trauma that might be thought to have been relatively insignificant. Clinically, it is characterised by persistent, burning pain. Joints are red and swollen, and later the skin becomes shiny and atrophic. Radiographs show patchy reduction in bone density.

Treatment is by having an index of clinical suspicion, and early institution of physiotherapy and elevation. If these measures are unsuccessful then treatments blocking sympathetic innervation to the area can be of benefit.

10 General anaesthesia

Introduction

Anaesthesia means absence of all sensation; analgesia means absence of pain. General anaesthesia is a state where all sensation is lost and the patient is rendered unconscious by drugs. Some anaesthetic agents have little analgesic effect whereas some analgesics produce little sleep. Combinations of drugs are, thus, commonly used in modern practice although, historically, an inhalational agent, such as ether or chloroform, was all that was available and was used as a single agent.

The administration of general anaesthesia used to be performed in a variety of settings, such as dental practices. Increased standards have now precluded this practice and general anaesthesia should be performed only by qualified anaesthetists in a hospital setting with access to appropriate medical support.

Some operations, such as cardiac surgery, are performed only under general anaesthesia. Other procedures, such as dental extraction, can often be performed under local anaesthesia with or without concurrent sedation, even in small children.

It is important, because of the risks of general anaesthesia alluded to below, that all methods of

---

Table 10.1 Aspects of general anaesthesia

Assessment of risk
Preoperative assessment and premedication
Induction of anaesthesia
Maintenance of anaesthesia
Maintenance of the airway
Inhalational anaesthetic agents
Anaesthetic gases
Intravenous agents
Drugs used to supplement anaesthesia
Monitoring during anaesthesia
Postoperative care

---

providing pain-free surgery are explained and the patient or guardian allowed to give informed consent to the methods of analgesia or anaesthesia to be employed (see Ch. 22).

The surgeon and the anaesthetist have a shared responsibility for the patient's wellbeing, and so an understanding of general anaesthesia is important for all surgeons. General anaesthesia will be considered here, as described in Table 10.1. Local anaesthesia for dental procedures is considered in Chapter 24.

Assessment of risk

The patient should first be made as fit as possible for operation in the time available. Second, the anticipated benefits of surgery should outweigh the anaesthetic and surgical risks involved. The overall mortality rate attributable to anaesthesia itself is approximately 1 in 100 000, whereas a broad average of surgical mortality is more than 1 in 1000. Factors that have been shown to contribute to this mortality include poor preoperative assessment, inadequate supervision and monitoring in the intraoperative period and inadequate postoperative care.

Audits of operative mortality commonly use the American Society of Anesthetists' (ASA) physical status scale (Table 10.2). Fitness for operation is always relative to the urgency of the proposed procedure.

Preoperative assessment and premedication

The anaesthetist must see and assess the patient preoperatively; failure to do so can be regarded as negligent. Many patients will be seen the night before surgery. With increasing economic pressures to admit patients on the

Table 10.2   The American Society of Anesthetists' physical status scale

Class I : A normally healthy individual
Class II : A patient with mild systemic disease
Class III: A patient with severe systemic disease that is not incapacitating
Class IV: A patient with incapacitating systemic disease that is a constant threat to life
Class V : A moribund patient who is not expected to survive 24 h with or without operation
Class E : Added as a suffix for emergency operation

Table 10.3   Aspects of the preoperative visit

Evaluation of history and physical examination
Ordering of special investigations
Institution of preoperative management
Risk assessment
Discussion regarding anaesthetic management which will involve patient consent
Prescription of premedication

day of operation, a screening process must be used to identify suitable patients. Preassessment clinics with a combination of nursing and medical input are increasingly being developed to improve efficiency and streamline 'the patient journey'. They must run to carefully designed protocols.

After a preoperative visit there should be no surprises for either patient or anaesthetist. The visit should establish rapport with the patient and should allow time for the various factors listed in Table 10.3.

History

A comprehensive history is important. It can reveal diseases, particularly of the cardiovascular and respiratory systems (for which breathlessness and chest pain are especially relevant). The identification of pregnancy is important because it is a contraindication to elective surgery in the first trimester due to the risk of teratogenicity. Later in pregnancy the patient faces the risks of regurgitation and aspiration of gastric contents.

Past medical history

This should elicit evidence of asthma, diabetes, tuberculosis, seizures or any chronic major organ dysfunction.

A past history of HIV infection or other infective agents can affect both patients and their carers. A history of previous anaesthesia can highlight problems of drug allergy, deep venous thrombosis or postoperative nausea and vomiting. Anaphylaxis is the most serious of these.

Drug history

Many interactions can be potentially dangerous, for example, anticoagulants might be a contraindication to spinal, epidural or other regional techniques; anti-convulsants might increase the requirements for anaesthetic agents and enflurane, a volatile anaesthetic agent, should be avoided as it might precipitate seizures. Beta-blockers have negative inotropic effects and can cause hypotension. They can also mask a compensatory tachycardia, concealing evidence of blood loss. Plasma potassium concentration should be checked in all patients taking diuretics because they might have hypokalaemia and careful monitoring of plasma glucose can be important in patients receiving insulin. Such measures may require a special perioperative regime. Corticosteroids have many well-known complications and extra corticosteroid cover to compensate for a relative lack might be needed.

Social history

Ceasing smoking 12 h before surgery can improve the oxygen-carrying capacity of the blood, although abstinence for a longer period is required to reduce the incidence of postoperative respiratory morbidity. Excessive alcohol can result in both hepatic and cardiac damage. Acute withdrawal in alcoholics can result in delirium tremens, which will require both a sedative such as a benzodiazepine agent and thiamine (vitamin B_1).

Family history

The anaesthetist must be aware of hereditary traits such as haemophilia and porphyria. Cholinesterase abnormalities can lead to prolongation of muscle relaxants such as suxamethonium.

Physical examination

A full physical examination is important to complement the history but the anaesthetist will also pay particular attention to the upper airway with a view to assessing the ease of tracheal intubation. This will involve assessment of the teeth and extent of mouth opening and flexibility of the neck.

Preoperative investigation of elective patients

Healthy patients less than 40 years old do not generally require any preanaesthetic investigation. Only relevant tests should be ordered and these will reflect age, comorbidity and complexity of the surgery. Circumstances where investigation would be important are listed in Table 10.4.

Other investigations, such as radiography of the cervical spine or lung function tests, will be undertaken for specific indications.

Table 10.4   Indications of preoperative investigations

Full blood count
  anaemia
  females post menarche
  cardiopulmonary disease
  possible haematological pathology, e.g.
    haemoglobinopathies
  likelihood of significant intraoperative blood loss
  history of anticoagulants
  chronic diseases such as rheumatoid disease
Clotting screen
  liver disease
  anticoagulant drugs or a history of bleeding or
    bruising
  kidney disease
  major surgery
Urea and electrolyte concentrations
  major surgery >40 years
  kidney disease
  diabetes mellitus
  digoxin, diuretics, corticosteroids, lithium
  history of diarrhoea and vomiting
Liver function tests: these will be carried out when there is any suspicion of liver disease
ECG
  >40 years asymptomatic male or >50 years
    asymptomatic female
  history of myocardial infarction or other heart or
    vascular disease
  <40 years with risk factors e.g. hyperlipidaemia,
    diabetes mellitus, smoking, obesity, hypertension
    and cardiac medication
Chest radiography
  breathlessness on mild exertion
  suspected malignancy, tuberculosis or chest infection
  thoracic surgery

Preoperative therapy

Patients with respiratory disease can be improved by physiotherapy or bronchodilator therapy. Prophylactic antibiotics are required in those at risk of subacute bacterial endocarditis. Hypertensive patients can sometimes require adjustment of their drug therapy to obtain optimal control, but it is usually reasonable to proceed with surgery if their diastolic pressure is below 110 mmHg.

Postponement of surgery

If time allows, it is not sensible to anaesthetise a patient with an acute upper respiratory tract infection and operation might also have to be delayed for patients with cardiac or endocrine diseases that are not yet under optimal control. Likewise, resuscitation and restoration of circulating blood volume can require delay in anaesthesia. Elective surgery should not be undertaken unless the patient has fasted for 6 h for solid food, infant formula or other milk, 4 h for breast milk or 2 h for clear non-particulate and non-carbonated fluids

Premedication

Whereas reassurance and explanation remain the most important components of the preoperative visit, drugs can be used to obtain one or a combination of the effects listed in Table 10.5.

Anxiolysis is most commonly achieved with the use of benzodiazepines such as diazapem or lorazepam, and these drugs also cause a degree of anterograde amnesia. Excessive secretions in the airway are less of a problem with modern anaesthetic agents but can be reduced with anticholinergic drugs either given before or at operation. Three drugs commonly used in this circumstance are the anticholinergic agents atropine, hyoscine and glyco-pyrronium. Vagal bradycardia, such as occurs with the

---

Table 10.5   Effect of premedication

Reduction in anxiety and fear
Amnesia
Reduction in secretions
Potentiation of the effects of general anaesthetics
Reduction in the volume and acidity of gastric contents
Reduction in postoperative nausea and vomiting
Attenuation of both the sympathetic and vagal reflexes

---

oculocardiac reflex, can be severe and atropine is protective of all the above. Antiemetics such as metoclopramide, ondansetron or antihistamines are administered preoperatively from time to time; metoclopramide also enhances gastric emptying. If it is desired to reduce gastric acidity this can be achieved with sodium citrate, H_2 blockers such as ranitidine or proton pump inhibitors. Alleviating the patient's anxiety is most important.

Preparation for anaesthesia

Preparation and communication are vital. Armed with information from the previous section and after discussion between surgeon and anaesthetist, a plan of action should be formed that will include the assembly of the necessary staff, equipment for airway care and monitoring, intravenous fluids and arrangements for proper postoperative and recovery facilities. The 'preflight' check of the anaesthetic machine must be carried out and the nature of the operation to be performed and consent checked with the patient. The patient must be on a tilting bed or trolley. Trained and dedicated anaesthetic assistance is essential.

Induction of anaesthesia

Anaesthesia can be induced by inhalational agents or by drugs administered intravenously.

Inhalational induction

Inhalational induction is more commonly proposed for either young children or those with an obstruction somewhere in their airway (e.g. epiglottitis or a foreign body). Rapport and patient confidence are important to ensure the patient's cooperation, and a gentle and gradual approach should be used. An anaesthetic mask should be held gently on or very near the face and the patient should be talked to calmly and reassuringly while being encouraged to breathe normally. It is common for nitrous oxide 70% in oxygen to be used; anaesthesia is gradually deepened as the anaesthetist introduces a volatile anaesthetic agent by increments. Patient monitoring will have been attached before induction and the patient is observed carefully for skin colour; the pattern and rate of ventilation and the patient's pulse, blood pressure ECG and arterial oxygen saturation by pulse oximetry (SpO_2) should all be observed. End tidal carbon dioxide

concentration ($ETCO_2$) can be monitored; this is mandatory in intubated patients. As consciousness is lost, the airway will require increasing support, which will usually involve pulling up the patient's chin. It can also require insertion of an artificial airway. This might be an oral or nasopharyngeal airway. A laryngeal mask airway (LMA) or an endotracheal tube can be inserted if required. For endotracheal intubation without muscle relaxants the patient must be at a much deeper level of anaesthesia. Airway obstruction is the most commonly encountered difficulty. Scavenging systems are usually employed to reduce environmental pollution from expired gases.

Intravenous induction

Induction of anaesthesia with an intravenous agent is used for most routine purposes and is the most appropriate technique for most patients undergoing emergency surgery. A cannula should be sited in a vein in the back of the hand or forearm to avoid the structures in the antecubital fossa or risk of intra-arterial injection of the brachial artery. Sterility should be maintained and local anaesthesia used if a large cannula is required for infusion of fluids. Prior to induction, the patient should breathe 100% oxygen with a tight-fitting mask for 3 min or, alternatively, be asked to take four deep breaths to vital capacity.

Emergency/rapid sequence induction

This is most commonly employed for patients with a full stomach and a risk of regurgitation and aspiration of gastric contents, provided preoperative evaluation indicates no major difficulty with airway or intubation. With all preparations made, intravenous access secured and suitable assistance, the patient breathes 100% oxygen for 3 min on a tilting trolley. The assistant on the right of the patient applies firm pressure over the cricoid cartilage with thumb and index finger. This posterior pressure compresses the oesophagus between the cricoid cartilage and the vertebral column. It is applied either just before administration of the intravenous induction agent or as soon as consciousness is lost. A predetermined sleep dose of induction agent is followed immediately by a paralysing dose of suxamethonium. As soon as the jaw begins to relax, laryngoscopy is performed and the endotracheal tube placed. Cricoid pressure is maintained until the cuff of the tube is inflated and correct placement is confirmed. This is intended to prevent regurgitation and aspiration. Further muscle relaxants are not normally given until control of the airway is secured, but this technique balances the greater risk of aspiration against the risk of losing control of the airway. Although this technique is commonly used for general surgical emergencies, it should not be used where there is any obstruction to the upper airway from trauma or inflammation and, in these circumstances, an inhalational technique or awake intubation is more appropriate.

Positioning of the patient for surgery

Patient safety is paramount and the patient should be positioned carefully, taking into account requirement for both surgical and anaesthetic access. The anaesthetist must be aware of the varying effects of different positions. Local pressure effects on nerves can result in postoperative morbidity. Intraoperatively, the head-down or prone positions will make abdominal breathing difficult. The sitting position requires careful support of the head and can result in cardiovascular instability from pooling of blood in the leg veins. The supine position is used for the majority of surgery. Aortocaval compression in pregnant patients or those with large abdominal masses can result in hypotension.

Maintenance of anaesthesia

Several options are available to maintain anaesthesia. Inhalational agents, intravenous anaesthetic agents or intravenous opioids can be used, either alone or in combination. Muscle relaxants are commonly used to facilitate tracheal intubation and subsequent ventilation of the lungs. Regional anaesthesia can be used to supplement any of these techniques.

Inhalational anaesthesia with spontaneous ventilation is appropriate for superficial operations where profound muscle relaxation is not required. The patient is allowed to breathe spontaneously and a volatile anaesthetic agent such as halothane, enflurane, isoflurane or sevoflurane is used with carrier gases nitrous oxide and oxygen. Most anaesthetic machines will not deliver less than 30% oxygen and have an interlocking device to ensure this. These volatile agents are delivered from vaporisers, which are specially calibrated containers that will deliver a constant percentage of agent irrespective of the gas flow through them, temperature or pressure. Analgesia as determined by the patient's response might also be required.

Minimal alveolar concentration (MAC) is the minimal alveolar concentration of an inhaled anaesthetic agent that prevents reflex movement in response to surgical incision in 50% of subjects. This value is commonly used as an index of relative potency and may be affected by the patient's age and concomitant use of other drugs.

Signs of anaesthesia

The signs and stages of anaesthesia were originally described by Guedel in patients premedicated with morphine and atropine and breathing ether and air. With newer agents the stages are less clearly differentiated but they remain a useful general guide.

Stage 1 – analgesia

This can be attained using nitrous oxide 50% in oxygen and provides 'relative analgesia'.

Stage 2 – excitement

This is seen with inhalational induction but with intravenous induction it is commonly bypassed. The eyelash reflex is often lost at this stage. Breathing is irregular and laryngeal and pharyngeal reflexes are still active. Patients might hold their breath and any instrumentation of the airway can produce laryngeal spasm.

Stage 3 – surgical anaesthesia

The patient develops rhythmic regular breathing and as they descend through the four plains from light to deep, respiratory reflexes are progressively abolished. Patients can no longer protect their own airway. The pupils become central and are classically large, although, with the newer agents, they are often much smaller than with the older agents.

Stage 4 – stage of impending respiratory and circulatory failure

In this stage, anaesthesia is too deep and brainstem reflexes are depressed by high anaesthetic concentrations. Anaesthetic agents should be withdrawn and oxygen administered.

Maintenance of the airway

Maintenance of the airway and of oxygenation is the cornerstone of safe anaesthesia. Inhalational agents can be administered with a face mask, a laryngeal mask airway (LMA) or an endotracheal tube.

Face mask

Face masks come in various shapes and sizes and should be chosen for the individual patient to provide an adequate seal. Nasal masks are used during dental anaesthesia. The mask is held against the patient's face and the mandible is held forwards because pressure on the submental soft tissues can exacerbate airway obstruction by pushing the tongue backwards. The reservoir bag on the anaesthetic circuit should be seen to be moving in and out with the respiratory movement of the patient. There should be no indrawing of the suprasternal and supraclavicular areas – this indicates obstruction. Breathing should be quiet; noisy ventilation or stridor provides further evidence of obstruction. It should be always remembered that total obstruction is silent as there is no movement of air. An oropharyngeal or Guedel airway can be used to assist in maintenance of the airway (Fig. 10.1).

Laryngeal mask airway

Laryngeal mask airways (LMAs) can be considered a halfway house between a face mask and an endotracheal tube (Fig. 10.2). They avoid the need for tracheal intubation during spontaneous ventilation while at the same time providing a clear airway without the need to hold on a mask. They can also occasionally be used to assist with difficult intubation.

They should not be used in patients who are at risk of regurgitation of gastric contents because an endotracheal tube is required to provide secure protection and there will be occasions when surgical access could be obstructed by the bulk of the cuff on the LMA.

Endotracheal intubation

An endotracheal tube provides the most secure airway short of tracheostomy. It is passed via the mouth or nose and between the vocal cords into the larynx. The cuff on the tube lies below the cords and when it is inflated with air protects the respiratory tract from blood, secretions or inhalation of gastric contents. Likewise, the cuff prevents leakage of air travelling upwards during controlled ventilation. The tube also allows access for suction of the respiratory tract. Cuffed tubes are used in adults, whereas uncuffed tubes provide an acceptable seal in children.

There are a multitude of designs for laryngoscopes. The McGill laryngoscope is favoured for children because their epiglottis is floppy. It has a straight blade and is designed to lift the epiglottis anteriorly, exposing the larynx. The McIntosh laryngoscope, which has a curved blade, is designed so the tip lies anterior to the epiglottis in the vallecula and pulls the epiglottis anteriorly to expose the vocal cords.

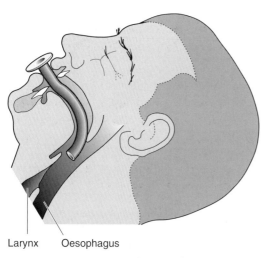

Larynx   Oesophagus

Fig. 10.1   Guedel airway in place.

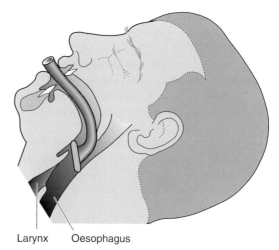

Larynx   Oesophagus

Fig. 10.2   Laryngeal mask airway covering the glottis but not occluding the opening to the oesophagus.

Laryngoscopy

The position of the patient's head and neck is important and was classically described as 'scenting the morning air'. The neck is flexed by raising the patient's head on a pillow and the head is extended. The laryngoscope, which is a left-handed instrument, is inserted into the right side of the mouth and pulls the tongue to the left as it is advanced slowly downwards. With the patient on his or her back, the laryngoscope is thus pulled upwards and away from the anaesthetist, avoiding levering against the upper teeth. This should reveal the dark, almost triangular orifice of the glottis. External pressure on the thyroid cartilage can allow better visualisation. The tube is placed through the glottis and its position within the airway should be confirmed by auscultation and monitoring of expired CO_2.

For nasal intubation, slightly smaller tubes are used after the introduction of vasoconstrictor into the nostrils to reduce bleeding.

Tracheal intubation can be undertaken under general anaesthesia but, where difficulties are anticipated, a tube can be inserted over a fibreoptic endoscope under local anaesthesia.

Extubation

Patients can be extubated supine if there is no risk of regurgitation but it is often safer to remove the endotracheal tube with the patient in the lateral recovery position. Prior to extubation the patient is given 100% oxygen and suction is performed to remove secretions from the endotracheal tube and from the mouth. After extubation the patient's clear airway, ability to breath, cough and clear secretions are carefully assessed while oxygen is continued by face mask. Laryngeal spasm occurs if the vocal cords come together as a result of irritation. A 'crowing' sound is heard and the patient will show signs of airway obstruction. This is treated by clearing secretions and applying positive airway pressure with oxygen. Occasionally, reintubation might be required.

Inhalational anaesthetic agents

The range of inhalational anaesthetic agents is listed in Table 10.6.

An ideal inhalational agent should be pleasant and non-irritant to breathe. It should also be potent and yet produce minimum depression of cardiovascular and respiratory systems. It should be safe for repeat

Table 10.6   Inhalational anaesthetic agents
Diethyl ether
Halothane
Enflurane
Isoflurane
Sevoflurane
Desflurane

administration and it should be neither flammable nor explosive.

Diethyl ether

Diethyl ether has been abandoned in the West because of its flammability, but it remains in widespread use in less developed countries. As it has a higher therapeutic ratio than more modern agents, it is relatively safe for administration in the hands of unskilled individuals. Its use is limited because it is highly irritant to the respiratory tract and can cause coughing, breath holding and profuse secretions. However, at deeper levels it was at one time a recommended treatment for bronchospasm.

Halothane

Halothane is again less commonly used, having been in widespread use for over 30 years. There has been concern because of the rare occurrence of hepatic toxicity after repeated administrations and it is also a depressant of myocardial contractility. Arrhythmias are also very common during halothane anaesthesia. Myocardial excitability is seen, particularly in the presence of hypercapnoea, hypoxia and with increased circulating catecholamines. Halothane should not be used in combination with local infiltration of adrenaline.

Enflurane

This is a clear, relatively pleasant-smelling agent. In common with the other agents it produces a dose-dependent depression in ventilation and tidal volume. It produces less depression of the cardiovascular system and is associated with fewer arrhythmias than halothane. It should be avoided in people with epilepsy.

Isoflurane

Isoflurane produces less myocardial depression than halothane or enflurane. It is rather pungent and less suitable for inhalational inductions. A large multicentre study in North America showed no significant outcome differences between these three agents.

Sevoflurane

Sevoflurane, popular for some time in Japan, was only introduced to the west in the 1990s. It is now the most commonly used agent for inhalational induction as it is pleasant and non-irritant, and might have a less depressant effect on breathing. Solubility characteristics allow a more rapid induction of anaesthesia. Recovery is also usually rapid.

Desflurane

Another new agent, desflurane, is the most recent addition to the volatile agents. It has to be given via a heated vaporiser and allows very rapid alterations in the depth of anaesthesia with recovery being faster than with any of the other agents.

Anaesthetic gases

Nitrous oxide

Nitrous oxide delivered via a pipeline or from blue cylinders is used with oxygen as a carrier gas for these potent volatile agents. As the MAC value for nitrous oxide is over 100%, it cannot be used with oxygen as an anaesthetic agent without the addition of a potent volatile agent, but it has proved safe over a long period in use. It is important that a high inspired oxygen concentration is given when nitrous oxide administration is discontinued. Nitrous oxide has also been incriminated in altering vitamin B_{12} synthesis by inhibiting the enzyme methianine synthetase, and excessive occupational exposure can result in myeloneuropathy. This condition is similar to subacute combined degeneration of the spinal cord and has been reported in individuals addicted to nitrous oxide.

Oxygen

Although oxygen is life-giving, there are some dangers associated with its use. It is flammable, it can cause a rise in the partial pressure of CO_2 (Pa_{CO_2}) in patients with chronic obstructive airways disease and, in high concentrations, it can lead to loss of pulmonary surfactant. On

occasion, toxicity of the central nervous system can be seen. Hyperbaric pressures result in convulsions. Retrolental fibroplasia is retinal damage with new vessel formation seen in infants exposed to high concentrations.

Intravenous agents

Induction of anaesthesia with intravenous agents is usually more rapid and smoother than with inhalation agents (Table 10.7). The ideal agent should have a rapid onset and recovery time with little hangover effect. It should be free of side-effects such as nausea, vomiting, cardiovascular and respiratory depression or toxicity to any major organs and it should also, if possible, be analgesic in low doses.

After intravenous administration, plasma concentrations rise rapidly and the drugs diffuse across the blood–brain barrier into the brain producing their effect. Reduced plasma concentrations and drug effects occur predominantly as they are distributed to other tissues. Metabolism occurs mostly in the liver but contributes relatively little to the recovery of consciousness.

Thiopentone sodium

Thiopentone sodium is one of a group of barbiturate agents and has proved safe in practice for over 50 years. It is important as a hypnotic but has an antianalgesic effect that can result in a reduction of pain threshold and restlessness in the postoperative period. On induction, consciousness is rapidly lost and in the absence of other agents is not regained for 5 to 10 min. As it does not depress airway reflexes to the same extent as other agents, laryngeal spasm can be precipitated by stimulation of the airway. There is usually a moderate tachycardia and reduction in blood pressure. It is a relatively long-acting drug and a hangover effect is common. This length of action makes it unsuitable as a drug for use by infusion in total intravenous anaesthesia (TIVA). It is an anti-

Table 10.7	Intravenous induction agents
Agent	*Induction dose (mg.kg^{-1})*
Thiopentone	3–5
Etomidate	0.3
Propofol	1.5–2.5
Ketamine	2

convulsant and can be used in the treatment of status epilepticus but must never be given to patients with porphyria, who might show severe cardiovascular collapse or neurological sequelae.

Etomidate

This is a rapidly acting general anaesthetic agent with a duration of action of 2–3 min. It produces less cardiovascular depression or vasodilatation than other agents and is most commonly used in patients with a compromised cardiovascular system. It causes more excitatory phenomenon on induction, which, on occasion, can be troublesome. Etomidate depresses the synthesis of cortisol by the adrenal gland even as a single bolus dose. Its use in intensive care has been abandoned as infusions resulted in increased infection and mortality probably related to reduced immunological competence.

Propofol

Propofol has become a very popular agent. It has rapid recovery characteristics and gives rise to a lower instance of postoperative nausea and vomiting than most other agents. It is formulated as a white aqueous emulsion, which contains soya bean oil. Loss of consciousness is rapid but blood pressure tends to decrease to a greater degree than with other agents. Respiratory reflexes are suppressed quite markedly and there is a low incidence of coughing and laryngospasm. Many regard propofol as the agent of choice where a laryngeal mask airway is to be inserted. Recovery is rapid, with little hangover effect. The drug is redistributed rapidly and probably metabolised not in the liver but in extrahepatic sites. The elimination remains constant, even after infusions lasting for several days, and it is thus the most suitable current agent for total intravenous anaesthesia (TIVA). It is also used by infusion for sedation in intensive care and is increasingly used as a form of relative analgesia and sedation during surgical procedures. Computer-operated infusion pumps are available, which aim to deliver a target plasma concentration based on patient's weight and age.

Ketamine hydrochloride

This differs from the other agents in producing a dissociative state rather than generalised depression of the central nervous system. Blood pressure might, in fact, increase with this agent and there is little respiratory depression. It is used in high-risk shocked patients and has, therefore, a place in anaesthesia and analgesia in times of war and at the scene of accidents. It can be given intramuscularly in low doses to produce analgesia. It has also been used in less developed countries, where equipment and staff are not readily available. Its use, however, is limited by the occurrence of restlessness, disorientation and often unpleasant nightmares or hallucinations, which can recur for up to 24 h.

Drugs used to supplement anaesthesia

Analgesics

Morphine

Morphine, produced from the poppy *Papaver somniferum*, and codeine are naturally occurring opium alkaloids. Morphine is the gold standard of analgesics affecting both the pain threshold and the psychological components of pain. Although it has little effect on the cardiovascular system, depression of ventilation is common; the cough reflex is also depressed. However, administration can be limited by distressing nausea and vomiting and it greatly reduces gut motility.

Pethidine

Pethidine is a synthetic opioid that, as it tends to relax the tone of smooth muscle, can be useful in renal colic; it can also be used to control postoperative shivering. Pethidine, however, should not be given to patients taking monoamine oxidase inhibitors (MAOI).

Buprenorphine

This can be useful on occasions as it can be administered sublingually. However, nausea and vomiting may be troublesome and subsequent use of other opioids, for example, morphine may be compromised as the drugs antagonise at opioid receptors.

Other opioids

Progressively shorter-acting synthetic agents are fentanyl, alfentanil and remifentanil. Remifentanil is sufficiently short acting to be useful administered by infusion.

Opioid antagonists

Naloxone is the drug of choice for reversing opioid-induced ventilatory depression. It should be titrated slowly because convulsions can occur occasionally and it reverses not only respiratory depression but also the analgesia.

Other analgesics

Non-steroidal anti-inflammatory drugs such as diclofenac, ketorolac and indomethacin can be used as analgesia in a balanced anaesthetic technique. The new alpha$_2$ adrenergic agonist dexmedetomidine is currently proving promising because it results in profound analgesia with less sedation.

Benzodiazepines

Benzodiazepines such as diazepam and midazolam can also be used as anaesthetic agents, but they have a longer duration of action than other agents. These drugs can be reversed with flumazenil, which is a competitive antagonist and again should be given in small titrated increments.

Neuromuscular blockade

Muscle relaxation is the third of the triad of anaesthesia that includes narcosis and analgesia. Neuromuscular blocking agents are classified into depolarising (or non-competitive) and non-depolarising (or competitive) agents.

Depolarising agents

The only depolarising agent now available in clinical practice is suxamethonium. After administration it results in an initial depolarisation of muscle cells. Muscular contractions can be seen and are known as fasciculation. Repolarisation does not occur and the muscle becomes flaccid. It produces a profound neuromuscular block within a minute and is useful to achieve rapid tracheal intubation in a patient who may have a full stomach. Recovery usually begins to occur within 3 min. It is metabolised by the enzyme cholinesterase and recovery can be delayed if this enzyme is either structurally abnormal or reduced in quantity. This is usually genetically determined and might require the patient to be ventilated until muscle function returns. Suxamethonium can give rise to muscle pains after operation. A rise in the plasma potassium can occur, which can be dangerous particularly in patients with burns or in those with neuromuscular disease.

Non-depolarising neuromuscular blocking agents

These compete with the neurotransmitter acetylcholine at the postsynaptic junction to prevent the threshold for an action potential being reached, and so the muscle does not contract. Tubocurarine (curaré) was used for centuries by native South Americans as an arrow poison and was the first agent to be used in humans. It has, however, been superseded. Atracurium degrades spontaneously in plasma and is therefore very safe for patients with liver or renal dysfunction. Such drugs have a longer duration of action of around 30 min. Vercuronium is also used and, because it releases less histamine, many consider it to be the drug of choice in asthmatics. Pancuronium, and more recently rocuronium, are aminosteroids. The advantage of rocuronium is its very rapid onset, which provides good intubating conditions within 90 s. Neuromuscular blockade can be monitored with a nerve stimulator intraoperatively and at the end of operation this block can be reversed by the administration of the anticholinesterase neostigmine in combination with either atropine or glycopyrronium. The addition of atropine or glycopurronium reduces respiratory secretions and prevents bradycardia.

Monitoring during anaesthesia

The word monitor is derived from the Latin verb *monere* 'to warn'. No device can replace the requirement for these warnings to be observed, interpreted and acted upon.

Monitoring the circulation

Monitoring of the circulation is necessary to maintain perfusion of vital organs (Table 10.8).

The pulse can be palpated and blood pressure measured either indirectly or, if necessary, directly from an arterial cannula. Electrocardiography gives information regarding heart rate, rhythm and ST changes produced by left ventricular ischaemia. It should be remembered that it is an index of electrical activity only and does not measure the mechanical activity that sustains life.

Table 10.8 Monitoring of the circulation

Heart rate and pulse
Blood pressure
Arterial oxygen saturation
ECG
Peripheral perfusion
Urine production

Pulse oximetry assesses the integrity of the components of the oxygen-delivery system to the tissues (see Ch. 11). It therefore assesses the oxygen supply to the patient, the oxygen uptake by the lungs and oxygen delivery to the tissues by the heart and circulation.

Pulse oximeters provide a non-invasive measurement of the arterial oxygen saturation (SpO_2). The principle involves the proportion of light absorbed by blood. This depends on the wavelength of the light and the ratio of oxyhaemoglobin to deoxyhaemoglobin. The wavelength of light known as the isobestic point is where absorption is the same for oxyhaemoglobin and deoxyhaemoglobin. At other wavelengths the absorption differs. The proportion of haemoglobin that is saturated with oxygen can, therefore, be calculated by measuring the absorption of light at two different wavelengths. As the electronics are capable of detecting a pulsatile component only the saturation of arterial blood is recorded. Because of the sigmoid shape of the oxyhaemoglobin dissociation curve arterial oxygen tension falls rapidly with saturations below 90%. The lower alarm limit is usually set at this level.

Cyanosis requires 5 grams of reduced haemoglobin. This represents an arterial oxygen saturation of 50% in a patient with a haemoglobin of $10 \, g/dl$. Oximetry, therefore, is a much more sensitive indicator of hypoxia than cyanosis. More intense monitoring of the cardiovascular system may involve insertion of a central venous pressure line. Pulmonary artery catheterisation will allow both measurement of filling pressure which reflects volume status and measurement of cardiac output. Newer Doppler systems also allow monitoring of these last two variables. Blood loss should also be monitored.

Monitoring the respiratory system

Clinical monitoring is most important. The patient should be observed for colour, respiratory rate, adequacy of respiratory movement and the movement of the reservoir bag or ventilator. Auscultation can detect intubation of a bronchus, the presence of secretions or the occurrence of a pneumothorax. It is important to detect respiratory obstruction, which can be revealed by tracheal tug or paradoxical abdominal movement with the absence of movement in the reservoir bag. The inspired oxygen concentration should always be monitored. When patients are ventilated there should also be capacity to measure airway pressures, volumes and both the inspiratory and end tidal concentrations of oxygen, carbon dioxide and volatile anaesthetic agents. Ventilator systems should also be fitted with a disconnection alarm. Capnography measures the end tidal carbon dioxide tension ($ETCO_2$) and provides the most reliable evidence of correct placement of an endotracheal tube. $ETCO_2$ will rise with rebreathing or underventilation and can fall rapidly with pulmonary embolism arising from air, fat or thrombos.

Monitoring the central nervous system

At the present time this is done clinically. The signs of sympathetic overactivity such as lacrimation, sweating, increasing pupil size or increase in heart rate or arterial pressure indicate that anaesthesia is too light. These signs are, however, not reliable but cerebral function monitors (CFM) are not at present in widespread practice. The depth of anaesthesia is often assumed from the measurement of end tidal volatile anaesthetic concentrations. It is only since the advent of neuromuscular blockers and the abolition of patient movement that undetected awareness has become a potential complication.

Other monitoring

Peripheral and central temperature measurement, neuromuscular blockade, together with haematological and biochemical variables may all be measured. Blood gas and acid-base status can be measured accurately from a sample of arterial blood and the patient's coagulation status may also require to be assessed.

There is strong evidence that there has been a reduction in intraoperative critical incidents and patient morbidity as a result of the adoption of higher routine standards of patient monitoring.

Postoperative care

The patient must be supervised and monitored closely at all times and should not be discharged from the recovery ward to the surgical ward until they are fully awake and maintaining their own airway, ventilation is adequate, the cardiovascular system is stable and they are not bleeding excessively.

Central nervous system – conscious level

The patient's airway must be carefully maintained until they are awake. If the patient is not awake in a reasonable time then other factors should be considered. Hypo- or hyperlgycaemia may occur particularly in diabetics and intracranial pathology may occur. The following, most particularly, should be excluded: hypoxaemia, hyper-capnoea, hypotension and hypothermia.

Confusion and agitation may occur at this time particularly in the elderly. This may be associated with anticholinergic drugs such as atropine or hyoscine but pain may also be a contributory factor. Bladder distension may be covert. If neuromuscular blockade has not been adequately reversed the patient may appear agitated and distressed with uncoordinated movements.

Oxygen

Particular care should be given to the patient's require-ments for oxygen which should be monitored by oximetry. All patients should be given oxygen postoperatively.

Intravenous fluids

They may also require fluids as a result of either intra-operative blood loss or preoperative fluid depletion.

Analgesia

Good pain control starting in the intraoperative period should be established in the recovery ward before return to the ward. This may be achieved with opioids which if the patient is sufficiently awake can be administered by a patient-controlled infusion device. Non-steroidal anti-inflammatory drugs and local and regional techniques may also be very valuable.

The recovery ward should have the staff, equipment and monitoring to deal with the full range of compli-cations. Problems are as liable to arise there as in the anaesthetic room or operating theatre.

Patients should be closely watched for a number of surgical complications which may include haemorrhage and blockage of drains or catheters. This high intensity environment should allow the patient to return to the appropriate level of ongoing care in the optimum condition.

11 Conscious sedation techniques

Introduction

The use of conscious sedation has risen dramatically in recent years. There are many circumstances responsible for this change including reduced general anaesthetic numbers as a result of its potential morbidity (see Ch. 10), regulation by the General Dental Council and increased patient education and expectations. The General Dental Council's definition of conscious sedation is:

> A technique in which the use of a drug or drugs produces a state of depression of the central nervous system enabling treatment to be carried out, but during which communication can be maintained and the modification of the patient's state of mind is such that the patient will respond throughout the period of sedation. Techniques should carry a margin of safety wide enough to render unintended loss of consciousness unlikely.

This definition gives some flexibility regarding drugs used and specific procedures chosen yet it emphasises the guiding principle of sedation: the patient is, by definition, conscious. Sedation as described here is an inherently safe method of anxiety control.

Sedative agents

Several currently available drugs are useful in sedation. In practice, however, conscious sedation usually involves the use of inhalational nitrous oxide or the newer anxiolytics, the benzodiazepines.

Nitrous oxide

At room temperature, nitrous oxide is a colourless gas with, arguably, a sweet smell. It is contained in blue cylinders as a mixture of gas and liquid.

Nitrous oxide is a weak anaesthetic with a minimum alveolar concentration (MAC) of 110% (see Ch. 10). This represents the concentration of gas required to anaesthetise 50% of subjects and is clearly impossible unless the gas is given in a hyperbaric atmosphere. Nitrous oxide has a blood gas solubility of 0.47, which makes it highly soluble in blood. This allows rapid onset of sedation and equally rapid recovery.

Benzodiazepines

Benzodiazepines were discovered by accident in the 1950s in Switzerland by researchers at Hoffman-LaRoche. They were first marketed in 1960 with the introduction of Librium. Benzodiazepines have a number of clinical effects: anxiolysis, sedation, amnesia, muscle relaxation and eventually anaesthesia. They produce this action by two main routes.

- First, and principally, benzodiazepines act in the central nervous system (CNS) via the gamma-amino butyric acid (GABA) network. GABA is an inhibitory neurotransmitter found in the brain and spinal cord. Benzodiazepines act by attaching to specific receptors close to the GABA receptors, prolonging the time the GABA is attached and producing a sedative effect.
- Second, benzodiazepines can attach directly to receptors for glycine (another inhibitory neurotransmitter) in the brainstem and spinal cord, producing anxiolysis and relaxation.

All benzodiazepines produce respiratory depression to some degree by a combination of CNS depression and thoracic muscle relaxation. They also produce mild hypotension as a result of muscle relaxation decreasing vascular resistance. As a result, the heart rate often rises as the body compensates for the reduction in blood pressure.

Assessment

Case selection is important when considering conscious sedation. An assessment visit prior to sedation is imperative. This visit is used to explain the procedure fully, to assess the patient's level of anxiety and to select an appropriate sedation method. It should be done in an environment that is pleasant and unthreatening. The assessment includes the history, examination and treatment planning.

History

An assessment of the patient's anxiety levels and discussion of specific phobias will inform the practitioner about the patient's likely behaviour and cooperation during the operative procedure.

A comprehensive medical history is required, with specific enquiry regarding previous general anaesthetics and sedation.

A number of drugs interact with particular intravenous sedation agents and can prolong sedation considerably. These include alcohol, opioids, antidepressants, other benzodiazepines and recreation drugs.

All intravenous sedation agents cause some level of respiratory depression and therefore patients with chronic obstructive airways disease are at risk. Upper respiratory tract infections are relative contraindications to both inhalational and intravenous sedation and if the treatment can be put off it should be to allow the patient time to recover. Asthma is often worsened by stress and anxiety and patients who can be treated without anxiety often display better control of their asthma throughout the procedure.

In general, patients in classes I and II of the American Society of Anesthetists (ASA) physical status scale (see Table 10.2) can be treated safely in the primary care sector, but ASA class III patients require management in a hospital environment.

Patients will require an escort to take them home if they are having intravenous sedation and will not be able to drive or to take responsibility for children or relatives

for 12 h; they will not be able to return to work that day. It is therefore important to assess the patient's family and employment circumstances.

At the assessment visit, it is important to record vital signs as baseline readings prior to treatment; these should include blood pressure and heart rate. Some practitioners advocate taking the patient's weight, although the dose of most intravenous sedation agents does not relate in any reliable way to weight.

Treatment planning

Conscious sedation offers a spectrum of anxiety control and the appropriate method for each patient can be decided only after a full history and examination is undertaken. Consent should be obtained from the patient or the patient's guardian. This should be written, witnessed and understandable.

Written instructions telling the patient what he or she can and cannot do before and after the operation should be given at this visit. These should include the following:

- You must be accompanied by a responsible adult who must remain in the waiting room throughout your appointment, escort you home afterwards and arrange for you to be looked after for the following 12 hours.
- You must not eat or drink anything for 2 hours prior to your appointment time; before this you should have a light meal e.g. toast and tea.
- If you are taking any medicines these should be taken at the usual times and should also be brought with you.
- You must not drive any vehicle, operate any machinery or use any domestic appliance for 12 hours after sedation.
- You must not drink alcohol, return to work, make any important decisions or sign any legal documents for 12 hours after sedation.

There should also be a discussion of the amnesia that often occurs in intravenous sedation.

Table 11.1   Ideal properties of a sedative agent
Anxiolytic
Easy to administer
Cheap
No side effects
Quick onset and recovery
No respiratory depression

Sedation methods

The ideal properties of a sedative agent are listed in Table 11.1. No single sedative agent possesses ideal properties and each of the following methods has distinct advantages and disadvantages.

Oral sedation

Oral sedation is the least specialised of the sedation methods. It presents a relatively simple way of providing mild preoperative sedation. It is often described as premedication and can be used alone or in conjunction with another sedation method. It is used principally to alleviate fear and anxiety, allowing the patient to tolerate either deeper sedation or further procedures. Oral sedation is almost universally acceptable because it requires very little patient cooperation.

The main disadvantage of oral sedation is the considerable individual variation in response. This is due to different absorption and metabolism of the drugs by individual patients. Benzodiazepines are the most commonly used drug for oral sedation. These are considered below.

Diazepam

Diazepam has been the most commonly used oral sedative for many years. The response to the drug varies; a suitable adult regime may be 5 mg the night before the treatment, 5 mg on waking and 5 mg 1 h before the procedure. This will not produce profound sedation but will allow the patient to approach the procedure with more confidence and less anxiety. Diazepam does have a relatively long half-life and therefore patients should not drive or operate machinery for 24 h after the operation, and there is even a risk of some remaining sedation after 2–3 days, due to the production of active metabolites. Patients taking diazepam, or other benzodiazepines long term, become tolerant to the drugs and therefore sedating these individuals with further benzodiazepines is very difficult.

Temazepam

Temazepam has advantages over diazepam because of its much shorter half-life of approximately 4 h. The dose for a normal, healthy 70-kg patient should be 20 mg approximately 30 min before the procedure. This dose can vary between 10 and 40 mg, according to the patient's weight, age, medical history and level of anxiety. Temazepam is a class 2 restricted drug.

Midazolam

Midazolam is the principal drug used in the UK for intravenous sedation, however it can be used orally and experimental results are very encouraging, particularly in children and special needs patients. The drug, however, is not licensed for oral use in the UK. It is used at an oral dose of 0.5 mg/kg.

A number of other drugs besides the benzodiazapines give varying degrees of sedation when given orally; however, most are unsuitable for general use. They include opiates and antihistamines, which are used particularly in children.

Inhalational sedation

The use of inhalational sedation has increased in recent years as a result of the reduced number of general anaesthetics and its usefulness when treating anxious children. It is often said that inhalational sedation is 50% drug and 50% behaviour management.

History

In 1884 the American Horace Wells attended a local fair and received what was known at the time as 'laughing gas'. He was intrigued by its effects and later had his third molar removed with 100% nitrous oxide anaesthesia. Later in the nineteenth century, this method was used by the American anaesthetist and inventor Gardner Colton, who gave over 121 000 100% nitrous oxide anaesthetics and reported no deaths. The first anaesthetic machine for nitrous oxide was introduced in 1887 but, by 1945, after local anaesthetic was introduced into dentistry, general anaesthesia was no longer necessary for dental extraction. A mixture of nitrous oxide and oxygen was first taught in the undergraduate curriculum in the United States in the 1960s.

Clinical application

The clinical effects of sedation with nitrous oxide can be described within the stages of anaesthesia first used by Guedel (see Ch. 10). The first stage in Guedel's classification is called analgesia, and this is split into three planes, the first two of which can be obtained by concentrations of 5–25% nitrous oxide and 25–55% nitrous oxide, respectively, and represent the so-called relative analgesia phases. It is in these planes that the most useful sedation is found. Going beyond these planes produces increased dissociation, which most patients find unpleasant. There is, however, considerable variation from patient to patient and therefore, the dose of the drug is given incrementally.

Inhalational sedation has a number of indications. As well as simple anxiolysis it is also useful in patients who have a hyperactive gagging reflex because it can often reduce this sufficiently to allow dental treatment that was previously impossible to be carried out. It is also useful in patients with physical and mental special needs, although there does have to be some level of under-standing and communication because it must be possible to undertake the behaviour management required to allow the agent to fulfil its potential. It is also useful in patients with mild medical problems worsened by anxiety, such as well-controlled asthma and epilepsy.

The relative contraindications to the use of inhalational sedation include upper respiratory tract infections that make nasal breathing difficult. The procedure should, if possible, be postponed in these circumstances. Particularly in children, it can be a problem when the tonsils and adenoids are enlarged, again making nasal breathing difficult. Difficulty communicating or understanding the nasal breathing required makes inhalational sedation very difficult in children, certainly under the age of three and in patients with severe special needs.

Inhalational sedation has a number of distinct advantages over other methods:

- it is non-invasive
- it only requires a nasal mask
- it has rapid onset and rapid recovery
- no fasting is required
- it produces anxiolysis and analgesia (it is said that 50% nitrous oxide gives analgesia similar to 10 mg of intramuscular morphine)
- it requires no electronic monitoring
- it is acceptable to most patients
- it produces no amnesia of any kind and therefore the whole procedure is remembered.

The principal disadvantage is pollution. The nitrous oxide that is expired into the atmosphere and consequently breathed in by the staff in the surgery has been related

to a number of medical problems (described in Ch. 10). This has led to a number of safety recommendations based around the Health and Safety Executive's 1996 decision to set a maximum dose of nitrous oxide of 100 parts per million in a time-waited 8-h period. These safety recommendations include active scavenging, which removes the expired gas as opposed to passive scavenging resulting from open windows and fans, the use of closed circuits so that the expired gas is exhausted away from the clinical environment rather than into the room and the monitoring of pollution levels.

Procedure

The importance of behaviour management to the technique cannot be overemphasised. Written consent is mandatory, as is a second appropriate person as a chaperone. The Quantiflex MDM machine is the standard machine used in the UK and it allows a variable mixture of nitrous oxide and oxygen to be given to the patient via a nasal mask. The machine is marked in 10% increments allowing a minimum of 30% oxygen. The manufacturers report a 5% error in either direction and therefore the absolute maximum is 75% nitrous oxide, which is rarely necessary. This still provides more oxygen than in standard room air.

Gas leaves the two active cylinders at the front of the machine (there are two full reserve cylinders on the back of the machine) and is mixed in the flow control head. The facemask is introduced and the patient is allowed to breathe 100% oxygen at approximately 5–6 L/min for 2 or 3 min. The flow rate can be adjusted according to the reservoir bag, which is on the machine. The flow rate will vary according to the size of the patient and the frequency of respiration. Nitrous oxide concentration is then slowly increased in 10% increments, approximately every 60 s, until the patient begins to report signs of sedation. It is important at this stage to ensure nasal breathing only, and the patient should be encouraged to speak only when absolutely necessary.

It requires considerable skill on the part of the operator to maintain a calm and pleasant environment. As the dose increases, the patient will report sensory changes including paraesthesia in the extremities, tinnitus and a general feeling of warmth. This is a result of peripheral vasodilation and can be seen in the flushing of the facial features. As the sedation level increases, patients often begin to report visual disturbance and a feeling of remoteness or disassociation. This is the stage at which maximum useful anxiolysis and analgesia has been obtained; beyond this level patients begin to feel light-headed and then restless and even nauseous. It is important to stop before reaching this stage, particularly in children because they will become uncooperative and it will be very difficult to persuade them that bringing the concentration down will make them feel better again.

With increased use of the technique, the operator becomes very adept at assessing the level of sedation from the sensory changes and from the reaction of the patient. The procedure can then be carried out, including the local anaesthetic, which will be significantly easier to administer because of the analgesia obtained from the nitrous oxide. It is possible to increase and decrease the concentration according to the procedure that is taking place, for instance it might be necessary to increase the concentration for the local anaesthetic injection and reduce it then for the procedure itself. At the end of the procedure it is important to let the patient breathe 100% oxygen for 2–3 min, to prevent the theoretical risk of diffusion hypoxia as nitrous oxide moves in significant quantities from the blood back into the alveoli and is rebreathed, therefore diluting the oxygen available for respiration producing hypoxia. In reality this is rarely a problem. The patient should be recovered until they feel fit enough to leave. Approximately 20 min after the procedure adults can leave unescorted; children require the same escort arrangements as they would after local anaesthetic.

Intravenous sedation

Intravenous sedation is, at present, the best method for conscious sedation and is the technique of choice for most adult patients. It requires considerable training and experience but rewards this with excellent operating conditions in a calm and relaxed environment even when dealing with severely phobic patients.

History

The first time intravenous drugs were used for sedation, rather than full anaesthesia, was in 1945 when the so-called 'Jorgensen technique' was introduced. This consisted of the intravenous injection of a barbiturate, an opioid and scopolamine. By most standards nowadays this would be considered deep sedation at best and dangerous at worst. In the 1960s, however, the discovery of benzodiazepines revolutionised the practice of

intravenous sedation. Initially in dentistry, intravenous conscious sedation was done using diazepam but this had a number of disadvantages, most importantly its elimination half-life of 43 h and the production of active metabolites. Patients were therefore sedated to some extent for up to 2 days and there was a risk of rebound sedation. Diazepam is insoluble in water, which means it has to be either given as a solute dissolved in propylene glycol, which is painful on injection, or emulsified in soya bean oil, which is the most common formulation.

The next generation benzodiazepine, midazolam solves many of the problems presented by diazepam. It is a water-soluble imadazobenzodiazepine. Usefully, it is water-soluble at a pH of less than 4 and lipid-soluble at physiological pH, making it painless on injection. It is available in two preparations: 10 mg in 2 mL of fluid or 10 mg in 5 mL of fluid. The latter is used for intravenous sedation because it is easier to control the incremental dosage. It acts more rapidly than diazepam and has a much more reliable patient response. It has an elimination half-life of between 90 and 150 min – considerably shorter than that of diazepam – and is metabolised in the liver.

Clinical application

There are a number of indications for intravenous sedation with midazolam. Psychosocial indications are often the most common reason for a patient to present for intravenous sedation. This group of patients includes those with anxieties and phobias related to dentistry including needles and drills. There is a specific group of patients who have considerable difficulty with vasovagal attacks prior to and during dentistry and intravenous sedation can often help.

There are a number of medical indications for intravenous sedation, particularly if the patient has a condition that is aggravated by stress. This group includes those with asthma, epilepsy, hypertension and those with mild ischaemic heart disease. Intravenous sedation can also be useful in those with mental and physical special needs.

Other indications for intravenous sedation include difficult, long or unpleasant procedures and patient preference.

There are a number of relative contraindications to intravenous sedation. Social contraindications include those who are unwilling to consider this mode of treatment or are extremely uncooperative. It is not possible to provide intravenous sedation for an unaccompanied patient and it is also difficult with extremes of age. The use of intravenous midazolam is controversial in children under 16 years.

Medical contraindications include severe systemic disease, particularly respiratory disease such as severe chronic obstructive airways disease, and severe mental or physical special needs. A number of drug interactions contraindicate the use of intravenous benzodiazepines, particularly if a patient has a history of psychiatric treatment or has been prescribed benzodiazepines over a long period of time, thereby making the patient very tolerant to the drug. Intravenous sedation should be avoided wherever possible in patients who are either pregnant or breast-feeding.

The topping-up of midazolam sedation is not recommended except in very skilled hands and, therefore, any procedure lasting longer than an hour is really unsuitable for this treatment method.

Procedure

An indwelling cannula is mandatory for all forms of intravenous sedation. It is useful to provide topical anaesthetic. This can be either Emla® or Ametop®, which are readily available and allow the painless insertion of intravenous cannulae.

As with inhalational sedation, it is essential that there is a second competent person in the room at all times during intravenous sedation. This person should be trained in both monitoring the sedated patient and assisting in the event of an emergency.

The patient should have blood pressure monitored and a pulse oximeter attached (Fig. 11.1). Midazolam is given routinely as a 2 mg bolus and then 1 mg increments every 60 s to a standard endpoint. Patients become gradually more comfortable with their surroundings, their speech begins to slow and slur, they respond to commands in a sluggish fashion and – most importantly – they become willing to accept treatment that they previously would have found unacceptable.

Verrill's sign occurs when the upper eyelid covers the upper half of the patient's pupil. This sign is not reliable with intravenous midazolam and often indicates over-sedation. Eve's sign occurs when the patient is asked to touch his or her nose with the forefinger and is unable to do so, invariably touching the upper lip instead. This is a more reliable sign for the endpoint for midazolam sedation.

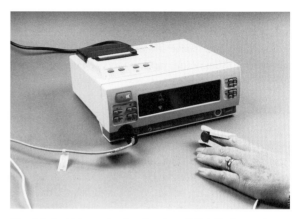

Fig. 11.1 Pulse oximeter showing digital display and finger probe.

It is important not to lose verbal communication with the patient at any point and, although response to commands will be slower than normal, this should still be possible. The total dose required varies considerably as a result of many factors, including anxiety, sleep deprivation, alcohol consumption in the previous 24 h and other drugs, both prescription and recreational. It is difficult to be prescriptive about a maximum dose but considerable thought should be given before increasing the dose above 10 mg.

Intravenous midazolam gives approximately 45–60 min of useful sedation, during which most procedures can be carried out. When the procedure is finished the patient should be given time to recover, either in the same room or in a designated recovery area, and should be monitored continuously. The patient's escort can be invited to sit with the patient during this period. The patient can be discharged approximately 1 h after the last increment of drug is given, but this varies from individual to individual and requires assessment of each case. It is important to remove the cannula before discharge. Postoperative instructions should be given to the escort, although they should already have been given to the patient at the assessment visit. The escort should be provided with a telephone number in case any problems arise.

Monitoring

Patients who are sedated have a reduced perception of their surroundings and of their own body. The staff around them, therefore, assume responsibility for their vital signs. Monitoring allows early intervention before injury takes place and is used to minimise risk to the patient. Clinical monitoring is most important and requires observation of the colour of the patient and their respiration. Electronic monitoring via a pulse oximeter is mandatory for intravenous sedation.

In normal, healthy patients the oxygen saturation of arterial blood will be between 96 and 100%. The oxygen saturation alarm should be set at 90% to allow remedial action to be taken prior to any injury. The oximeter also provides a constant reading of the patient's heart rate (see Ch. 10).

The principal side-effect of intravenous benzodiazepines is respiratory depression. If this occurs, as indicated by a reducing oxygen saturation, the first step is to talk to the patient and perhaps to shake him or her gently, asking them to take deep breaths. This will usually wake the patient from the light sleep he or she has drifted into and allow them to take a number of deep breaths, thereby, increasing the oxygen saturation to normal. A patient who is unable to carry this action out unaided is over-sedated and the operator must assist the process of respiration by lifting the patient's chin upwards, thrusting the jaw forwards and tilting the head backwards. This allows the airway to be straightened and makes respiration considerably easier. The next stage, if necessary, is to give oxygen via a mask, or more commonly via a nasal cannula. Oxygen should be given at approximately 2 to 3 L per minute via a nasal cannula or at 5 to 6 L per minute via a mask. If these measures are unsuccessful, the next step is reversal of the sedation agent.

Flumazenil is a benzodiazepine antagonist. It was discovered in 1978 and, although some practitioners have advocated its routine use, it should be used for emergencies only. It belongs to the benzodiazepine group of drugs but lacks the active benzene ring that makes benzodiazepines sedatives. Because it has a higher affinity for receptors than midazolam, flumazenil reverses the action of midazolam without having any sedative action of its own. It is available in vials of 500 µg in 5 ml of fluid and the standard dose is 200 µg (2 ml) initially then 100 µg increments every 60 s until recovery. It has a shorter half-life (50 min) than midazolam and should therefore be used with care because there is a theoretical risk of resedation once the flumazenil wears off and the midazolam reattaches to the receptors.

Section B
Specialist Surgical Principles

12 Fractures of the facial bones

Introduction

Fractures of the facial bones are common and present in Accident and Emergency departments and to medical or dental practitioners. Physical violence tends to be the most common aetiology in the UK, followed by road traffic accidents and falls; sports and industrial injuries are relatively uncommon. Most assaults result in low-energy injuries and are associated with excess alcohol consumption, most frequently in young males. They can be accompanied by soft tissue injuries. The majority are caused by fists and boots, glass bottles and knives and, in recent years, baseball bats. When associated with drug addiction, gunshot wounds are an increasingly common factor.

Most high-energy injuries are traffic related. Despite the increased use of safety belts and drink driving regulations, severe injuries are still regularly seen; high-speed accidents often result in fatal or very severe injuries, although improved car design has lessened the risks to the front-seat passenger and driver. Other less common causes of isolated fractures are industrial and sports injuries, which mostly affect the upper and mid face. War injuries tend to be high velocity injuries caused by a mixture of exploding bombs, shells and gunshots, often leading to extensive damage to the soft tissues and facial skeleton.

Falls commonly cause injury to the nose or the malar complex, but less so the mandible. They tend to occur under 10 years of age and in the elderly infirm patient with brittle bones.

The general examination

The general examination of the patient should take account of the presence of alcohol and drugs before examination of the facial injuries. Inspection and palpation of the various parts of the face will pick up

Table 12.1 Fractures of the facial bones
Mandibular
Middle third
lateral
zygomatic (malar)
central
nasal
nasoethmoidal
maxillary

obvious asymmetry, often masked when there is swelling present. This examination should be gentle but organised and precise.

The ears and eyes need to be fully examined and, where an ophthalmic injury is suspected, early ophthalmic consultation is advisable. At least 12% of all orbital injuries are associated with severe ocular injury, which is often unrecognised. The injuries should be recorded and further information sought from accompanying persons at the incident. Other life-threatening injuries must be excluded. Although conventional radiography is helpful in identifying fracture sites, obtaining good films requires a cooperative patient, and where this is in doubt, radiography should be postponed.

Fractures of the facial bones affect either the mandible or the middle third of the face, or both (Table 12.1). These will be discussed in turn.

Mandibular fractures

The mandible is essentially a bone with three joints, both condyles and the dental occlusion, and it is important that the condyles remain in their fossae and that the occlusion is correctly maintained. Simple approximation of fractures with intermaxillary fixation can lead to respiratory and masticatory difficulties and is being superseded by open reduction and plating. The intraoperative use of intermaxillary fixation to fix the occlusion is valuable but, after plating mandibular fractures, this can usually be released. Semirigid fixation with miniplates is widely employed and although titanium is probably the metal of choice, other alloys and stainless steel are also used. The last is likely to require removal and they are an occasional cause of metal allergy.

Clinical features

There is usually swelling and pain at the fracture site. Where there is significant displacement, malocclusion is likely with an inability to bring the teeth correctly together. Loosening of teeth commonly occurs at the fracture site, often accompanied by partial avulsion of teeth and root fractures. Early recognition is essential as delay can contribute to later infection at the fracture site. Grossly mobile and fractured teeth should be removed. In the younger child where the apices are open, they may be retained. All fractures where the teeth are involved are compound into the mouth and there is some risk of infection.

There will usually be some asymmetry of the mandible with unilateral fractures. With condylar neck fractures there is likely to be shortening of the mandibular ramus and an anterior open bite (Fig. 12.1). Where there is gross displacement at a fracture site there is often another fracture elsewhere (Table 12.2).

Whenever a fracture arises in the tooth bearing area, such as in the mandibular body between the lingula and mental foramen, disruption of the inferior dental nerve is likely, and with wide separation of fragments the nerve may be torn and require repair. The accurate repositioning, stabilisation of fragments and reconstitution of the canal

often results in some recovery of lower lip and chin sensation. Pain and crepitus may be present at the fracture site but should not be elicited, although there should be a check for mobility. Trismus is common, irrespective of the site of the fracture, as mouth opening will increase discomfort. Similarly, dysphagia and lack of control of saliva (which may be blood stained) may be due to discomfort when approximating the teeth on swallowing.

Bruising in the floor of the mouth is a pathognomonic sign of a mandibular fracture in the edentulous patient. Almost the only other way this can occur is with a penetrating injury. More rarely, the fractured or intact condyle, with severe force applied to the chin area, may pass backwards tearing the external auditory meatus. This tear tends to occur through the anterior or inferior part of the ear canal, often accompanied by leakage of clear synovial fluid or bleeding. If there is a tear on the superior or posterior wall or tympanic membrane it is highly likely that there is a fracture of the petrous temporal bone accompanied by hearing loss and a CSF leak.

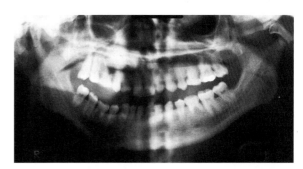

Fig.12.1 Orthopantomogram showing fractures of the mandibular condyles.

Table 12.2	Possible clinical features of common mandibular fractures with displacement	
	Angle	*Subcondyle*
Pain, swelling bruising	At angle of jaw	Preauricular
Sublingual haematoma	Yes	No
Trismus	Yes	Yes
Mental anaesthesia	Yes	No
Occlusal disharmony	If fracture through or adjacent to standing tooth	Premature contact on affected side
'Step' palpable	Yes: at lower border	Difficult to palpate
Bleeding from ear	No	Possible
Condyle palpable in fossa	Yes	No: if fracture and dislocation
Intraoral bleeding	Possible	No
Compound	Commonly	Very rarely

Displacement of the mandibular fracture is very much related to its site. Extensive fractures of the mandibular ramus often remain undisplaced because they are splinted by the masseter and pterygoid muscles. Fractures in the angle region of the mandible, however, are subject to pull from the elevators, pterygoid and suprahyoid muscles and displacement may well occur, especially when the fracture is bilateral leading to posterior displacement of the distal segment and an anterior open bite with loss of chin prominence. A careful note needs to be taken of these in the semiconscious or unconscious patient, because airway obstruction can occur. If plating techniques are not available it is important to identify the direction of the fracture in the angle region. If, on the orthopantomogram (OPT), it runs obliquely from the external angle to the third molar tooth, the proximal fragment tends to displace superiorly. If, on the posteroanterior view, the fracture runs obliquely from the angle region forwards, the proximal fragment will again tend to displace but in this case medially as a result of pterygoid muscle action (Fig. 12.2). The doubly unfavourable fracture will need stabilisation with a wire at the lower border of the mandible or plate or it will tend to torque apart when in intermaxillary fixation. These considerations tend to disappear with good plating techniques that encourage accurate fragment inter-digitation to take place (e.g. with a strong upper border plate placed along the external oblique ridge). Accurate stable repositioning avoids the necessity for postoperative intermaxillary fixation.

Radiography

Imaging of the mandible is largely through plain radiographs taken in two planes. The orthopantomogram (OPT) is essentially a lateral view of the whole mandible, which visualises clearly body and ramus fractures but is less effective in the parasymphyseal region (Fig. 12.3). Both condylar heads and necks must be included. A posteroanterior (PA) view at right angles to this is essential. A reverse Towne's view will often show anteromedial displacement or dislocation of the condyle when not seen on a standard PA view. Dental and occlusal intraoral views are particularly valuable and should be taken routinely for suspected dental injuries and alveolar fractures in the tooth-bearing area. They demonstrate the relationship of the teeth to the fractures and their involvement in the fracture line. Lower occlusal views are helpful in picking up sagittal fractures in the anterior mandible.

Imaging of the mandibular condyle is sometimes difficult in young children, especially those under five years where there is comminution of the condylar head in intracapsular fractures, and also where there is suspected condylar displacement through the glenoid fossa. Here, computerised tomography (CT) scanning is particularly

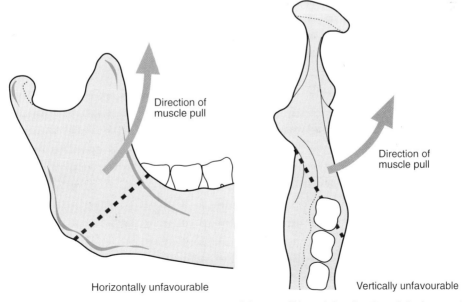

Direction of muscle pull

Direction of muscle pull

Horizontally unfavourable

Vertically unfavourable

Fig. 12.2 Unfavourable fractures at the angle of the mandible and the direction of displacement.

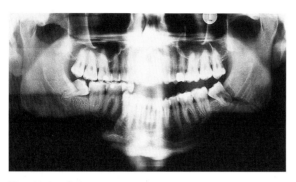

Fig. 12.3 Orthopantomogram showing a fracture at the angle of the mandible.

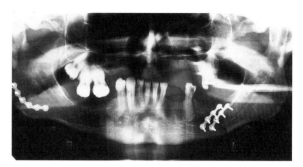

Fig. 12.4 Radiograph showing bilateral fractures of the mandible fixed with titanium plates.

helpful in identifying the nature of the injury and the extent of comminution present. This is important in the young child where there is always a risk of disturbance of growth and possibly ankylosis. If the patient is unconscious or has sustained injuries such as severe neck or skull fractures or other spinal injuries then CT scanning is essential. Good views of the temporomandibular joints should be obtained and are best seen on coronal views.

Treatment

Preliminary treatment includes maintenance of the airway by clearance of foreign bodies from the area. Local bleeding needs to be stopped by suturing or pressure. Temporary support at the fracture site is given when there is any delay in treatment using a wire around adjacent teeth at the fracture site to hold the fragments together or by supporting the jaws in occlusion with a head bandage. In the unconscious patient the passage of a suture through the tongue to hold this forward with any symphyseal bone fragments may also be necessary. All compound fractures require early antibiotic therapy.

The general principles of fracture treatment are reduction, fixation, immobilisation, prevention of infection, and restoration of function. These need to be considered in the management of mandibular fractures.

Manual reduction of the fracture by repositioning the fragments can be carried out under either local or general anaesthesia. For late-presenting fractures the application of arch bars to the teeth both upper and lower will allow elastic traction to be applied bringing the fragments into occlusion.

Fixation, in the dentate patient, can be by a variety of attachments made to the teeth. These include arch bars or eyelet wiring around individual teeth, cast silver cap splints and when teeth are missing the use of modified dentures or Gunning splints.

With the establishment of rigid fixation as the method of choice for stabilising facial fractures the principle of intermaxillary fixation for a significant period after reduction of the fractures has become less important. Whereas in the past fractures were fixed with intermaxillary fixation and interosseous wiring, or various combinations of special wiring techniques, nowadays the majority of fractures are fixed with titanium or occasionally steel alloy plates (Fig. 12.4). Various forms of miniplates are available; usually a 2 mm thickness plate, with appropriate screws, is required. Most fractures can be fixed with a single plate provided at least two monocortical screws are placed on each side of the fracture. In certain areas of the mandible additional fixation is required, principally in the symphyseal region where two plates are advantageous in preventing torquing of the bone fragments at the lower border. Bone plates are normally inserted through an intraoral approach. Where there is gross comminution of bone or there are missing bone fragments then the use of a heavier, thicker reconstruction plate should be considered. These heavy plates are more difficult to mould to the bone and are usually inserted through a skin incision just below the lower border of the mandible. Additional corticocancellous iliac crest bone graft is needed when there is bone loss.

The angle region is a common fracture site and here a single plate along the external oblique ridge is normally adequate. Teeth in the fracture line can be left if they are undisplaced and intact. If the blood supply at the apex has been destroyed, if infection is present or if the fracture is treated late, consideration should be given to early extraction. Teeth not requiring to be retained, such as an impacted third molar, can be removed at the same time unless this tends to disrupt the fracture line when they should be temporarily retained (see Ch. 27).

The condylar segment in severe trauma may displace posteriorly, leading to rupture of the external auditory meatus; only occasionally is it fractured in this situation.

Certain fractures require special treatment: the grossly infected fracture and the fracture where there is significant bone loss can be stabilised by the insertion of pins into the major fragments joined together with a bar holding the fragments as far as possible in their correct position. Following this, the infection will usually settle and any bone loss can be replaced with iliac crest bone graft.

For the atrophic mandible, especially in the elderly where perhaps the main body of the mandible is less than 6–8 mm in height, primary bone grafting of the fractured mandible with split ribs is often the best solution. The ribs are split lengthwise and shaped to the mandible on the lingual and buccal sides and held in place with at least two circumferential wires on each side of the fracture line. Additional small screws can be helpful for stabilisation.

The condylar neck is commonly fractured and is difficult to treat. Low condylar neck fractures, especially bilateral and displaced or dislocated tend to develop an anterior open bite. Open reduction and fixation with one or two miniplates is often the treatment of choice. For simple single condylar neck fractures, the use of arch bars and light elastic traction may be all that is required but, when accompanied by fractures elsewhere (e.g. in the parasymphyseal region, body or angle), or by mid-face fractures, it is safer to reduce and fix the condyle.

Fractures in young children should be managed conservatively under the age of 12. No condylar fracture requires operative treatment as they will all remodel and reform. Comminuted condylar fractures in the young child are usually intracapsular and can lead to ankylosis; they require early but gentle mobilisation and generally should not be explored. Minor degrees of irregularity in the occlusion may be acceptable because remodelling occurs and malocclusions tend to resolve. Simple splinting devices for pain relief may be required.

Certain general principles need to be mentioned, such as the provision of adequate analgesia. The semifluid diet given should be high in protein and calories. Good oral hygiene should be maintained using chlorhexidine and saline mouthwashes and a toothbrush.

Good healing requires stabilisation for an adequate length of time. Indirect reduction of fractures with inter-maxillary fixation alone, although successful, often takes 6 weeks to unite. For most fractures, callus provides an osteoid mass of tissue around the fracture site giving it some stability. Conventional miniplates allow for excellent repositioning of the fractures provided they are correctly adapted to the surface of the mandible and they provide the necessary immobilisation across the fracture.

Care needs to be taken to avoid the insertion of miniplate screws into the inferior dental canal or the roots of the teeth. With accurate reduction of the fracture, any sensation lost due to separation of the fracture usually recovers, but this may be incomplete when there has been extensive damage to the inferior dental nerve or considerable delay in treating the fracture.

Complications

Complications associated with mandibular fractures are not uncommon and, although they can be related to the fixation used (e.g. plates), are often due to infection or exposure of the plate into the mouth. It does not necessarily follow that a plate has to be removed immediately if there is infection, only if infection persists and there is a lack of bony union will this be necessary. Minor infections do not necessarily prevent union when there is adequate drainage and the fractures are well fixed. Delayed union may result from infection arising from the teeth, bone or a breakdown of the soft tissues. It might also be caused by a poor reduction of the fracture, interposition of soft tissue into the fracture line and mobility of fragments. These problems run a high risk of delayed or non-union. Complicating local pathology such as a cyst or tumour may be present but even then most fractures unite. Malunion is the result of poor reduction of fragments, rarely seen with modern open techniques. It can occur with late-treated or untreated fractures. Osteotomy of that malunion may be required to achieve a normal occlusion and symmetry of the mandible.

There is some argument about the retention of teeth in the fracture line. If very loose or displaced, they may well be lost at the time of injury, shortly afterwards or later if there is extensive exposure of the root surface. A very mobile tooth in the fracture line is likely to be non-vital and is best removed to prevent delayed union even though there is plate fixation at the fracture site.

In fractures around the condyle, angle region and ramus there may be late onset trismus after much trauma to both muscle and bone or comminution in that area. More rarely, ankylosis will result, or bony hyperplasia of either the coronoid or condylar processes, typically in young children. Early mobilisation of fractures in young children is essential as union occurs quickly, often within 3–4 weeks. It is essential to keep the condyle moving with comminuted condylar head fractures and haemarthroses. Condylar remodelling occurs over a period of months and symmetry usually returns in childhood fractures.

Persistent mental anaesthesia can occur as a result of damage to the inferior dental or mental nerves or occasionally at the site of the lingula. Severe damage or section of the nerve in the body of the mandible may require nerve repair and consideration should be given to this. Anatomical reduction of the fracture must be obtained so that the inferior dental canal is maintained.

Middle third fractures

The middle third of the face consists of nasoethmoidal complex, the maxillae and smaller bones attached to it together with the malar complexes. It lies between the

mandible and the cranial cavity and calvarium, in particular the frontal and sphenoid bones. Fractures, when of some severity, are likely to involve the cranial cavity especially following high-velocity or high-energy injuries associated with road traffic trauma or gunshot wounds. Cranial involvement should be excluded at an early stage as this may require neurosurgical intervention or a combined approach.

Classically, middle third fractures are divided into central and lateral middle third fractures, the lateral middle third being essentially the malar or zygomatico-maxillary complex. Central middle third fractures include nasal, nasoethmoidal and maxillary fractures. The original descriptions of Le Fort in 1901 divided maxillary fractures into the Le Fort I fracture, which is a subzygomatic fracture separating the dentoalveolar complex from the nasal and antral cavities passing through the pterygoid plates (Fig. 12.5).

The Le Fort II fracture is a pyramidal fracture, again subzygomatic, which may involve the cranial cavity in the cribriform plate area. There may be significant

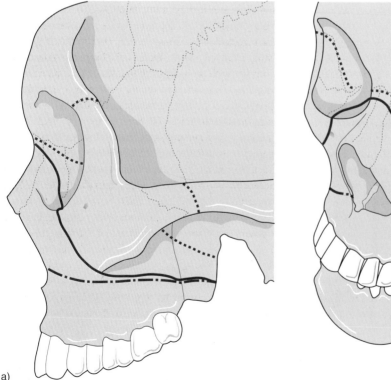
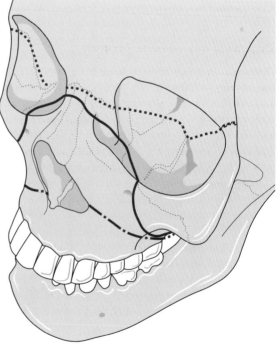

a)
b)

Fig.12.5 (a) Lateral view of skull showing middle third fractures; (b) Oblique view of skull showing middle third fractures. ---·---·--- position of Le Fort I fractures. ———— position of Le Fort II fractures. ---------- position of Le Fort III fractures.

damage to the orbit involving the infraorbital nerves, nasolacrimal apparatus and medial canthal ligaments often associated with blowout fractures of the orbits. The Le Fort II fracture passes across the bridge of the nose, not always at the frontonasal junction but through the nasoethmoid and lacrimal bones, then usually between the nasolacrimal duct and infraorbital nerves and around the zygomatic buttress to the pterygoid plate area, where there may also be fractures (Fig. 12.5). The nasal septum will be separated.

The Le Fort III fracture is a craniofacial dysjunction separating the whole of the midface structures from the cranial bones. This extends from the frontozygomatic sutures across the sphenoid bone into the inferior orbital fissure and through the ethmoid, lacrimal bones, nasal septum and frontonasal junction and then across to the other side often with some comminution. The zygomatic arches will be fractured and there will be separation or fractures of the pterygoid plates (Fig. 12.5).

Displacement of all midface fractures tends to be downwards and backwards, thus creating an anterior open bite appearance, with lengthening of the midface as the solid structure of the basisphenoid prevents upward displacement.

Zygomatic (malar) bone fracture

The malar complex or zygomatic bone constitutes the lateral middle third of the face and it is commonly fractured in isolation. Fractures occur close to the suture lines often with comminution of the anterolateral wall of the maxilla and sometimes at the zygomatic arch or infraorbital margin. The masseter muscle exerts some pull on the malar and there is a tendency for it to displace if not adequately fixed.

Clinical features

These include swelling, circumorbital ecchymosis and sometimes surgical emphysema, as a result of blowing the nose often after an epistaxis (Table 12.3). Infection may spread from the nasal cavity into the sinus and soft tissues. Unilateral epistaxis commonly occurs except in zygomatic arch fractures.

Subconjunctival haemorrhages are common and tend to be in the inferior and lateral aspect in malar fractures.

Diplopia is not uncommon. In the initial phase it may be due to swelling or bleeding around the inferior extra ocular muscles causing restriction of upward gaze.

Table 12.3 Possible clinical features of zygomatic (malar) fracture

Swelling: periorbital and over prominence of cheek
Haematoma
    periorbital (black eye)
    in buccal sulcus
    subconjunctival
    epistaxis (via blood in air sinus)
Anaesthesia
    infraorbital ± anterior and middle superior
    dental
    zygomaticofacial, zygomaticotemporal – these are rare
Eye problems
    loss of acuity/blindness (rarely)
    diplopia
    enophthalmos
    drop in interpupillary line level
    exophthalmos (proptosios) – rare after injury but
      possible on reduction
Trismus: obstruction of coronoid process
Step palpable: possible at: frontozygomatic suture, infraorbital margin, zygomatic arch

---

Occasionally, the inferior rectus or inferior oblique muscles are damaged by bone fragments and, more rarely, their nerve supply is damaged. True trapping of the muscle can sometimes occur between bone fragments. Much more commonly there is displacement of the orbital contents with prolapse of orbital fat into the antrum. This is known as a blowout fracture. Within the orbital fat there are fine fibrous tissue bands attached to the muscle sheaths which catch on bone fragments and restrict normal eye movements. Where there is a very large defect, gross displacement of the orbital contents can occur into the antral cavity. This may be accompanied by a medial wall blowout, which must be identified and treated.

Whenever there is a floor blowout enophthalmos (retraction of the eyeball within the orbital cavity) is likely to be present usually with a drop in pupillary level. This must be identified because it might not be immediately evident because of intraorbital bleeding and oedema. It is crucial that the bony orbit is fully restored and the walls rendered intact, otherwise enophthalmos will persist.

Occasionally, the malar is grossly displaced medially with severe proptosis of the eye, which can need early release, there being a risk of damage to the cornea from exposure and of a retrobulbar haemorrhage with – ultimately – loss of vision. Careful examination of the eye itself, and appropriate referral for an ophthalmic opinion, is mandatory when eye injury itself is suspected.

Rarely, with severe lateral middle third injuries there is crushing of the superior orbital fissure resulting in a superior orbital fissure syndrome with ophthalmoplegia, a dilated pupil, ptosis, supraorbital anaesthesia and proptosis; when there is associated blindness from damage to the optic nerve or optic foramen this is called the orbital apex syndrome. Vision is rarely recoverable when the optic nerve is damaged but pressure can be relieved where there is gross proptosis by drainage of any retrobulbar haemorrhage reducing the risk of visual loss. A strict protocol should be adopted for the management of orbital injuries, with frequent reassessment of the at risk patient. In most cases the superior orbital fissure syndrome recovers spontaneously. Structures in the narrowest upper part of the fissure recover most slowly, the abducent and the lower branch of the oculomotor nerve recover more quickly; surgical intervention is not normally required.

Asymmetry from displacement of the malar complex may not be apparent immediately because of the swelling. An examination of the patient from above and below, palpating the cheek prominences and orbital margins, will usually show any flattening or asymmetry. If there is any doubt about this, waiting up to 10 days will clarify the position and any aesthetic need for treatment. Separation of the frontozygomatic suture can lead to inferior displacement of the malar complex and globe but an intact periosteum will prevent this. Infraorbital margin displacement is usually posterior and inferior or a combination of both, when the arch is displaced. The pupillary and canthal position should be noted and the zygomatic arch checked for any step deformity.

Infraorbital anaesthesia is common with malar fractures, because the fracture line passes close to or through the infraorbital foramen or canal. The anterior superior dental nerve branch may also be damaged, causing numbness of the incisor and canine teeth. If the nerve is crushed or severely damaged, full recovery is unlikely. In severe injuries damage to the zygomaticofrontal and zygomaticotemporal nerves will result in numbness over the cheek prominence and temporal region. Accurate reduction of the malar assists recovery of infraorbital sensation.

Trismus is common with malar fractures often due to the impingement of the malar complex on the coronoid process or its fracture with bleeding into the masseter, temporal and pterygoid muscles. This should recover

with reduction of the fractures and haematoma absorption. Ecchymosis in the buccal sulcus due to bleeding at the fracture site is frequently seen.

Radiography

Imaging of the malar has become contentious in recent years. The 10° and 30° occipitomental views show displacement of the malar complex and the submentovertex view, the zygomatic arch and malar prominence (Fig. 12.6). Other views have been abandoned as a result of CT scanning. It also provides clear information on soft tissue changes in suspected blowout fractures. For simple displaced fractures of the malar with no obvious orbital floor damage, a single 15° occipitomental radiograph is acceptable. MRI scanning has a small place in the diagnosis of blowout fractures. B scan ultrasonography can be used for detecting the medial wall blowout when CT scanning or MRI are not available.

Treatment

If there is gross swelling it is usually worth waiting up to 10 days for it to reduce for a better assessment of the orbit, its contents and its position. If, however, there are compelling reasons for early treatment then often the earlier the treatment the simpler the fixation can be.

In the UK, the Gillies temporal approach is widely used for reduction. A Rowe's or Bristow elevator is passed under the temporal fascia from a hairline incision and is used to lift the malar forward and slightly laterally. Occasionally, the malar remains stable but more commonly additional fixation is required.

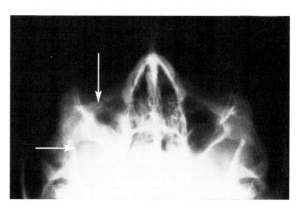

Fig. 12.6 30° occipitomental view showing displacement of the malar complex (fracture lines arrowed).

It is possible – under local anaesthesia – to elevate a simple malar fracture with a hook through a small cheek incision, lifting it anterolaterally into a stable position. However, for most unstable fractures additional fixation is required. Usually, fixation with one or two miniplates for low-energy injuries at the zygomatic buttress or frontozygomatic suture where there is separation, is required. At the infraorbital margin a microplate provides the most aesthetic fixation.

Following malar repositioning, the orbital floor needs to be checked and any significant defect needs to be repaired. Calvarial bone graft is best for large defects but for small defects silicone sheeting with dacron mesh has been widely used. It works well, but there is a complication rate and around 12% are eventually lost or require removal; a medial wall defect can be similarly repaired. Microplate fixation is used for simple orbital rim fractures. For comminuted complex fractures, fixation at the frontozygomatic suture and – intraorally – the buttress, are the minimum requirements. Additional plates may be required at the infraorbital margin, across a main body fracture and along the zygomatic arch (Fig. 12.7).

Nasal and nasoethmoidal fractures

Nasal bone fractures are the most common facial bone fracture caused by direct violence. They may be laterally displaced or anteriorly depressed. Many are simple requiring minimal treatment but where there is bony displacement then reduction is required with straightening of the septum.

Clinical features

The clinical features depend on the extent of violence and displacement of the nasoethmoid and adjacent structures. Typically, there will be bilateral periorbital haematomata, oedema and nasal obstruction with a tendency to mouth breathe accompanied by epistaxis. Nasal obstruction can be caused by septal displacement, which needs to be identified. Lateral displacement is common and may be associated with damage or separation of the cartilages and fractures of the nasal bridge. With more severe trauma, the nose becomes saddle shaped, shortened and broadened. With upwards force there may be telescoping of the nasoethmoidal complex into the frontal sinus and then intracranially through the cribriform plate. There is likely to be telecanthus and separation of the medial canthal attachments. Damage to the nasolacrimal apparatus can occur and penetrating injuries can tear the nasolacrimal duct. Obstruction of the canaliculae and duct stenosis at the lacrimal sac can lead later to drainage problems. Damage to the cribriform plate area may result in persistent cerebrospinal fluid (CSF) rhinorrhoea. This needs to be recognised early and managed appropriately. It is sometimes difficult to ascertain whether the clear discharge from the nose is CSF or mucus. Once bleeding has stopped it is possible to identify this by testing the fluid for glucose or transferrin, which will not be present in mucus. Other tests, such as radioisotope studies, can be used to identify difficult and intermittent CSF leaks.

Radiographs

Radiographs of the nasal bones or nasoethmoidal complex are usually unsatisfactory, with around 50% of the fractures not adequately shown. Marked displacements can be seen on 10° and 30° occipitomental views where there is displacement of the septum, but this is usually clinically obvious. Nasal bone fractures can often be seen on a soft tissue lateral view. The detail of a nasoethmoidal injury can only be ascertained from good CT scans. MRI can also be helpful where there is a CSF leak, as this is likely to show rather better than on CT scans. Medial wall blowout fractures, comminution of the nasoethmoidal complex and involvement of the

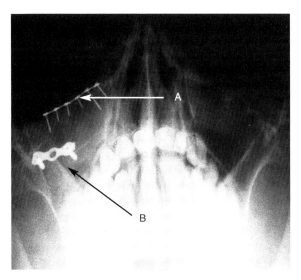

Fig. 12.7 Radiograph showing a reduced malar fracture fixed using microplate (A) and miniplate (B).

frontal sinus will be well demonstrated on CT scans taken in the coronal and axial planes.

Treatment

Simple nasal bone fractures can be repositioned with Walsham's forceps. In addition, the nasal septum needs to be straightened with Asche's forceps and the lower portion of the septum relocated in its groove on the nasal floor. Where there is doubt about the support for the nasal bones and the septal position, gentle packing with Vaseline® gauze is usually all that is required. The use of an external splint is controversial; some feel it helps to hold the complex in place, others use Steri-strips® to support and maintain the position.

In the past, when there has been a degree of telecanthus present, various forms of external fixation using transnasal wires with lead plates or acrylic buttons have been used to bring the canthal attachments into position. This has sometimes proved successful but it depends on the size of the bone fragments. In most cases where there is significant telecanthus, exploration and open reduction is necessary. Any damage to the nasolacrimal system needs to be repaired before closure of the soft tissues. Additional support of the soft tissues in the medial canthal area is valuable. A nasal plaster may be applied and sometimes a small nasal pack. Early treatment is essential for severe nasoethmoidal injuries, ideally within 10 days of the injury.

Maxillary fractures

The Le Fort I, or Guerin's, fracture is the simplest low-level fracture; Le Fort II and III fractures frequently can involve the cranial cavity. Some symptoms of each fracture are common but others are individual. It is not unusual to see combinations of Le Fort fractures, with perhaps a Le Fort I or Le Fort II on one side and a Le Fort III on the other, depending on the force applied to the midface. There may be a midline split of the palate, which, if wide, will require repair.

Clinical features

Bilateral periorbital ecchymosis and oedema are typically seen with Le Fort II and III fractures, and sometimes with Le Fort I fractures. Subconjunctival haemorrhages are usually seen with Le Fort II and III fractures but where there is good drainage of blood into the antrum

they may be absent; they are limited by the corneal attachment and extend into the fornix and tend to be segmental rather than complete. There is a flattened dish face appearance to the face and often an increase in the midface height with extensively mobile fractures.

The midface may be foreshortened and impacted upwards and posteriorly with an accompanying telecanthus but in general there is an anterior open bite with gagging of the bite posteriorly and trismus. A check should be made for a split of the palate by gently springing the molar teeth apart on their palatal surface. Sometimes this split is obvious but there may be just bruising in the midline. A check on the mobility of the teeth and fragments should be undertaken.

In the Le Fort II fracture, typically, there is dense bilateral infraorbital anaesthesia. A mild degree of anaesthesia may be present in the Le Fort I and also in the Le Fort III fractures, with numbness in the cheeks, upper lip and lower half of the nose.

The orbits are involved in Le Fort II and III fractures and diplopia and restriction of eye movements may be evident. There may be marked proptosis of the eyes due to intraorbital bleeding and oedema. The eyes must be examined carefully to exclude any serious globe damage; the incidence of which varies in different case series but around 20% is a likely figure, with around 10% permanent visual loss. In craniofacial injuries there may be visual field changes. Retinal detachments and other intraocular injuries must be excluded to avoid their deterioration during mobilisation of the midface or intraorbital surgical intervention. Usually, if 7–10 days are allowed to elapse it becomes safe to operate on the orbit. Careful examination of the lids and surface of the eye will identify lacerations and other injuries; an early ophthalmic assessment is advisable.

CSF rhinorrhoea and bleeding from the nose are commonplace in Le Fort II and III fractures. Patients should be questioned for any discharge or a salty taste at the back of the throat. They should be sat up and leant forwards, placing a filter paper strip under the external nares. If after 15 min there is no staining then it is unlikely that leakage is present. The CSF leak usually stops after fixation of the midface. In the absence of any intracranial injury, early reduction of the facial bone fractures is advised. A persistent CSF leak beyond 10 days after jaw fixation is an indication for dural repair. Neurosurgical views are mixed on the repair of dural leaks: some insist on repair of all, others feel that only persistent leaks beyond 10 days need repair. Small defects will be plugged by brain tissue and fibrosis and the defect seals off in the cribriform plate area, however CSF leaks elsewhere may persist, especially in the frontal sinus area.

Where there is insignificant displacement of the midface then the dental occlusion can be maintained. A check on the mobility of the midface by supporting the head and feeling with a finger in the palate will indicate any movement there. Tapping of the teeth of a fractured maxilla will give a hollow percussion note. With significant displacements and an anterior open bite usually the midface is easily repositioned but in late fractures there may be a degree of impaction and mobility may be difficult to ascertain.

With major midface injuries the rest of the craniofacial skeleton should be examined fully to exclude mandibular condylar and skull fractures. Intracranial involvement in major Le Fort II and III fractures often gives rise to anosmia. Early anosmia may be due to oedematous thick nasal mucosa, which settles over a few weeks. Disruption of the olfactory nerves can lead to permanent anosmia.

Radiography

Imaging in the midface has radically changed in recent years with the availability of excellent CT imaging, however certain basic radiographs may be taken in Accident and Emergency departments (i.e. 10° and 30° occipitomental views and a true lateral facial bone view, including the anterior skull). If the lateral radiograph is taken with the patient horizontal, any intracranial air will become obvious. Posterior maxillary displacement will be seen, as will damage to the pterygoid plates. In major injuries, mandibular and skull imaging should be undertaken with appropriate intraoral views. Neck injuries must be excluded and the cervical spine should be appropriately imaged. Coronal and axial CT scans are taken for nasoethmoidal injuries. MRI has only a limited place in midface injuries. However some blowout fractures are rather better seen on MRI and for all forms of brain injury this form of imaging is superior. To avoid repeat scans, patients with cranial injuries should if possible have their midface imaged at the same time.

Treatment

Emergency treatment of severe injuries is primarily that of troublesome bleeding and respiratory problems. Shock, which can result from blood loss or related cranial or other injuries, needs to be identified (see Ch. 4). Careful examination will ascertain the reason for this. Relief of pain is not usually a major issue with midface injuries. Narcotics should be avoided as they can confuse neurological examinations and interfere with the conscious level.

It is usual to give antibiotic prophylaxis for potential craniofacial communications, aerocoeles and CSF leaks, although recent guidelines suggest this is unnecessary (see Ch. 19). In the past, penicillin and sulphonamides were given; more recently, cephalosporins have replaced them. If antibiotics are given they should cross the blood–brain barrier, but in the presence of injury this presents no problem. Extensively compound dirty fractures may require additional antistaphylococcal antibiotics.

Reduction and fixation of fractures is normally carried out under general anaesthesia. Care should be taken to ensure an intact airway in the pre-, peri- and postoperative periods.

High-energy injuries should be differentiated from low-energy injuries. The latter usually have a simpler fracture pattern with less displacement and often minor soft tissue injuries. The essence of reconstruction is to ensure that the facial projection is correct, that the facial width is not increased and that the facial height is correctly maintained.

With low-energy injuries, relatively simple forms of fixation for Le Fort I and Le Fort II fractures are often effective. When there is minimal displacement, sandwiching techniques can be used with external pins into the supraorbital ridge, attached by bars to the dentition of the maxilla or mandible with intermaxillary fixation. Additional malar complex fractures can be individually explored and fixed after the central midface.

A greater degree of surgical intervention is required for high-energy midface injuries. In recent years the concepts of treatment and protocols have radically changed. Vertical strutting may be identified in the anatomy of the midface with three principal buttresses on each side – nasomaxillary, zygomaticomaxillary and pterygomaxillary (at the junction of the maxillary tuberosities and pterygoid plates) – extending up to the skull base. Comminution in those areas is uncommon and it is usually possible to plate those sites.

Access to the upper midface is obtained through the coronal scalp flap and to the inferior orbit through a lower eyelid or transconjunctival incision. The subciliary approach tends to yield more complications than a mid-lower lid incision made through a skin crease. The transconjunctival approach is also widely used, with a crow's foot extension at the lateral canthus. This gives good access to the inferior orbit but is limited for the medial and lateral orbit the latter being better approached bicoronally. A buccal vestibular incision is used to give good access to the buttress areas. Reconstitution of the zygomatic arch requires a bicoronal incision, taken well down and extended around the tragus or in a preauricular skin crease.

The general principles for management are to expose all fracture sites or at least have good access to them and to apply fixation with miniplates. Where there are small fragments (e.g. at the infraorbital margin), the use of microplates is advantageous. Where there are sizeable missing fragments, primary bone grafting with calvarial bone graft is the best solution. All bone fragments should be preserved and used. Projection of the midface is obtained by reconstruction and fixation of the zygomatic arches, frontozygomatic sutures and by nasoethmoid reconstruction to complete the orbit. The maxillary dentoalveolar segment is realigned at an occlusal level and plated at the malar buttress. The junction of the greater wing of sphenoid and malar complex intra-orbitally needs no fixation but should be checked for any malpositioning. The dental occlusion, intact mandibular dental arch and rest of mandible are critical for accurate three-dimensional fixation of the middle third.

The principles are to obtain first projection of the face, then the width followed by the vertical dimension. Care needs to be taken to avoid overclosure of the jaws; hence the necessity for the mandible to be rendered intact. Facial width is corrected by plating the zygomatic arches and frontozygomatic sutures and by reconstruction of the nasoethmoidal complex and infraorbital margin. Finally the height of the face is settled with buttress plating.

There is always some conflict over management of the soft tissues. If they are completely stripped off the bone they tend to sag, not only as a result of their own weight but because of oedema and haematoma present. It may be possible to leave portions attached to large bony fragments. This should be done if it is without detriment to repositioning bone fragments, otherwise reattachment of the soft tissue by suturing periosteum at various sites is essential to avoid displacement of, for example, the malar fat pads. Finally, orbital wall defects especially in the floor and medial wall are repaired and when necessary the superior and lateral walls. After medial canthal recon-struction the lateral canthi are checked and if necessary

stabilised with light wires to the supraorbital ridges. Incision lines should be closed in layers with appropriate attention to suturing the galea prior to skin closure with clips or sutures. Large scalp areas should have suction drainage for at least 24 h. Small facial incisions are closed in layers with subcuticular or small interrupted sutures. The intraoral vestibular incision is sutured with a resorbable material.

Blowout fractures

Certain classic signs present notably diplopia, a lowering of pupillary level and enophthalmos, which are pathog-nomonic of this injury. There is often accompanying infraorbital anaesthesia. The diagnosis is confirmed by CT scanning. Treatment is based on persistence of diplopia and enophthalmos greater than 3 mm or a marked loss of orbital contents out of the orbit. Surgery should ideally be done within 10 days to achieve a good result.

Access for the pure blowout with no significant orbital rim fracture is best through a transconjunctival approach. If there are other fractures, a lower lid blepharoplasty incision is effective but in the elderly an infraorbital skin crease incision is safer. For reconstruction, cranial bone or cartilage grafts or an alloplastic material such as a silicone rubber with dacron mesh are widely used.

Craniofacial fractures

Serious craniofacial injuries require early recognition and joint management with a neurosurgeon. The head injury takes precedence in the management of the patient and with a deteriorating conscious level early evacuation of a blood clot can be lifesaving. Facial injuries and their investigation take second place. Major high-energy injuries should be treated relatively early, preferably 7–10 days from time of injury to obtain a good result. CT scanning and an ophthalmic assessment of cranio-orbital injuries will be needed.

With injuries of this severity, cervical spine injuries and their management must be considered. Fractures of the odontoid peg may be seen in association with cranio-facial injuries. When presenting to the maxillofacial surgeon, regular checks on eye opening, best verbal response and best motor response (Glasgow Coma Scale) are necessary; any deterioration requires neurosurgical assessment. A careful visual check on acuity, eye move-ments and visual fields is needed. Sensory changes need to be identified and the cranial nerves should be fully tested. The external auditory meati should be inspected for any sign of a petrous temporal fracture, noting any CSF otorrhoea or haemotympanum. CSF rhinorrhoea needs to be identified. Isolated cranial nerve injuries (e.g. to the abducent nerve) are not uncommon. Fractures passing through the frontal sinus area may involve the trochlea and lead to a superior oblique paresis (Brown's syndrome). Gross periorbital swelling can make the assessment of telecanthus or traumatic hypertelorism difficult and CT scanning is essential to distinguish these.

Whenever there is displacement of the cranial components in craniofacial injuries a combined neurosurgical approach is required, and frequently when a CSF leak persists (see Ch. 19).

Complications

Cranial

The most common cranial complication is a persistent CSF leak. Failure to recognise this can lead to late onset meningitis. This should be searched for pre- and post-operatively.

Frontal aerocoeles are not uncommon and arise as a result of air being forced into the extradural or subdural spaces at the time of injury, often when there are airway difficulties. They can usually be managed expectantly provided the airway is well maintained with oral endotracheal intubation or a tracheostomy. Intracerebral aerocoeles are an acute emergency and require immediate neurosurgical intervention.

Occasionally, there is infection postsurgically, with loss of the frontal bone flap necessitating late aesthetic reconstruction with a titanium plate.

Postconcussional headaches are common following craniofacial injuries and may be persistent. Post-traumatic epilepsy from local brain injury or surgical repair requires anticonvulsant therapy.

Ophthalmic

Blindness can occur with severe pressure on the optic nerve or from its avulsion in major trauma. Fundal examination is essential, to detect this and injuries such as retinal detachments, choroidal tears and lens dislocations. Persistent diplopia can result from damage to muscles or persistent trapping and failure to reposition prolapsed orbital contents. Enophthalmos persists following loss of orbital contents or an increase in orbital size following poor surgery.

Proptosis is much less common; it can be due to an inward repositioning of one of the orbital walls. Corneal exposure is a risk when there is marked proptosis. It can occur following operative treatment of orbital injuries. The eye should be lubricated with chloramphenicol drops and ointment.

Nasolacrimal

Nasolacrimal damage occurs with severe midface injuries, often from penetrating objects or gross comminution. Early assessment after the injury is worthwhile and immediate reconstruction of the ducts and sac should be carried out if at all possible. The nasolacrimal duct and sac is kept patent with a drainage tube. Initial epiphora occurs but usually settles with adequate drainage. Poor drainage will lead to infection and dacryocystitis and recurrent infections will require treatment and dacryocystorhinostomy. Careful evaluation with appropriate imaging can be helpful in identifying the site of the obstruction.

Neurological

Neurological deficit is not uncommon with midface injuries. In the orbit, damage can occur to the optic nerve. Total or partial loss of sight is not so uncommon (around 10–12%). Persistent ophthalmoplegia occurs most often in relation to the abducent nerve with a lateral rectus palsy, less commonly from oculomotor or trochlear nerve damage. There may be sensory loss from supraorbital, supratrochlear or infraorbital nerve damage. Most commonly there is numbness of the upper lip, cheek and side of nose. Damage to the zygomaticofrontal and zygomaticotemporal nerves may lead to persistent pain in their distribution but this is uncommon.

Nasal

Oroantral and oronasal fistulae occasionally occur and these are easily treated by appropriate flap closure. Persistent antral infection when there is an obstruction to the orifice in the lateral nasal wall may necessitate some form of antrostomy, but modern endoscopic surgery is often effective.

Dental

Malocclusions may result from failure to reduce the maxillae they usually present with an anterior open bite or retropositioned maxilla. Only osteotomy can satisfactorily correct this (e.g. a Le Fort I osteotomy). Occasionally, there is trismus and ankylosis from fusion of malar to the coronoid process. This requires operative intervention with separation of the fragments, best carried out via a bicoronal and intraoral approach.

Late deformity

Severe craniofacial injuries in children can lead to a lack of development of the midface, especially the frontonasal area with a resulting saddle nose. Reconstruction with a cantilever bone graft may be helpful but it is difficult to achieve adequate nasal lengthening. There may be a pseudohyperteloric appearance with canthal drifting. Late correction is difficult but if there is adequate nasal projection a slight increase in width of the nasal bridge may be acceptable. Much scarring around the medial canthus makes later surgery difficult. A failure to reduce the midface at the Le Fort II and III levels will result in major dishing of the face. At the Le Fort III level there is an increased breadth of the face and vertical shortening only correctable with a major osteotomy. Hollowing in the temporal regions, usually following repeated bicoronal flaps being taken down, can be corrected by inserting an alloplastic material in the temporal fossa. Irregularities of the frontal bone and supraorbital ridges can be corrected by onlaying cold-curing acrylic. A major displacement of a segment requires osteotomy surgery with or without bone grafting; minor degrees of deformity require onlaying or masking procedures using cranial bone graft or alloplastic materials. High quality early corrective surgery almost always produces a better result.

Current developments

The development of resorbable bone plates may well result in their replacing metal plates. This would avoid the doubtful necessity for metal plate removal, considered essential in some countries. Polylactide and other similar materials are being used for this purpose.

Where there has been non-union the use of substances such as bone morphogenic protein with its insertion at that site might well prove valuable and where there has been extensive bone loss again it may be possible to use bone morphogenic protein at the site of interpositional fibrous tissue or muscle.

There is also the possibility of using distraction osteogenesis in the mandible to create missing bone following gun shot wounds. These techniques are now available and should be considered for more complex fracture situations.

13 Orthognathic surgery

Introduction

Orthognathic surgery is widely carried out for the correction of dentofacial deformities. Until the early 1970s there were relatively few techniques available for this correction but since that time great advances have been made, with regard to assessment, preparation for surgery (which is often accompanied by orthodontic treatment) and surgical technique.

A proper assessment of the patient must be carried out in the first instance. The reason for the request for elective surgery needs to be ascertained. In most cases there is a concern about appearance. However, other factors, such as mastication, speech, temporomandibular joint symptoms and occasionally other features (e.g. ocular problems) in relation to craniofacial deformity may need to be considered. Proper patient selection is mandatory for a successful outcome.

Preoperative assessment

As part of the preparation for orthognathic surgery, the patient must undergo assessment and treatment planning (Table 13.1).

Assessment

Psychological

A psychological and social assessment is required for patients with unreal expectations and dysmorphophobia. The patient's personality may be affected by the facial deformity and they sometimes present in an aggressive way, or they may be withdrawn. However, the majority are able to give a clear indication of their concerns. Patients with significant deformity may be improved by relatively simple surgery that allows them to be accepted

---

Table 13.1   Preoperative assessment, treatment planning and preparation in orthognathic surgery

Assessment
  psychological
  aesthetic
  orthodontic
  clinical
  radiographic
Treatment planning
  cephalometric
  dental casts
  photographic
Preparation
  photocephalometric
  orthodontic
  splint construction

---

in society. The type of job that the patient has, and his or her home background and social position may have an effect on the type and extent of surgery; the expectations from surgery for those in the public eye, who often demand a perfect dentition and occlusion, is often greater than for others, for whom the simple correction of major jaw deformity and a minor discrepancy in the occlusion will be acceptable.

It is important to have an assessment of the family situation during the planning process and time should be taken for identifying and prioritising a problem list, discussing the issues not only with the patient but also the family. With treatment being essentially elective, risk–benefit needs to be taken into account.

Aesthetic

An understanding of facial aesthetics is essential. Measurements are only a guide to a pleasing and acceptable profile, they do not necessarily make one.

103

The balance of the facial parts needs to be considered, particularly identifying that part which is out of balance. There may be an apparent proclination of the upper incisors in association with gross mandibular retrusion. The latter needs to be corrected and the former does not need to be changed.

Orthodontic

It is essential to have a good orthodontic assessment and preparation prior to surgery to obtain a sound interlocking postoperative occlusion. To prevent relapse, presurgical orthodontic treatment is, in most cases, required and a refusal to participate in this needs to be taken very seriously when deciding upon surgery. It is important to recognise that orthodontic treatment alone can rarely correct a significant discrepancy in jaw size. Pressures to correct discrepancy in jaw size early in childhood need to be resisted. Although severe retrusion of the mandible and maxilla may be an indication for this, when extreme protrusion is corrected early in adolescence, growth is likely to continue and further surgery will be required at the end of the growth period.

In the next decade it is likely that many severe deficiencies in jaw size will be corrected by distraction techniques, with osteotomy surgery being largely reserved for the end of the growth period (see p. 102).

Clinical

The first step in treatment planning must be the correct diagnosis of the deformities present and the associated dental problems. Measurements of the face need to be taken from both full face and profile views followed by an oral examination and assessment of nasal and temporomandibular joint function. This will need to be evaluated radiographically, photographically and with dental casts. Additional investigations such as computerised tomography (CT) scanning, full speech assessment and in some cases a full ophthalmic and neurological assessment will be needed where changes to the jaws also involve the upper midface.

Radiographic

There are two basic aspects of appropriate imaging for orthognathic surgery. Conventional radiographs are required for the diagnosis of pathology and to show detail of the jaws and teeth. These will include panoramic radiographs, intra-oral views, occipitomental views to exclude infection in the midface and views of the temporomandibular joints where there is a likelihood of changes occurring there. Radiographs are also required which are used essentially for planning purposes. These include the lateral and posteroanterior (PA) cephalogram and sometimes the submentovertex view to show asymmetry.

The lateral and PA cephalograms need to be taken in a standard position with the head in the natural position and the Frankfort plane horizontal. The soft tissues need to be imaged and it is therefore necessary to use appropriate intensifying screens for the lateral cephalogram.

Treatment planning

The basis of planning for the correction of jaw deformity is through cephalometry. The skeletal, soft tissue and dentoalveolar relationships are taken into consideration in the three dimensions of anteroposterior, vertical and transverse, and various analyses can be used for the identification of the discrepancy in jaw size.

Cephalometric

To assess the projection of the maxilla and the mandible in the anteroposterior dimension, SNA, SNB and Pogonion points and angles are measured on a cephalogram. The vertical dimension is assessed, not only in relation to the maxilla but also the mandible. The occlusal plane and the upper and lower incisal angulations and the relationship of the lips and soft tissues to the dentition and to the jaw bones are measured.

Dental casts

A clinical study of the patient's occlusion is helpful but a proper analysis of the dental occlusion can only be obtained by assessment of the study casts and these should normally be placed on an anatomical articulator.

Photographic

Although it is customary to take photographs for record purposes, a lateral profile photograph may also be produced life size on an acetate sheet and superimposed on the cephalogram. If they are matched carefully to the soft tissues on the cephalogram, 'surgery' can be carried out on the photograph. This form of photocephalometric planning has provided a reliable way of demonstrating to the patient the changes that can occur following surgery and predictions using this method are helpful when making a decision as to precisely what changes should be made and whether these are acceptable to the patient. It is essential that the photographs are taken in the natural head position and that there is no posturing. Colour transparencies of the head and neck, both lateral profile positions, full face and with close-ups of the dental occlusion and in a smiling position are desirable. Various tracing methods are used for the photocephalometric planning and the exact method chosen and the cephalometric points used will depend on the orthodontist and surgeon.

Preoperative preparation

Photocephalometric

In the process of photocephalometric planning the osteotomies are carried out on the lateral profile as they would be at the time of surgery. That is, the lines drawn should be as for the osteotomy cuts. For bimaxillary surgery, especially when height changes are involved, it is usual to move the maxilla first so that the upper anterior teeth are placed in their optimal position. The mandible can then be rotated appropriately to achieve a satisfactory interincisal relationship. The posterior part of the maxilla can then be adjusted to complete the occlusion.

It is essential to remember that the soft tissues do not move the same amount as the hard tissues. When the maxilla is advanced using a Le Fort I osteotomy the upper lip is likely to move forwards only half of that distance and the tip of the nose by one third. For Le Fort II osteotomies, this changes to two-thirds movement, and for the middle third at the Le Fort III level the movement is approximately 1:1, whereas an advancement genioplasty will move the soft tissues approximately 85–90% of the bony advancement. Vertical changes of the chin as they affect the soft tissues are close to 1:1. These changes are estimated and recorded photocephalometrically.

Orthodontic

Orthodontic treatment can take 18 months or more to obtain the optimal position for surgery. It is generally better to complete orthodontic treatment prior to surgery; only minor realignment should be left until after surgery as any need to open the occlusion postoperatively may lead to a degree of relapse.

Splint construction

Following completion of photocephalometric planning, the precise movements need to be transferred to the appropriately articulated casts so that a good occlusion is obtained. The precise jaw movements need to be defined when an ideal occlusion has been found.

Once the casts are set up on an articulator, and following the measurements from photocephalometric planning, each jaw movement is carried out. From this optimal position, thin acrylic occlusal splints can be made to record each movement. Each splint needs to be checked individually in the mouth with the upper teeth and lower teeth after any occlusal equilibration has been carried out. They should be made within 1–2 days of surgery because minor changes in the occlusion in the postorthodontic period are not uncommon. The positional changes of the casts are transferred to the jaws at the time of surgery and appropriate markings made on the upper and lower portions of the maxilla.

Mandibular surgery

Mandibular surgery can be divided into several sections:

1. surgery in which the jaw is moved in an antero-posterior direction by an osteotomy either in the ramus or body of the mandible
2. surgery to the dentoalveolar area, such as segmental surgery to shift teeth and alveolus but maintaining the integrity of the lower part of the mandible
3. surgery to the chin, moving it in a superior, inferior, posterior or anterior direction sometimes accompanied by levelling and reshaping.

The best operation should be chosen for the patient by a surgeon proficient in all forms of jaw surgery.

Mandibular prognathism

Mandibular prognathism is probably the most common deformity that requires surgical treatment. It may be corrected in several ways.

Vertical subsigmoid

The vertical subsigmoid osteotomy, (vertical ramus osteotomy) is currently done through an intraoral approach sectioning the ramus from sigmoid notch to mandibular lower border. The coronoid processes may

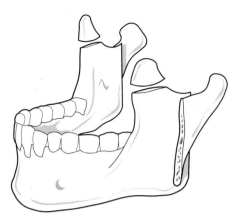

Fig. 13.1 Vertical subsigmoid osteotomy. The ramus is sectioned from the sigmoid notch to the lower border of the mandible and the fragments are overlapped.

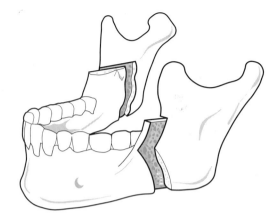

Fig. 13.3 Diagram showing a sagittal split osteotomy.

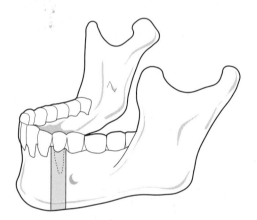

Fig. 13.2 Diagram showing body osteotomy of the mandible with the segment of bone to be removed along with the first premolar (hatched).

also be sectioned (Fig. 13.1). This is followed by overlapping the proximal fragment and shaping it to lie flat against the posteriorly repositioned ramus and mandibular body in its optimal position. Usually this particular operation is stabilised by keeping the teeth in occlusion with intermaxillary fixation for at least 4–6 weeks.

If intermaxillary fixation has to be avoided then it is possible to use the sagittal split osteotomy (see below), taking the distal fragment posteriorly with removal of bone followed by screw or plate fixation.

Body osteotomy

It is also possible to carry out a body osteotomy when there is spacing in the lower jaw or a single tooth can be removed (e.g. in the premolar region; Fig. 13.2). This is often helpful in correcting vertical changes in the mandible and can produce a very good occlusion. Surgery tends to be carried out in front of the mental nerve, if at all possible, by removing the first premolar and adjacent bone, although it is acceptable to take the inferior dental and mental nerves out of the canal and foramen and reposition them if this produces a better occlusion. This allows both height changes and some tipping of the distal segment. It does, however, require careful planning and some expertise. Fixation will be with bone plates accompanied by light intermaxillary fixation with elastics in the first instance.

Mandibular retrusion

Sagittal split osteotomy

Mandibular retrusion is most commonly corrected with an Obwegeser sagittal split osteotomy. The Obwegeser dal Pont osteotomy splits the ramus and angle region of the mandible sagittally and then slides the segments apart maintaining the integrity of the inferior dental bundle (Fig. 13.3). Fixation is usually by means of three screws or a plate sometimes accompanied in the early stage by light intermaxillary fixation. The sagittal split osteotomy has been modified to produce better contact with less risk of fragmentation and an improved blood supply reducing the risk of aseptic necrosis at the angle of the mandible.

Most surgeons now fix the mandible with semirigid fixation. This reduces the relapse rate, ensures bone contact and a correctly aligned occlusion.

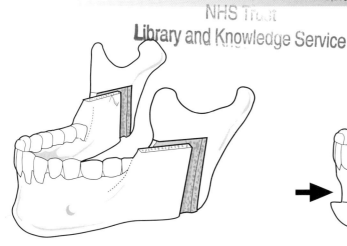

Fig. 13.4   Inverted L osteotomy (hatched area bone grafted).

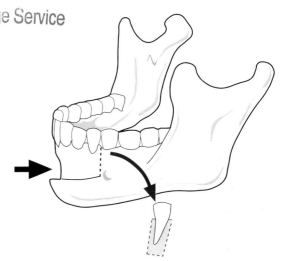

Fig. 13.5   Segmental osteotomy. The first premolar and a wedge of bone have been removed (red arrow) to allow the segment to be repositioned back (black arrow).

Inverted L osteotomy

The inverted L osteotomy is used for lengthening the ramus of the mandible and is particularly helpful in syndrome and congenital deformity patients (Fig. 13.4). This can be done either through an intraoral or extraoral approach but if a considerable amount of bone graft is required then it is usually easier to do this through an extraoral submandibular approach. Rigid fixation with plates can be used to stabilise the segments.

Segmental osteotomy

Segmental procedures are largely carried out in the anterior mandible. It is essential that the blood supply is maintained through the genial muscles on the lingual side and these must not be detached from the bone or necrosis of the whole segment will occur. The approach to the lower anterior segment is with a mucosal lip incision (Fig. 13.5). If the segment has to be significantly raised then some form of interpositional material such as bone or hydroxyapatite may need to be placed in the space accompanied by good plate fixation.

Chin deformities

The chin deformities of retrogenia and progenia are corrected by advancing or retruding the lower border segment of the mandible at the chin. Fixation is normally by means of wires or screws or occasionally plates. Changes in the chin for vertical reduction, require a piece of mandible to be removed 5 mm below the level of the teeth. Fixation is applied to the upper and lower segments usually with wires or alternatively screws and plates. Vertical augmentation of the anterior mandible requires a bone graft into the space created and care needs to be taken to avoid retropositioning the chin point when this procedure is carried out.

Maxillary surgery

Maxillary osteotomies can be divided up into three principal types. The first involves the dentoalveolar component of the maxilla at a low level, the Le Fort I osteotomy. This parallels the low level fracture of the maxilla that occurs in association with trauma. The Le Fort II and III osteotomies involved are at a higher level and involve the nasoethmoidal complex and, for the Le Fort III, the whole midface. Essentially, this becomes a craniofacial dysjunction (see Ch. 12).

Le Fort I osteotomy

By far the commonest procedure carried out in the midface is the Le Fort I osteotomy, which corrects discrepancies in jaw size involving the lower half of the maxilla and the dentoalveolar component. Thus the Le Fort I osteotomy is used for advancement of the lower midface and for inferior and superior repositioning. Any form of setback of the maxilla involves removal of a portion of the dentoalveolar segment because it is not possible simply to set back the maxilla in its entirety because it impinges on the pterygoid plates. It is often difficult to obtain a satisfactory occlusion, usually due to narrowness of the maxilla, especially in secondary cleft deformities where there is scarring and collapse and in this situation the maxilla should be expanded prior to surgery. Small degrees of expansion can be carried out orthodontically and in children rapid expansion is often a way of separating the two halves of the maxilla through the midline palatal suture. In the older age group segmental surgery or alternatively surgical expansion of the maxilla is required. Presurgical planning is essential to detect any discrepancy in the arch size and any problems with the occlusion following repositioning of the maxilla.

Any verticomaxillary excess in the lower face height can be corrected by raising the maxilla through removal of a segment of bone on both sides, which includes the lateral nasal walls and nasal septum. In the reverse situation where there is shortness of lower face height, this can be corrected by an inferior repositioning Le Fort I osteotomy, with bone grafting of the space created. Superior repositioning tends to be a stable procedure, whereas inferior repositioning has a reputation for some degree of relapse and therefore appropriate compensations might be needed. The tooth position must be related accurately to the upper lip at rest. Any shortness of the upper lip will not allow for major inferior repositioning nd likewise raising the maxilla excessively with a short upper lip can similarly give an ugly appearance.

Complications

Complications with this surgery include haemorrhage, a failure to reposition the segments, damage to the teeth (especially the roots) and loss or damage to the blood supply of the segments; all of these are avoidable. The patient needs to be warned of the potential risks of this type of surgery. Residual oronasal or antral fistulae can occur but these are uncommon. Fortunately, complete necrosis of the segment occurs only rarely, usually when the soft tissue flaps have been damaged extensively. Hyperbaric oxygen therapy is sometimes helpful in this situation.

Le Fort II osteotomy

The Le Fort II osteotomy has a unique place for patients with central midface hypoplasia extending into the nasoethmoidal area. It allows a certain amount of lengthening of the midface, especially of the nose with a complete advancement of the central midface.

Various modifications of the Le Fort II osteotomy have been carried out in the past, simply advancing the infraorbital margins, leaving the nose behind or advancing the malars and infraorbital margin leaving the nose behind (Kufner osteotomy). These have a small but useful place in the armamentarium of osteotomies. With rigid plate fixation intermaxillary fixation postoperatively is not required.

Complications

The complications associated with Le Fort II osteotomy are similar to those associated with a Le Fort I; occasional orbital complications or damage to the infraorbital nerve or nasolacrimal duct can occur, but this is unusual. There is a slight tendency to vertical relapse anteriorly and this is important when maxillary inferior repositioning is being carried out and account needs to be taken of this when planning. If onlaying of the maxilla especially over the malar prominence is required then cranial outer plate bone graft is best, fixing this to the anterior maxilla and malar bones with small screws.

Le Fort III osteotomy

The subcranial Le Fort III osteotomy and its variants are used primarily for correction of total midface hypoplasia, usually of craniosynostotic origin, typically in the Apert and Crouzon's syndromes. In this situation there is usually significant proptosis of the eyes, severe malar and maxillary hypoplasia and a class III malocclusion with a short midface height. This can be accompanied by other problems such as sleep apnoea, postnasal choanal atresia and sometimes a cleft deformity. There is often a skull deformity that may require correction either at the same time or at a later date. It may be necessary to carry out bimaxillary surgery in this situation, with the advancement of the midface as well as its vertical repositioning. A Le Fort I osteotomy may be needed at the same time for vertical repositioning and to achieve a good occlusion.

Careful preoperative assessment is essential, particularly with CT scanning to exclude any prolapse of cranial contents into the naso-orbital areas. Preoperative ophthalmic assessment is also important because changes will occur within the orbits themselves and it is not uncommon to see some diplopia following surgery, which usually settles spontaneously but sometimes requires extraocular muscle surgery. The approach to the upper midface is through a coronal flap, which is extended down into the preauricular areas on both sides, together with an intraoral approach through vestibular incisions. The latter allows for a Le Fort I osteotomy to be carried out at the same time. Sometimes it is possible to do all the surgery through these two incisions, but in other cases it is preferable to use the transconjunctival approach to the orbital floors, which allows accurate cutting and repositioning in that area. Fixation with multiple miniplates is required and orbital floor repair.

The Le Fort III osteotomy is occasionally used for post-traumatic cases and rarely for secondary clefts. It can also be used in Treacher–Collins syndrome and other conditions. There is an increasing tendency to think that this type of osteotomy surgery is becoming outmoded and advancement through distraction may well be the answer because this avoids the extensive bone grafting.

Complications

A number of complications can arise from this complex surgery. Immediate complications associated with the surgery are a cerebrospinal fluid leak if an inadvertent communication with the cranial cavity has occurred. Troublesome bleeding can occur probably from damage to the maxillary vessels or from the pterygoid veins. There can be airway problems and iatrogenic damage to the endotracheal tube; rarely, blindness has been reported and occasionally postoperative infections associated with the bone grafting procedure. Later problems are meningitis and postinfective epilepsy. In addition to blindness, diplopia, residual exophthalmos or the development of enophthalmos, ptosis of the lids or corneal ulceration can complicate the orbital surgery. There may be an inferior and lateral medial canthal drift. Nasolacrimal damage has been reported, including dacryocystitis and epiphora, the latter normally recovers spontaneously. Nasal obstruction and paranasal sinus infections rarely occur. There may be damage to the supra and infraorbital nerves and rarely to the oculomotor nerves and muscles, or facial nerve and occasionally anosmia. Dental malocclusion with an anterior open bite deformity is occasionally seen, as well as trismus. Residual deformity can result from relapse or asymmetric correction and temporal hollowing. Speech is occasionally affected, with the development of hypernasality.

Distraction osteogenesis

Distraction osteogenesis is now being widely practised as an alternative approach to osteotomy surgery. Whereas most mandibular and midface osteotomies are carried out towards the end of the growth period, distraction therapy is possible from infancy. An osteotomy is carried out, gently mobilised and then gradually separated with a distraction apparatus at a rate of 1 mm a day. This can be carried out in the mandible for vertical repositioning, for horizontal advancement and for transverse changes. It is used in the maxilla, principally for advancement and inferior repositioning and this can be at Le Fort I, II and III levels. It avoids the necessity for bone grafting and seems to be a stable process. There are a significant number of reports on the various osteotomies and their distraction but there have been no long-term comparisons between conventional osteotomy surgery and distraction osteogenesis.

14 Salivary gland surgery

Introduction

Saliva is produced by the three pairs of major salivary glands – the parotid, submandibular and sublingual glands – as well as the many hundreds of small salivary glands scattered throughout the buccal and pharyngeal mucosa. The majority of surgical pathology affects the parotid or submandibular gland, with the sublingual and minor salivary glands being less frequently affected. Both the anatomy and physiology of salivary gland function is important in surgical pathology and these will be discussed first.

Anatomy

Parotid gland

The parotid gland is the largest of the salivary glands. It lies just in front of the ear extending from the zygomatic arch downwards to between the angle of the mandible and the mastoid process. This inferior portion is also known as the tail of the parotid gland. The anterior border corresponds approximately to the ascending ramus of the mandible (Fig. 14.1). It is important to appreciate that the tail of the parotid gland extends into the neck and that lesions in this area can affect the parotid gland and are sometimes mistaken for lymph nodes in the neck. Swellings in this area should be assumed to be arising from the parotid until proven otherwise (see below).

The facial nerve is intimately associated with the parotid gland and runs through the gland, dividing it into a superficial lobe, which arises lateral to the facial nerve, and a deep lobe, which arises deep to the facial nerve. This is an artificial division and no true anatomical plane exists between the superficial and the deep lobe. A normal parotid gland consists of 80% superficial lobe and 20% deep lobe. The facial nerve enters the parotid

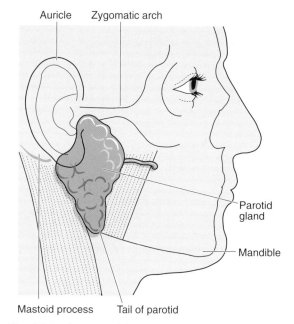

Fig. 14.1   Anatomy of the parotid gland.

gland from the stylomastoid foramen and, shortly after entry, divides into an upper and lower division. The upper division gives off a temporal branch that supplies the muscles of the forehead and eye, a zygomatic branch that supplies the muscles of the eye, and occasionally a buccal branch that supplies the muscles of the nostril and upper lip. The lower division gives off a mandibular branch that supplies the muscles of the lower lip and a cervical branch that supplies platysma in the neck. The lower division often also gives off the buccal branch. (Fig. 14.2). The facial nerve controls the muscles of facial expression.

The parotid gland is drained by the parotid duct, which opens into the mouth opposite the second upper molar tooth.

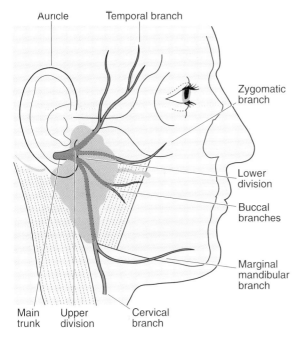

Fig. 14.2 Branches of the facial nerve.

superficial and deep part, the superficial being the largest. The superficial lobe lies superficial to the mylohyoid muscle, whereas the deep lobe lies deep to the mylohyoid muscle and is drained by a duct that drains forwards and upwards to open close to the frenulum in the floor of the mouth (Fig. 14.3). Three nerves are closely linked to the submandibular gland – the marginal mandibular branch of the facial nerve, the lingual nerve and the hypoglossal nerve. As mentioned above, the marginal mandibular nerve supplies the muscles of the lower lip and damage to this nerve will leave the patient with deformity. The lingual nerve supplies sensation to the anterior two-thirds of the tongue whereas the hypoglossal nerve supplies motor function to the tongue muscles.

Sublingual gland

The sublingual gland is the smallest of the major glands and lies beneath the mucosa of the floor of the mouth near the midline. It drains into the mouth by small ducts, as well as by ducts that open directly into the submandibular gland duct. It is closely associated with the lingual nerve.

Submandibular gland

The submandibular gland lies in the submandibular triangle bordered anteriorly by the digastric muscle, posteriorly by the stylomandibular ligament and superiorly by the mandible. This gland also has a

Physiology

Between 1 and 1.5 L saliva are produced a day. In the resting state, the submandibular gland produces most

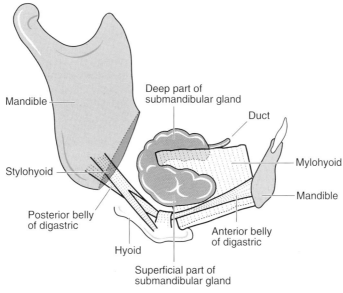

Fig. 14.3 Anatomy of the submandibular gland.

saliva but on stimulation most saliva is produced by the parotid gland. The parotid gland produces a serous secretion whereas the sublingual and submandibular gland produce two-thirds mucous and one-third serous secretion. Serous secretion contains amylase for digestion, whereas the mucous secretion contains mucin for lubricating purposes. Removing a major salivary gland has a negligible clinical effect upon saliva production.

Investigation of salivary gland disease

Radiological investigations

Plain radiography

Plain radiographs are usually only of use in diagnosing the presence of stones in the submandibular gland as the majority in this gland are radiopaque (Fig. 14.4). Plain radiography is of little value if parotid duct stones are thought to be present because the vast majority are radiolucent; sialography is of more use.

Sialography

Sialography consists of injecting radio-opaque contrast medium into the submandibular duct orifice or the parotid duct orifice, depending upon which gland is being investigated, and radiographs being taken. It is useful in the diagnosis of radiolucent stones and duct strictures. Sialography is of some value in sialadenitis where a 'tree in leaf' or 'snowstorm' appearance is often seen (Fig. 14.5). Sialography can also show tumours of the parotid gland indirectly by showing duct displacement but computerised tomography (CT) and magnetic resonance imaging (MRI) are much more useful for this. It should be noted that sialography is contraindicated in the presence of an acute infection as it may worsen the condition.

Ultrasound

Ultrasound is a relatively quick and easy way of identifying localised swellings of the salivary glands: usually tumours but also abscesses. It has the advantage of no radiation and can be easily combined with fine-needle aspiration cytology. Its disadvantage is that it is not always easy to define deep lobe involvement of the parotid gland and is also operator dependent.

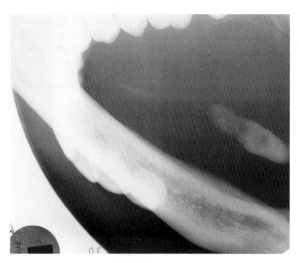

Fig. 14.4 A lower occlusal radiograph showing a sialolith in the submandibular duct.

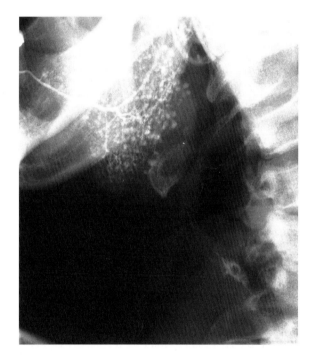

Fig. 14.5 A parotid sialogram showing the 'snowstorm' appearance of punctate sialectasis in a patient with Sjögren's syndrome.

CT scanning

CT scanning is useful in defining tumours of the salivary glands as it usually locates the tumour well and defines extension outside the gland. It also shows lymphadenopathy in the neck, which is useful in assessing malignant tumours as well as possible bone invasion (Fig. 14.6). Its disadvantage is that it involves a substantial dose of radiation to the patient and it does not always detect tumours in the deep lobe of the gland if they have the same radiological density as the gland.

MRI scanning

MRI scanning is probably the best investigation of salivary gland tumours as it gives excellent detail of size and position and there is no radiation (Fig. 14.7). Its disadvantages include availability, and some patients can't tolerate it because of claustrophobia especially as it takes a lot longer to perform than CT, and bony detail is not as well seen.

Radioisotope scanning

At one time, radioisotope scans were used to help differentiate different types of tumours in, especially, the parotid gland. The procedure was unreliable and now with the advent of fine-needle aspiration is no longer performed to investigate salivary gland tumours, although it is still occasionally used in assessing function of the salivary glands.

Fine-needle aspiration

Fine-needle aspiration is a very valuable tool in the diagnosis of salivary gland tumours. It is an easy procedure and can be performed in the outpatient clinic. With the aid of an experienced cytologist its yield is good. However, it is sometimes not always possible to differentiate one type of tumour from another. The diagnostic success rate for malignant tumours is about 70% whereas for benign tumours it is about 90%. The risk of tumour seeding following fine-needle aspiration is more hypothetical than real and, if it does occur, is exceedingly rare. Its use in non-neoplastic swellings is less well defined as interpretation of these specimens is difficult even for experienced cytologists.

Salivary gland biopsy

Open biopsy of a parotid swelling should be performed only if it is certain that the lesion being biopsied is not

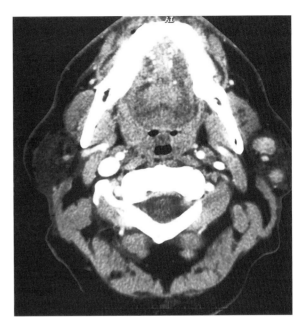

Fig. 14.6 Computerised tomography (CT) scan of a parotid Warthin's tumour.

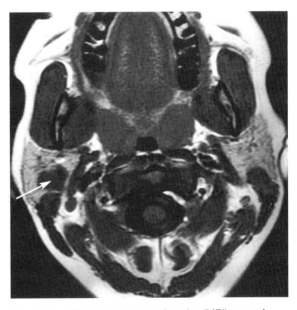

Fig. 14.7 Magnetic resonance imaging (MRI) scan of a parotid pleomorphic adenoma.

a tumour, as biopsy of a tumour risks seeding it and making subsequent management more difficult. It is sometimes useful when the cause of a diffuse salivary gland enlargement remains obscure, or if the diagnosis of

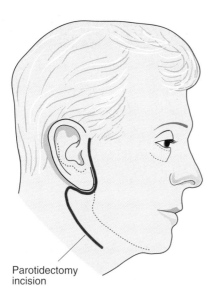

Fig. 14.8 Incision for a biopsy of the parotid gland. The biopsy incision should be placed in part of the standard parotidectomy incision as shown above, depending on the part of the gland to be biopsied.

lymphoma is suspected. Very occasionally, an open biopsy is necessary to make the diagnosis of a tumour involving a salivary gland. If this is the case, the specimen should be sent for frozen section to confirm or deny the presence of a tumour and, if tumour is confirmed, then the definitive surgical procedure should be performed at the time of the frozen section. The site of skin incision is important when performing a biopsy of the parotid gland and its correct position is shown in Fig. 14.8. It is also very important to be aware of the position of the facial nerve when performing a biopsy of the parotid gland so as not to damage it. Biopsy of minor salivary glands is discussed in Chapter 34.

Salivary gland swellings

Most surgical pathology of the salivary gland presents as a swelling in the associated gland and it is helpful clinically to characterise the swelling as one that affects the whole of the gland or as a discrete swelling that affects only part of the gland. Most discrete swellings are caused by a tumour, whereas swellings affecting the whole of the gland are usually caused by sialolithiasis, sialadenitis or sialadenosis (Table 14.1). There is obviously some overlap in this classification but it is helpful in the clinical context.

Table 14.1	Salivary gland swellings
Discrete	
tumours	
Diffuse	
sialolithiasis	
sialadenitis	
sialadenosis	

Sialolithiasis

Sialolithiasis, or salivary gland stone disease, is caused by the presence of stones either within the gland itself or in the duct that is draining the gland, symptoms being more common when the stones are found in the ducts. The presentation and diagnosis of these are considered in detail in Chapter 34.

Stones in the anterior part of the submandibular duct can be removed via the mouth by opening (and marsupialising) the duct (see Ch. 34) but if the stone is further back in the duct, or in the submandibular gland itself, then it is safer to remove the gland externally by a neck incision to avoid damage to the lingual nerve. Recurrent parotid duct stones are rare and if they cannot be removed through the mouth and are considered very troublesome then they require a parotidectomy, but this is very unusual. Dilatation of the parotid duct has been tried for parotid duct stones, especially when they are associated with a stricture in the parotid duct, and this is worth trying as it is a lot less invasive and has lower morbidity than a parotidectomy, but its effectiveness is doubtful.

Sialadenosis

Sialadenosis is defined as a non-inflammatory salivary gland disease due to metabolic and secretory disorders of the gland parenchyma, accompanied by recurrent, usually painless, bilateral swelling of the glands due to acinar enlargement.

Sialadenosis has an equal incidence in the two sexes and occurs most commonly in the fourth to seventh decades. The disease is suspected when there is recurrent enlargement of *both* pairs of the major salivary glands, usually the parotids (Fig. 14.9). The gland enlargement can persist from weeks to months. It is usually associated with an underlying condition. Sialadenosis has three major causes:

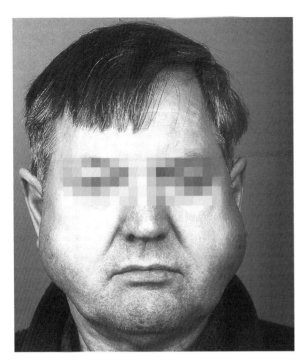

Fig. 14.9 Sialosis occurring in a patient with a history of alcohol abuse.

- *Endocrine*: gland enlargement has been described in most endocrine diseases but it is particularly linked to diabetes mellitus. It can also occur during pregnancy and lactation where its cause is thought to be endocrine in origin.
- *Dystrophic/metabolic*: this is most commonly seen in chronic starvation and is thought to be linked to the deficiency of proteins and vitamins. This is also the reason it is sometimes seen in alcoholics.
- *Neurogenic*: dysfunction of the autonomic nervous system can give rise to sialadenosis and this is most commonly seen in people taking drugs that affect the autonomic nervous system, such as some antihypertensive drugs, It may also be the reason it is seen in patients who are anorexic but there is probably also a nutritional element in this as well.

The diagnosis is made upon the history and clinical appearance associated with an underlying cause. A parotid biopsy is needed occasionally, and histology will then show acinar enlargement.

The underlying disease is treated but it is very rare that a parotidectomy will be needed for cosmetic reasons. Even with treatment of the underlying disease, it is common for the parotid enlargement to persist.

Table 14.2 **Sialadenitis**
Acute
bacterial
viral
Chronic
chronic recurrent parotitis
tuberculosis
radiation
Sjögren's
sarcoidosis

Sialadenitis

Sialadenitis is inflammation of the salivary glands, most commonly the parotid, and can be categorised into acute and chronic types (Table 14.2).

Acute sialadenitis

Acute sialadenitis may be bacterial or viral in nature. Viral sialadenitis is self-limiting and only bacterial sialadenitis will be considered here.

Bacterial infection usually presents with a sudden sense of swelling of the affected gland and there may be redness of the overlying skin. Pus is often seen exuding from the salivary gland duct into the mouth and the patient is unwell. Most acute bacterial infection is related to a reduction in the flow of saliva and this is commonly secondary to an underlying disease such as poorly controlled diabetes mellitus or renal failure and occurs in older patients. There is often an association with poor oral hygiene. It used to be a common postoperative finding but now, with the use of antibiotics and better fluid management and postoperative oral toilet, it has become an uncommon disease.

Treatment is usually with antibiotics and correction of the underlying disease processes if present. Sialogogues (e.g. citrus-flavoured sweets) are often given to encourage the flow of saliva. If an abscess develops it may need draining externally. Care must be taken not to damage the facial nerve when the parotid gland is affected.

Chronic sialadenitis

Chronic sialadenitis has several causes (see Table 14.2) and usually presents with persistent inflammation and enlargement of the affected gland.

Chronic recurrent parotitis

This presents mainly as a unilateral or alternating swelling of the parotid gland, which can be painful. It is mainly a disease of children and the saliva can be very milky or purulent. Attacks occur at variable intervals and in between attacks the child is totally symptom free. The underlying cause is not known but it is thought that duct ectasia may be a predisposing factor.

Diagnosis is again made from the history and sialography can be considered. Duct ectasia supports the diagnosis when seen on sialography.

Treatment is symptomatic as the underlying cause is not fully understood. It often involves antibiotics and analgesia and sialogogues are often given. Most cases in childhood disappear after puberty. If the attacks continue, ligation of the parotid duct or a tympanic neuroectomy can be recommended. It is very occasionally necessary to perform a parotidectomy.

Tuberculosis

Tuberculosis can present as a chronic sialadenitis, affecting mainly the parotid or submandibular gland. Its diagnosis may not be suspected if the patient is not known to have tuberculosis and is often diagnosed by biopsy when the cause of a unilateral parotid gland enlargement remains obscure. Occasionally the disease can cause a fistula to develop into the skin above the parotid and this is strongly suggestive of tuberculosis.

Radiation sialadenitis

The salivary glands are very sensitive to the effects of radiation and this is especially a common problem in patients who have been irradiated for head and neck cancer, as the major and minor salivary glands are often included within the field. They present with a dry mouth and the presence of thick tenacious saliva, which can be very distressing. Unfortunately the symptoms tend not to improve with time.

Treatment is symptomatic and although many types of artificial saliva are available on the market, their clinical effectiveness is not high.

Sjögren's syndrome

A consideration of Sjögren's syndrome is beyond the scope of this chapter. The significance of Sjögren's syndrome to surgical practice is that there is an increased incidence of malignancy associated with this condition, especially non-Hodgkin's lymphoma. If there is an associated parotid swelling with Sjögren's syndrome then there is a 70-fold increase in the development of a non-Hodgkin's lymphoma. In patients with no salivary gland swelling this decreases to a 10-fold increase in incidence of non-Hodgkin's lymphoma and these patients should therefore be followed-up to watch for this.

There is no specific treatment for Sjögren's syndrome apart from symptomatic treatment and treatment of the underlying connective tissue disease present. A rapidly enlarging salivary gland should be biopsied to rule-out a lymphoma.

Sarcoidosis

Sarcoidosis can effect the salivary glands, especially the parotid glands, causing them to enlarge. Treatment is usually with corticosteroids.

Tumours of the major salivary glands

Salivary gland tumours usually present as a discrete swelling or nodule in the associated gland. Over 90% of salivary gland tumours are epithelial in origin and most salivary gland tumours are benign. A classification of salivary gland tumours is given in Table 14.3. Eighty per cent of tumours arise in the parotid gland, 10% in the submandibular and 10% in the minor and sublingual glands.

Most tumours present as a slow growing swelling in the associated salivary gland and the patient may have noticed it for some time. It is important, especially in the parotid gland, not to confuse a swelling in the tail of the parotid with a swelling in the lymph node. Indeed, in this region it can be difficult to differentiate a salivary gland tumour from a lymph node on clinical grounds alone. This is where fine-needle aspiration and imaging are useful. When a patient presents with a lump in the parotid gland, it is important not only to examine the lump itself but also to document the function of the facial nerve. The oropharynx should also be examined, as in deep lobe tumours of the parotid gland they can often be seen projecting into the oropharynx and pushing the tonsil inwards. It is also important to examine the neck for any other associated lymphadenopathy.

Table 14.3 Salivary gland tumours

Benign
   pleomorphic adenoma
   monomorphic adenomas
      Warthin's tumour (adenolymphoma)
      duct adenoma
      basal cell adenoma
      oncocytoma
      other adenomas
Malignant
   intermediate
      mucoepidermoid
      acinic cell
   carcinomas
      adenoid cystic
      carcinoma expleomorphic
      adenocarcinoma
      squamous cell
   non-epithelial tumours
   metastases

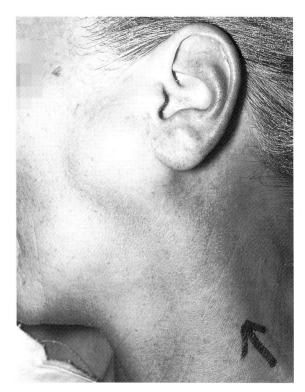

Fig. 14.10 Pleomorphic adenoma of the parotid gland.

The majority of salivary gland tumours are benign but malignancy should be suspected if there has been a rapid growth in the lump associated with pain or if there is an associated facial nerve paralysis, which is almost always indicative of malignancy. Malignancy should also be suspected if there is ulceration of the overlying skin or there is associated lymphadenopathy present in the neck.

Investigation of the salivary gland lesion should include fine-needle aspiration, which will help to differentiate a lymph node in the tail of the parotid from a true salivary gland tumour. It will also be able to give an indication of the type of salivary tumour present, although it is not 100% sensitive or specific, and indeed interpretation of parotid tumours by fine-needle aspiration can be difficult. CT scanning of a parotid swelling is also useful because it will indicate if there is any deep lobe involvement of the parotid gland and also show if there is any other associated lymphadenopathy in the neck. It may also help to differentiate a lymph node from a true parotid swelling.

Benign salivary gland tumours

Pleomorphic adenoma

The most common benign tumour is the pleomorphic adenoma (Fig. 14.10). This is a benign tumour that is most commonly seen in the parotid gland. Histological examination shows that there are two elements, an epithelial element and a stromal element. There is an incidence of malignant degeneration in pleomorphic adenomas of the order of 3%. This is usually in those tumours that are of longstanding and have been present for over 20 years. Also, on histological grounds, the greater the epithelial component of the pleomorphic adenoma, the greater the chance of malignant degeneration.

The treatment of pleomorphic adenomas is removal, providing the patient is fit enough. As most arise in the superficial lobe of the parotid gland this requires a superficial parotidectomy. The operation consists of removing the superficial lobe of the parotid gland (i.e. that part that lies lateral to the facial nerve), but leaving the deep lobe in situ. However, tumours that arise in the deep lobe require removal by a subtotal or total parotidectomy. This first involves performing a superficial parotidectomy and then carefully mobilising the facial nerve, to allow the deep lobe to be removed. The pleomorphic adenoma should not be enucleated as there is an increased chance of recurrence of the tumour with this. Although, macroscopically, the tumour appears to have a reasonably well-defined capsule, histological studies show that the capsule is incomplete and there is often breach of the capsule by tumour cells. The tumour should therefore be removed with a margin of normal parotid tissue. This is sometimes difficult if the tumour is itself lying against the facial nerve. As the surgical practice of lumpectomy has greatly reduced over recent years, the incidence of recurrence of pleomorphic adenoma has also equally reduced.

Adenolymphoma or Warthin's tumour (monomorphic adenoma)

This benign tumour often occurs in the tail of the parotid gland. It has a male predominance and usually occurs in the sixth and seventh decades. Ten per cent of these tumours are bilateral and present characteristically as a soft, fluctuant, mobile mass. The tumour is thought to arise histologically from duct epithelium. Again, providing the patient is fit and well, a superficial parotidectomy is the treatment of choice but if it is absolutely sure the tumour is an adenolymphoma (confirmed by fine-needle aspiration) then a lumpectomy will suffice because recurrence is unusual. Equally, malignant degeneration does not occur. In elderly patients, in whom this tumour is common, follow-up is wise to make sure there is no sudden change in the parotid swelling (which may indicate another pathology), rather then subject the patient to a parotidectomy.

Malignant salivary gland tumours

As indicated, malignant salivary gland tumours are uncommon. Interestingly, of all tumours occurring in the parotid gland, just 13% are malignant. The incidence increases in the submandibular gland, where of all tumours presenting, 32% are malignant. Malignancy is much more common in the sublingual and minor salivary glands, with the majority of salivary gland tumours being malignant (56%). The vast majority of malignant salivary gland tumours occur in adulthood and are very rare before puberty. The most common malignant tumour below puberty is the mucoepidermoid carcinoma. The aetiology of malignant salivary gland tumours is not known but malignant degeneration can occur in a pleomorphic adenoma.

The six most common types of malignant salivary glands tumour are acinic cell, mucoepidermoid, adenoid cystic, adenocarcinoma, squamous cell and carcinoma expleomorphic. The first two – acinic cell and mucoepidermoid – are often known as intermediate tumours because, depending on their histology, they can behave in a relatively benign or aggressive fashion.

The treatment of malignant salivary gland tumours is excision, if possible. Depending upon the size of the tumour, its position and its histology, this may require removal of the facial nerve and other surrounding structures, including the ear and petrous part of the temporal bone, and part of the mandible.

Postoperative radiotherapy may be necessary. Radiotherapy can be offered in tumours that are thought to be inoperable, but this is usually in a palliative role only.

Acinic cell tumour

This tumour is more common in males and tends to present as a well-localised lesion. Histologically, it is thought to arise from the boundary zone between the acinar and intercalated ducts. Overall, with resection, about 20% may recur. Pathology is very important as low-grade acinic cell tumours behave relatively benignly, whereas high-grade acinic tumours behave in a malignant fashion.

Treatment is excision and, in tumours that are histologically high-grade, postoperative radiotherapy is often given. If neck nodes are present at presentation then a neck dissection will also be included in the resection. Prognosis is generally good, with a 5-year survival of over 85%.

Mucoepidermoid tumour

The mucoepidermoid tumour is again similar to the acinic cell tumour in that it that it can be classified into histologically low-grade and high-grade types; the low-grade type is relatively benign whereas the high-grade type is a truly malignant tumour. The tumour is thought to arise from the ductal epithelium. Tumours with a high mucous content tend to have a low malignant potential whereas the highly cellular tumours tend to have a high malignant potential. Treatment is similar to that of the acinic cell tumour.

Prognosis is dependent on histological type, with well-differentiated tumours having a 5-year survival of over 90% but poorly differentiated tumours having a 5-year survival of only 20%.

Adenoid cystic tumour

Adenoid cystic tumours of the salivary gland are interesting in that they often present with a long history of a swelling of the affected salivary gland. They are characterised histologically by perineural spread and are often associated with pain. Seventy per cent of adenoid cystic tumours actually arise from the minor salivary glands. There are three histological types: one with a tubular pattern, one with a cribriform pattern and one with a solid pattern. The tubular has the best prognosis, whereas the solid pattern has the poorest prognosis. Cribriform has an intermediate prognosis. Interestingly, although it is sometimes very difficult to cure adenoid cystic tumours, they tend to be very slow growing and the patient can live a long time with this disease. Indeed, many patients have lung and liver metastasis but can live for many years even with these present.

Treatment is by excision and postoperative radiotherapy is often given as this is thought to increase local control of the disease. Whether the facial nerve should be sacrificed, because of its propensity for perineural spread in this disease, is controversial. Most surgeons would try to save the nerve because of the propensity of this tumour for distant metastases and also due to the difficulty in obtaining local control despite apparent adequate local excision. If neck nodes are present then a neck dissection will also be required.

Prognosis is again dependent upon histological type and also on length of follow-up. The tubular variety of adenoid cystic has a 5-year survival of over 95%, with the 10-year survival being only slightly less than this. The cribriform and solid types have a 5-year survival of 65% but at 10-year follow-up this drops to 15%, thus illustrating its propensity for late recurrence.

Adenocarcinoma of the salivary gland

This is a very aggressive tumour and has a poor prognosis. It is important to exclude metastasis of adenocarcinoma from elsewhere to the parotid gland before subscribing the tumour to the gland itself e.g. lung and breast. Treatment is by surgical excision, often combined with postoperative radiotherapy. Prognosis is poor, with a 5-year survival of 40%.

Squamous carcinoma

Again, this is usually a disease of elderly males, often in their eighties. It has a poor prognosis and it is important, as in adenocarcinoma, to exclude metastasis to the parotid gland often from the skin before subscribing it as a primary tumour of this area.

Treatment is usually by surgical excision if possible and, again, postoperative radiotherapy is usually given, especially if the tumour is large, the resection was incomplete or the margins were involved. Prognosis is poor, with a 5-year survival of 35%.

Carcinoma expleomorphic

This tumour arises from a pre-existing pleomorphic adenoma and presents as a sudden growth of a known pleomorphic adenoma. It has a poor prognosis and it is often associated with facial nerve palsy. Treatment is as for squamous carcinoma. Prognosis is poor, with a 5-year survival of 15%.

Complications of salivary gland surgery

Facial nerve function

The patient should be warned preoperatively about the risk of damage to the facial nerve. Permanent paralysis of the facial nerve should be less than 1% in experienced hands. Some degree of temporary paralysis is not too unusual after a parotidectomy, and is more common when the deep lobe has also to be removed, as this requires much more manipulation of the facial nerve. This represents a degree of neuropraxia of the facial nerve, which should recover fully over a period of 2–3 months.

Various devices are used to help locate the facial nerve and thus prevent injury, the most useful being the facial nerve monitor and stimulator, which warns the surgeon when he or she is working close to the nerve, and also allows the nerve to be stimulated for confirmation. It is important when using such devices that the patient is not paralysed, and the anaesthetist should be aware of this. Unfortunately, technology is not infallible and experience of parotid gland surgery is the best method of avoiding damage to the facial nerve. Stimulating the nerve and seeing the face twitch can confirm that the facial nerve is working after a parotidectomy.

In submandibular gland surgery it is important to avoid the marginal mandibular branch of the facial nerve that runs in the tissue superficial to the submandibular gland. If this is damaged it leaves the patient with an unsightly droop to the corner of the mouth. Other nerves at risk in submandibular gland surgery include the lingual nerve (supplies taste and touch to the tongue) and the hypoglossal nerve (supplies motor function to the tongue).

Greater auricular nerve

The greater auricular nerve is usually divided in parotid gland surgery and this leaves the patient with a numb feeling of the lower half of the ear lobe. This is of no great consequence to the patient as it will often recover, but the patient should be warned of it preoperatively. It is often possible to save a branch of the nerve, which sometimes prevents this from happening.

Frey's syndrome

Following a parotidectomy, the patient may complain of sweating of the skin over the area of the parotidectomy, especially on eating. The problem is quite common following a parotidectomy but is only troublesome in about 10% of patients. This is thought to occur because of the inappropriate regeneration of injured autonomic nerve fibres, which are misdirected and supply the sweat glands of the overlying skin. Elevating a thick skin flap when performing the parotidectomy can reduce its incidence. Most cases are not too troublesome and can be controlled by the use of an antiperspirant. More troublesome cases may require other procedures such as a tympanic neurectomy or the interposition of a tissue flap between the skin and the parotid bed, procedures that have a variable rate of success.

Salivary fistula

This occurs very occasionally after performing a superficial parotidectomy, and usually presents as saliva appearing from the wound several days after surgery. The most surprising thing is that it does not occur more frequently as functioning parotid tissue is left behind (the deep lobe). The vast majority settle with conservative treatment, which usually includes a pressure bandage and often the prescribing of an anticholinergic drug to suppress saliva production. It is sometimes confused with a seroma that can also occur, occasionally, after surgery. To distinguish a seroma from a salivary fistula, the fluid should be aspirated and its amylase content measured, this being very high in a fistula.

Other conditions of the salivary glands

Drooling

Drooling is a normal phenonomen when it is associated with teething in childhood, but at most other times it is abnormal. It is often seen in patients with cerebral palsy but it also may be seen in adults with neurological diseases such as Parkinson's disease. It can be caused by the overproduction of saliva or the presence of an abnormal swallowing reflex. Various surgical treatments have been described for the treatment of drooling, including rerouting of the submandibular ducts to drain into the tonsil fossae and also excision of the submandibular glands with rerouting of the parotid ducts, with varying degrees of success. Tympanic neurectomy also has been shown to be of benefit in the short term but, like all autonomic nerve surgery, its long-term results are disappointing.

Branchial cleft anomalies

First branchial cleft anomalies can present as a sinus, fistula or a cyst, usually in childhood or in the young adult. The sinus tract often has an external opening in or near the external auditory meatus. If a true fistula is present this has an internal opening into the pharynx near to the posterior tonsillar pillar. It is often seen in association with abnormalities of the ear. One-third of first branchial clefts are bilateral. They usually present as a cystic swelling in the region of the parotid gland and they have a variable relationship to the facial nerve Treatment is by surgical excision and this usually requires a superficial parotidectomy and exposure of the facial nerve for their complete removal.

Salivary duct cysts

These usually occur in the parotid gland and are more common in men often in their seventh or eighth decades. They present as a swelling in the affected gland, which on aspiration reveals a clear coloured fluid, and they often completely disappear on aspiration. Often the diagnosis is only made when the cyst is removed, as it is not always easy preoperatively to distinguish this from cystic degeneration in a Warthin's tumour.

Ranula

A ranula is a sublingual swelling. Most consist of a mucus filled cyst that lies under the mucosa, just lateral to the frenulum. It is thought to be a retention cyst that arises from the obstruction of one of the several ducts draining the sublingual gland. It presents as an asymptomatic swelling of the floor of the mouth, but occasionally can get so large that it interferes with speech or eating. Treatment consists of uncapping and marsupialising it. Very occasionally, the ranula can penetrate through the mylohyoid muscle and into the neck, when it is known as a plunging ranula. This requires excision, as does a simple ranula if it recurs after uncapping.

15 Plastic surgery

Introduction

Plastic surgery techniques are widely used to treat a variety of diseases and deformities in an effort to reconstruct both form and function. The basic principles are fundamental to all surgical practice involving the head and neck. Advances in plastic surgery techniques have opened up new possibilities for reconstruction in the head and neck. Many of these advances have arisen from an increasing understanding of the structure of tissues, their anatomy and their vascularity.

This chapter will concentrate on plastic surgery techniques that are applicable in the face and head and neck region. This area of the body is one of the most important in determining body image where deformities or disfigurement are clearly identifiable. It is also the area essential for communication with the outside world, allowing us to express emotions such as happiness or anger, which are transferred into visible changes in the face.

A description of the tissues, the skin and facial muscles will be followed by a consideration of incisions, lacerations, skin grafts and flaps (Table 15.1).

The skin

The skin of the head and neck has several unique features that differentiate it from other areas in the body. It communicates with the respiratory tract via the nostrils, the digestive tract via the oral cavity and the conjunctival lining of the eyelids. The skin of the head and neck has a rich blood supply via a complex network of intercommunicating vessels. These can dilate under physical or emotional stress, changing skin colour and appearance (e.g. blushing). This high intensity blood supply opens up plastic surgery techniques that are not routinely available elsewhere in the body.

Table 15.1 Plastic surgery techniques
Incisions
lines of election
surgical access
Treatment of lacerations
Management of scars
Wound closure
skin grafts
split thickness
full thickness
composite
skin flaps
local
distant
free
Novel methods
prefabrication
tissue engineering

The skin is also not a single entity. There are variations in skin thickness and in the distribution of hair growth, the latter being a sexual characteristic. There are differences in fixity and laxity of the skin with the eyelids being very thin and elastic to allow free mobility. Elasticity and mobility is seen in facial expression and in the development of creases and wrinkles associated with increasing age. There are also variations in skin colour, particularly in the face, partly as the result of exposure to the elements or related to skin diseases such as rosacea. In addition, the face has key landmarks such as the ears, the eyes, the nose and the lips. There are clear boundaries that separate cheek skin from eyelid skin or nasal skin. These separations have allowed the face to be divided into cosmetic units and have changed the thinking in facial reconstructive plastic surgery. Understanding the special characteristics of the skin of the face is an essential component of all surgery in this area.

Facial muscles

Muscles of the face can be divided into two broad groups. The first group concerns functioning of the jaws and is sometimes termed muscles of mastication. These include the temporalis muscle, and masseter. These muscles are innervated by the trigeminal nerve. The second group of muscles is known as the muscles of facial expression and forms an extensive network of interconnecting and interweaving fibres, joined together to produce a powerful composite muscle complex. The muscles of facial expression are innervated by the facial nerve. The muscles are separated from the skin and subcutaneous tissue by an extension of the superficial cervical fascia. This specialised layer is known as the superficial muscular and aponeurotic system (SMAS), which is continuous with the platysma of the neck inferiorly and the galia of the scalp superiorly. It is also attached to the periosteum of the zygomatic arch. This plane has become increasingly important in face-lifting procedures. Within this SMAS there are connections to the overlying skin, which aid the muscles of facial expression in creating creases and wrinkles and contributing to facial expression. The other importance of the SMAS is that the facial nerve lies deep to it, therefore the superficial surface provides an excellent plane for surgical dissection, without risk of damage to the facial nerve. The special characteristics of facial skin and the complexity of the underlying facial musculature, play an important part in all facial surgery.

Incisions

Incisions are used either for excision or for access to areas in the head and neck. Such incisions therefore have to be capable of extension should this be required, but should also give a good cosmetic result. Wherever possible, incisions should be placed in the line of election.

Lines of election

Wrinkle lines (lines of facial expression)

Wrinkling of the skin occurs in response to underlying muscular contraction, and therefore is noticeable in grimacing, showing the teeth, pursing the lips, closing the eyes tightly or in facial expressions of anger or joy. Such wrinkle lines are clearly identified in older people as permanent crease lines. Where the lines are not visible,

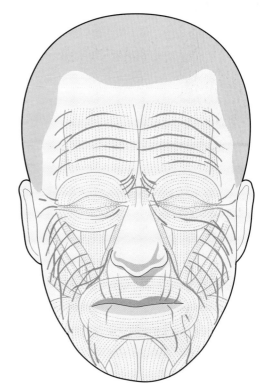

Fig. 15.1 Lines of election on the face.

as in young patients, the direction of the skin creases can be determined by considering the direction of the underlying muscle. The wrinkle line lies perpendicular to the long axis of muscle activity. An example is the frontalis, which works vertically to elevate the eyebrow but creates horizontal furrows in the forehead. The orbicularis oris, which runs horizontally along the upper and lower lips, produces vertical wrinkles in the skin (Fig. 15.1).

Contour lines

Contour lines occur at the junction of cosmetic units. Examples include the nasolabial crease, which separates cheek skin from nasal skin and cheek skin from the lips, and the mental crease, which separates the lower lip from the chin. Incisions should not cross cosmetic units and contour lines.

Surgical access

The head and neck has many hidden areas that are difficult to visualise and thus add to the problems of surgery. Advances in endoscopy equipment have certainly improved matters but in many tumour situations direct visualisation requires better access both for tumour excision and for reconstruction. Such access incisions should have minimal morbidity, in terms of function and cosmesis.

Maxillary sinus tumours may be effectively dealt with by endoscopic surgery, as in functional endoscopic sinus surgery (FESS) (see Ch. 18). Another approach is via the upper labial sulcus, which exposes the anterior part of the maxilla. When more exposure is required, a modified Weber Fergusson incision can be used. This essentially splits the lip in the line of the philtrum and extends along the nasal base and superiorly as a lateral rhinotomy at the junction between cheek skin and nasal skin. It can be further extended in a vertical direction to the gabella frown lines, or in a horizontal direction in a pretarsal line. This allows the soft tissue to be hinged laterally to expose the maxilla. This approach can also be used as a midline facial split by incorporating bone separation of the facial skeleton and palate which, like the upper face, is essentially split into two halves.

For the oral cavity, access can be improved by a lower lip incision placed in the midline in a vertical plane. This incision can also be extended to curve round the mental crease, keeping in the contour line and extending down into the neck, extending laterally in the crease line in the neck. This, combined with an access osteotomy of the mandible, allows the mandible to swing out, giving excellent exposure and access to the oropharynx.

Such incisions used for access stay within the lines of election, and give excellent functional and aesthetic results (Fig. 15.2).

Facial lacerations

The integrity of the skin can be broken as a result of sharp or blunt trauma or following abrasion. The extent of facial lacerations or wounding is often difficult to determine, partly because of profuse bleeding but also because of oedema, which distorts the anatomy. The history and mechanism of the injury are essential, and further investigations are often required (see Ch.12).

Wounds often require exploration under general anaesthetic to determine their extent and damage to underlying structures, notably nerves, vessels and muscles. There are some differences in the management of facial lacerations compared with wounds outside the head and neck area. Wound debridement is usually not as radical as elsewhere. This is because of the exceptional

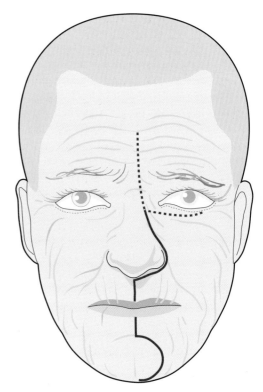

Fig. 15.2   Incisions for surgical access: bicoronal, upper lip and lateral rhinotomy, lower lip and chin.

blood supply to facial structures and because of the importance of maintaining specialised tissues (e.g. eyelid and lips). What is vital in debridement is to remove all foreign material such as gravel. Foreign bodies may cause problems subsequently and gravel appears as tattooing of the scar. It is essential that meticulous wound closure in layers matches anatomical structures (e.g. eyelids, lips, nostrils, ear), to avoid notching deformities and irregularities subsequently. It is important to repair all structures at the time of primary wound closure. If branches of the facial nerve are divided they should be repaired using an operating microscope. If the parotid duct is divided it should similarly be repaired or a stent inserted, with an approximation of the divided ends. All muscles should be repaired meticulously, paying particular attention to orientation of the fibres. The process of wound healing is covered in Chapter 3.

Management of scars

Scars in the head and neck are not only disfiguring and noticeable but often have a social stigma attached. Initial wounds can look quite satisfactory but, as healing progresses, scar formation develops. This appears as reddening and increasing size of the scar as it tends to become wider and raised from the skin surface. The scar becomes hard and can be associated with itch and pain. As the scar matures it should become softer paler and flatter. The final scar should look paler than the surrounding skin, flat and soft and have an atrophic appearance (i.e. look thinner than the surrounding skin), with no skin appendages such as hair or sweat glands.

This cycle of scar maturation can take 1–2 years, and patients often require support throughout this phase. Occasionally, intralesional injection of corticosteroids can accelerate the process of maturation; it can also be a useful treatment for itchy and painful scars. Cosmetically unsightly scars are usually those that cross the lines of election. The pull of the muscle tends to widen the scar with the passage of time and, as these scars do not lie in the relaxed tension lines, scar maturation tends to be poor. Cosmetically unsightly scars can require the direction of the scar to be altered, or the length of the scar to be broken up. A Z-plasty is a useful way of changing the direction of facial scars so that at least one limb of the scar lies in the line of election (Fig. 15.3) and also breaks-up the length of the scar. Sometimes, facial scars become soft and flat but retain a red colour; lasers can sometimes help in this situation.

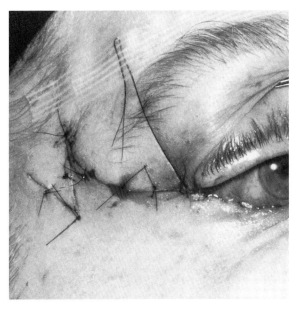

Fig. 15.3 A Z-plasty in lower eyelid reconstruction.

Wound closure

The details of wound closure and wound healing have been discussed previously (Ch. 3). As far as plastic surgery techniques are concerned, wounds may be closed directly by edge-to-edge apposition or by techniques that involve the import of tissues. Tissue can be imported either as a graft, which is a non-vascularised piece of skin, or as a flap, which brings with it, its own blood supply.

Skin grafts

Skin grafts have no blood supply and rely on survival by revascularisation from the surrounding tissue. A graft will therefore not survive in areas of poor vascularity, such as bare bone (without periosteum) bare cartilage (without perichondrium) or overexposed joints. Grafts are also not applicable where protection is required over major vessels and nerves.

Split thickness skin grafts

These grafts comprise the epidermis and some dermal elements but leave sufficient dermis to allow rapid healing with re-epithelialisation of the donor site. Large amounts of skin can be harvested and such grafts are useful for resurfacing large areas of skin loss, such as occurs following burn injuries. The thicker the graft, the more dermal skin appendages it contains, leading to less likelihood of subsequent contracture and a more normal appearance of the skin. Hypopigmentation and poor colour match in the skin of the head and neck is likely particularly with thinner grafts. Common donor sites for split thickness grafts include the thigh the upper arm and buttock. Due to the raw surface that remains prior to re-epithelialisation, donor sites can be painful in the early postoperative period.

Full thickness skin grafts

These include the full thickness of the skin and dermis down to the subcutaneous fat, therefore the donor site requires to be closed. Skin retains the characteristics of its donor site. To obtain a good colour and texture match, grafts have to be harvested from the head and neck region. Common donor sites include the postauricular skin, the preauricular skin and the supraclavicular skin, with direct closure of the donor site. Full thickness grafts, because they contain the dermis, are not prone to

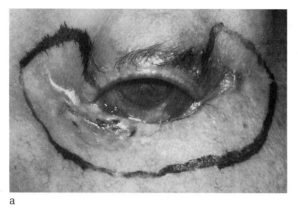

a

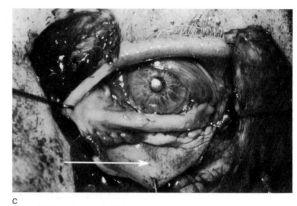

c

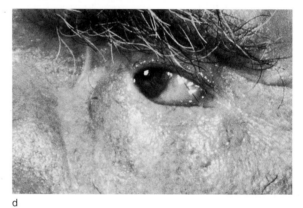

d

b

Fig. 15.4   (a) Extensive basal cell carcinoma eyelids;
(b) planned excision and cervical facial flap; (c) composite
chondromucosal graft (arrowed) from nasal septum;
(d) postoperative appearance.

contracture and give good quality pliable skin, with a
better colour match, when harvested from the head and
neck region.

Composite grafts

Composite grafts are peculiar to facial reconstruction and
are used in specific areas. Defects of the nostril, which
involve the skin, cartilage, nostril rim and nasal mucosal
lining, can be reconstructed using a composite graft from
the ear. Excising a wedge from the ear provides two skin
surfaces with a portion of cartilage in between. This can
be inserted to reconstruct the nostril providing skin for
lining for the nasal mucosa, cartilage to give support
and shape of the nostril and skin for external nasal
reconstruction. A similar wedge can be used for reconstruction of the columella and septal lining.

In lower eyelid reconstruction, lining and support can
be provided using a composite graft from the nasal
septum, comprising mucosa and underlying cartilage.

Table 15.2   Advantages and disadvantages of skin graft types

Graft	Advantages	Disadvantages
Thin split–thickness graft	Size – large grafts. Good graft take. Rapid re-epithelialisation and healing of donor site	Shrink and contract. Poor colour and texture match. Often unstable. Painful donor site
Thick split–thickness graft	Size – large grafts. Less contraction than thin grafts. Stable	Slow healing of donor site. Donor site hypopigmentation. Possible scarring at donor site. Poor colour match for face
Full thickness grafts	Good colour and texture match if harvested from head and neck. Not prone to contracture. Stable	Size limited by necessity to close donor site primarily
Composite grafts	Good tissue match. Composite tissue	Unpredictable graft take. Limited size

Graft success is unpredictable. In nasal reconstruction revascularisation has to occur from the edges of graft insertion, since there is no graft bed. Survival can be improved by enlarging the skin reconstruction element as a full thickness skin graft, to carry the composite tissue at its distal end. In eyelid reconstruction, a well vascularised flap is required to cover the graft and ensure revascularisation (Fig. 15.4). The advantages of the different types of grafts are listed in Table 15.2.

Skin flaps

Skin flaps carry with them their own blood supply and comprise both skin and subcutaneous tissue. Flaps adjacent to the defect requiring reconstruction are termed local flaps. Those from further away and not contiguous with the defect are known as distant flaps. Distant flaps, which remain attached to the body, are further termed pedicled flaps, whereas those that are detached from the body and revascularised by anastomosing the arteries and veins, are called free flaps.

The success of flaps is totally dependant on their vascularity. Where the blood vessels supplying and draining the tissue is known, flaps are given names, either based on the geographical area (e.g. delto-pectoral flap), on the vascular pedicle (e.g. deep circumflex iliac artery flap) or on the tissue types that the flaps contain (e.g. pectoralis major, myocutaneous flap). Flaps may therefore be skin flaps (which incorporate skin and fat), myocutaneous flaps (incorporating muscle and skin), muscle-only flaps or composite flaps, involving a wide variety of tissues that can include skin, fat, muscle, nerve, tendon and bone in any combination. Where the blood supply is not named or known, vascularity of the flap assumes an indeterminate pattern. These flaps are called random pattern flaps and are restricted to local skin flaps. They are particularly useful in the face because of the intense vascularity of this region.

Local flaps

By definition, these flaps are continuous with the defect to be reconstructed. Many in the face are random pattern flaps and are named according to their geometrical design (e.g. transposition flaps, rotation flaps, rhomboid flaps). Essentially, local flaps transfer tissue from an area where it is available into the defect that requires reconstruction. In the face, common areas of tissue availability are the glabellar region, the preauricular region and the neck. When designing local flaps, it is important to pay attention to the lines of election. Local flaps generally provide a good colour and texture match in the face but are limited by tissue availability (Fig. 15.4).

Tissue expansion

One method of increasing the role of local flaps is to use tissue expansion. An inflatable prosthesis is inserted – subcutaneously – and the tissue is gradually distended by inflating the prosthesis over a period of weeks. This increases the tissue availability for local flap transfer. It is most useful in tissues that can be readily expanded (e.g. forehead and scalp) because of the firm base of the cranium. In scalp reconstruction, in particular, it allows reconstruction of hair-bearing skin, thus replacing like tissue with like.

Distant flaps

These flaps have the disadvantage of often being outside the head and neck area, therefore they do not provide good skin colour and texture match. However, the deltopectoral flap, taken from the upper chest, can be used effectively to resurface the neck and will extend up to the zygomatic arch. It is certainly adjacent to the neck skin area and probably provides one of the best colour matches. This flap has to be taken up in two stages, with the pedicle divided at 3 weeks and subsequently returned to its original site (Fig. 15.5). This essentially means that the blood supply, which enabled the transfer of the flap, is divided, and the tissue has to survive from ingrowth of vessels from the original defect.

More useful flaps are those in which the vascular pedicle can be transferred to the head and neck in a single stage and maintained permanently in this transferred position. This retains the blood supply to the transferred tissue, promoting wound healing. One of the major flaps of this type is the pectoralis major myocutaneous flap (Fig. 15.6).

Free flaps

The advent of the operating microscope has opened up new possibilities in reconstructive surgery. The ability to revascularise tissue by anastomosing small vessels of 1–3 mm in diameter has enabled the transfer of specific tissue types. The golden rule of plastic surgery is to reconstruct like tissue with like. For example, the ability to reconstruct the jaw with vascularised bone has revolutionised head and neck cancer surgery (see Ch. 17) (Fig. 15.7). Similarly, facial paralysis can be improved by transferring a functioning muscle flap, reconstituting its vascular and neural supply. Large volumes of skin can be transferred to resurface defects for the head and neck, but here the problems of tissue type and colour match become apparent (Fig. 15.8). A notable feature of these well-vascularised distant flaps is that they maintain the characteristics of their original donor sites. A free skin flap placed for intraoral reconstruction remains as a free skin flap, with keratinising squamous epithelium, and does not change its character to mucosa.

Improved understanding of the anatomy of the body has provided an increasing number of donor sites for free tissue transfer and surgeons are no longer restricted by the need to raise flaps in close proximity to the head and neck. A variety of specialised tissues can now be transferred in an attempt to replace like with like.

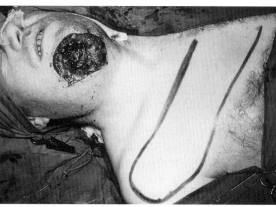

a

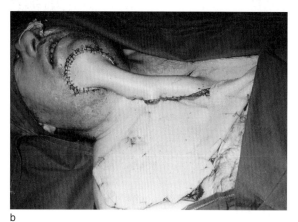

b

Fig. 15.5 A deltopectoral flap: (a) incision lines; (b) transposed flap in place.

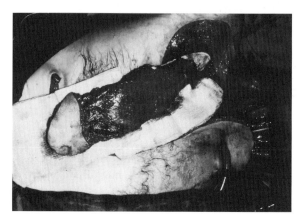

Fig 15.6 A pectoralis major flap isolated on its vascular flap.

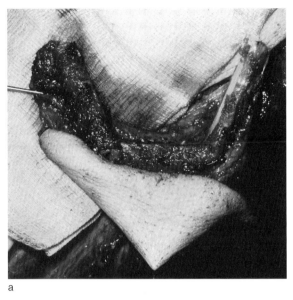

a

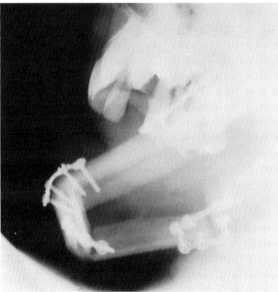

b

Fig. 15.7 (a) Fibula osteocutaneous flap; (b) radiograph showing flap restoring mandibular contour.

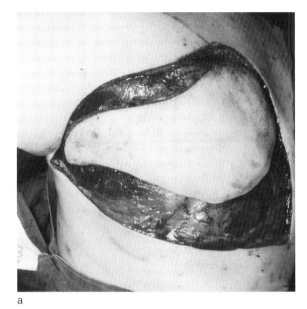

a

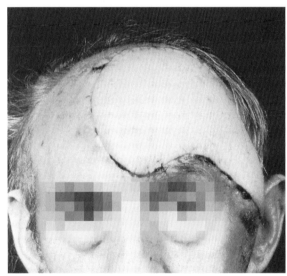

b

Fig. 15.8 A scapula flap: (a) flap elevation; (b) showing poor colour match.

Free flaps are designed on particular vessels and they tend to have a very good vascularity, which is dependent on a successful microvascular anastomosis of both artery and veins. There is significant evidence of the vascularity of free flaps, in their ability to heal wounds in the head and neck, and their ability to tolerate postoperative radiotherapy in cases of malignancy. Free flaps continue to have a major impact on the cosmetic and functional outcomes following major head and neck surgery.

Novel methods

Plastic surgery is concerned with excision and the creation of surgical defects and their subsequent reconstruction.

A wide variety of methods are now available but some specialised tissues in the head and neck are virtually irreplaceable and it is often difficult to replace like tissue with like. In an attempt to solve some of these problems, there has been a move towards prefabrication and tissue engineering.

Prefabrication

Prefabrication involves multistage surgery to create a purpose-designed flap to reconstruct a particular defect. A simple example of prefabrication is to harvest buccal mucosal grafts and insert these grafts under the skin and onto the fascia of the forearm. These grafts will take on the fascia and form a mucosal surface. The flap comprising the fascia and this new mucosa can be transferred subsequently as a radial forearm free flap, to provide mucosal reconstruction of the oral cavity.

Tissue engineering

Tissue engineering is in its infancy. Specific tissue types can be grown (e.g. epithelium or bone) under a variety of growth stimulators. Tissue engineering in essence creates new tissue, which can be of a specialised nature. These techniques are being developed in the laboratory and look promising in the reconstruction of the specialised tissues of the face and head and neck in the future.

16 Clefts of the lip and palate

Introduction

Clefts of the lip and palate are one of the most common congenital facial malformations described in humans. They remain, however, poorly understood and present a significant challenge for reconstruction.

Early records of successful repairs of clefts of the lip exist in Eastern texts and the earliest recorded case of a successful repair of a cleft lip appears to be around AD 390 in China. Over the centuries, many techniques have been reported to disguise the visible deformities of cleft lip or the occlusion with cleft lip and palate, as well as surgical techniques for their repair.

Surgeons dealing with clefts of the lip and palate today must recognise that although significant advances have been made in surgical and anaesthetic technology, the techniques of repair are far from perfect and remain an area of immense controversy and intense debate.

An understanding of the management of cleft deformities requires a knowledge of the embryology of the face and the classification of cleft deformity. The structural abnormalities that comprise the cleft deformity dictate the patient management and, in particular, the surgical procedures employed. These will be discussed in turn (Table 16.1).

Embryology

The embryological development of the face is a complex process but occurs very early in fetal life. The face develops from a central or frontonasal process, which grows forwards and over the developing brain. Two maxillary processes advance anteriorly between the optic vesicles and the primitive stomodeum and two mandibular processes advance beneath the stomodeum. The distal end of the frontonasal process is defined into medial and lateral nasal processes by the olfactory placodes (Fig. 16.1).

Table 16.1	Management of cleft deformities

Embryology
Classification of cleft deformity
Structural abnormalities of cleft deformity
Patient management
Surgical treatment
Surgical procedures
Philosophy

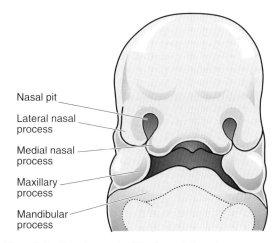

Fig. 16.1 Development of the face at 5 weeks.

Nasal pit
Lateral nasal process
Medial nasal process
Maxillary process
Mandibular process

Fusion of the maxillary processes with the frontonasal process results in the formation of the premaxilla, which bears the incisor teeth. Facial features become recognisable by the fifth to sixth week of intrauterine life. Fusion of the maxillary palatine processes with each other and the premaxilla (between the lateral incisor and canine teeth) commences at around the eighth week of intrauterine life at the area defined by the incisive foramen and progresses posteriorly to the uvula by the twelfth week.

It was initially believed that facial clefts occurred as a result of failure of fusion of the ectodermal processes

131

described above. However, patterns of presentation of clefts of the lip and palate have resulted in increasing support for theories suggesting that clefts of this region are likely to be due to a failure of migration of the ectomesenchymal cells responsible for the formation of the deeper tissues, such as the muscles and nerves, resulting in inadequate tissue support between the two epithelial layers and consequent breakdown.

The presentation of clefts of the secondary palate is consistent with failure of fusion of the margins of the palatal processes.

Clefting may arise as part of a syndrome. Non-syndromic clefting arises as a result of a genetic link combined with environmental insults in utero, although the mechanisms remain unclear.

Classification of the cleft deformity

The deformity in clefts of the lip and palate can range widely in severity and extent, rendering attempts to classify them into a limited set of patterns somewhat impractical. The various terms used to describe palatal clefts are defined in Table 16.2.

Clefts of the lip may be barely noticeable, with minimal surface abnormalities or asymmetry of vertical height indicating an underlying abnormality of muscle anatomy, a 'forme fruste' or microform cleft lip. The

deformity can range from this to a complete cleft of the lip, alveolus, primary palate and secondary palate.

Clefts of the palate alone may similarly manifest a wide range of severity. There may be no surface or visible evidence of clefting, but abnormalities of soft palatal function only displayed by features suggestive of velo-pharyngeal incompetence. This occult submucous cleft may occur in an otherwise intact palate with minimal surface evidence of an underlying abnormality of muscle anatomy. The clinical features of submucous cleft deformity are listed in Table 16.3.

Although clefts of the lip and primary palate associated with clefts of the soft palate and/or the posterior hard palate with an intervening bridge of intact hard palate are rare, they have been described. Similarly, clefts of the palate alone involving the bony palate may be unilateral with partial or complete attachment of the vomer to one side.

Structural abnormalities of cleft deformity

To fully understand the rationale for treatment of clefts of the lip and palate, it is essential to comprehend the complex nature of the underlying functional and structural abnormalities associated with this deformity. The components of the anatomical deformity are listed in Table 16.4 and these will be discussed in turn.

Table 16.2	Terms used to describe palatal clefts
Primary palate	Palate anterior to the incisive foramen
Secondary palate	Palate derived from the palatal shelves of the embryo (posterior to the incisive foramen)
Complete cleft palate	Cleft extending to the incisive foramen
Incomplete cleft palate	Cleft not extending to the incisive foramen
Submucous cleft	Cleft of the muscle layer only in the soft palate (usually with notch on the posterior border of the hard palate)
Unilateral palatal cleft	Vomer attached to one of the palatal shelves
Bilateral palatal cleft	Vomer totally separated from the palatal shelves

Table 16.3	Clinical features of submucous cleft deformity

Bifid uvula
Notching of the posterior edge of the hard palate
Midline translucency of the soft palate
Absence of musculus uvulae

Table 16.4	Anatomical components of a cleft deformity

Lip
Nose
Alveolus
Primary palate
Secondary palate
Maxilla
Mandible
Other

The lip

There is soft tissue discontinuity of the lip involving the vermilion and skin. Disruption of the orbicularis oris with abnormal attachments of the muscle to the skin, the lateral crus of the alar cartilage and the underlying bone occurs. Some authorities have proposed that the extent of muscular abnormality is far more extensive on the affected side and includes the muscles of facial expression and nasal sphincters, thus requiring a meticulous restoration of functional muscular anatomy.

The nose

The deformity of the nose is minimal or absent in clefts of the lip that are incomplete with a largely intact anatomy of the orbicularis oris. 'Forme fruste' nasal deformities may occur occasionally with otherwise intact lips, suggesting that components of the nasal deformity are related to abnormal insertions of the disrupted fibres of the facial muscles.

There is nasal deformity in more complete clefts of the lip. The alar cartilage is caudally displaced and the medial crura and alar domes are separated. This results in apparent shortening of the columella on the cleft side and deviation of the nasal tip towards the cleft side. The body of the cartilage may be elongated and rotated. The caudal edge of the septal cartilage may be dislocated. The nasal floor may be stretched and lower in incomplete clefts and absent in complete clefts. In addition, the nasal lining may be webbed with a band of skin across the upper lateral wall.

The alveolus

The premaxillary portion of the alveolus carries the incisor teeth and forms the primary palate, which is the part of the palate anterior to the incisive foramen. The gap in the alveolus usually occurs between the lateral incisor and canine teeth and extends obliquely towards the incisive foramen. The extent of alveolar clefting may range from barely visible notching of the gingiva to a complete cleft, but the visible manifestations may not correlate directly with the extent of underlying bony disruption.

The primary palate

Clefts of the primary palate extend posteriorly to the incisive foramen, resulting in a deficiency of the nasal floor. The alveolar arch component on the cleft side (referred to as the lesser segment) tends to be rotated mesiopalatally and the primary palatal component on the non-cleft side (referred to as the greater segment) is rotated outwards by the action of the abnormally attached facial muscles. The combination of these deformities can result in a virtual appearance of a significant tissue deficit at the site of the cleft. The septal cartilage is also deviated as the premaxilla is rotated out.

The secondary palate

The secondary palate extends posteriorly from the incisive foramen to the uvula and is composed of the bony hard palate and the soft palate. Unilateral clefts of the bony hard palate result in the separation of the palatal shelf on the affected side from the contralateral palatal shelf at the midline. The affected shelf is often smaller in length and width and may also be retrodisplaced. The transverse deficiency (in width) can be exaggerated by the cranial tilt of the shelf. The attachment of the vomer to the contralateral shelf may be variable in extent. The posterior palatal arch width is greater than normal because of lateral displacement of the maxillary tuberosities.

The soft palatal component of a cleft palate results in a midline deficiency that can be overt (e.g. in a complete cleft) or submucous, with continuity of the lining but a deficiency of the muscles in the midline. The muscles of the soft palate are attached abnormally to the posterior edge of the hard palate and the edges of the cleft. The anteroposterior length of the soft palate is reduced.

The maxilla

The maxilla on the affected side is deficient in vertical and anteroposterior dimensions.

The mandible

The dimensions of the mandible may be smaller in patients with clefts of the palate, especially as part of the Pierre Robin sequence and the potential for growth might be compounded by the existing maxillary deformity.

Other anomalies

The abnormal anatomy of the muscles of the soft palate, especially the tensor veli palatini, is believed to be responsible for interference with aeration of the middle ear due to failure of adequate eustachian tube opening during swallowing, yawning and other pharyngeal movements.

Patient management

The management of clefts of the lip and palate is multidisciplinary and requires the involvement of several specialities, which constitute a cleft team. In most centres, the minimum complement of a cleft team involved in the primary management would consist of a surgeon, orthodontist, speech and language therapist, ENT surgeon and audiologist. The participation of several other disciplines is also crucial in the management of the child with a cleft deformity, including paediatricians, geneticists, paediatric dentists, hygienists, prosthodontists, psychologists and specialist nurses and dieticians.

The initial management of the child born with a cleft deformity is essentially supportive. The birth of a baby with a facial deformity is often a traumatic experience for the parents and other members of the family. The staff involved in immediate perinatal care (the obstetricians, midwives and paediatric perinatologists) must be able to recognise and deal with the shock and distress of the parents, as well as with any medical problems that may arise. It is vital that the parents are visited as soon as possible by a member of the cleft team to discuss the long-term management of the condition. A considerable effort must be made to allay the fears and anxieties of the parents and relatives with detailed discussions to explain the nature of the problem and the long-term prognosis of treatment.

Parents of babies born with clefts are often overcome by feelings of guilt and self-accusations of punishment for past sins, as well as with a significant loss of self-esteem generated by feelings that the appearance of facial deformity in the baby is a manifestation of their own imperfection. The absence of perceptible emotional distress should not be considered as evidence of coping. It is essential to explore the parents' feelings, ideally with the support of a clinical psychologist, as rejection of the baby will have significant long-term consequences for both the parents and the child. Non-syndromic clefts of the lip and palate are unlikely to present any serious medical problems and the only immediate concerns are mainly related to potential airway problems and feeding.

Airways

Newborn babies are obligate nasal breathers and any evidence of airway obstruction should be assessed immediately by careful suction of secretions occluding the oropharynx, and by measures to prevent the tongue from blocking the airway.

The Pierre Robin sequence is associated with micrognathia (a small mandible with obvious lack of chin prominence), relative macroglossia (a tongue that appears disproportionately large) with a tendency to develop glossoptosis (falling backward of the tongue into the oropharynx) resulting in intermittent airway obstruction, and a cleft palate. Although originally labelled as a syndrome, it is now recognised that this combination of features may be associated with a variety of conditions. Feeding difficulties associated with the respiratory obstruction are also very common.

Various manoeuvres have been utilised to prevent the glossoptosis, which is the fundamental cause of the intermittent airway obstruction. These include nursing in the prone position in special harnesses, suturing the tongue to prevent retraction, nasopharyngeal or oropharyngeal airways, endotracheal intubation and tracheostomies. The problems of airway obstruction tend to be more pronounced when the baby is more relaxed or asleep and are unusual when awake, crying or in the upright position. Fortunately, severe problems of airway obstruction warranting a tracheostomy or other surgical procedures are relatively rare. However, it is essential to recognise the condition and institute early appropriate treatment. Failure to recognise the problem is potentially fatal because of the possibility of acute obstruction, progressive exhaustion or brain damage associated with chronic hypoxia. Pulmonary hypertension and cardiac failure may result from the chronic hypercapnia and hypoxia.

In mild cases, simple postural measures are often adequate and careful supervision with the judicious use of devices such as pulse oximeters and sleep apnoea monitors to detect episodes of airway obstruction are sufficient. The immense emotional and physical stress imposed on the parents or carers of the child must not be underestimated. It is essential to ensure that the child is kept in a suitable high-dependency or intensive care facility until it has been established that the risk of apnoea or cyanotic spells is minimal and the parents feel comfortable about the prospect of managing the problem at home.

It may be necessary to arrange readmission to hospital to 'wean' the infant from the apnoea monitor and demonstrate to the parents that the airway problems are unlikely to constitute a serious risk. A combination of establishing breathing patterns and the progressive growth of the mandible often results in fairly rapid improvement in the situation. In severe cases requiring surgical intervention such as tracheostomies, it may take a long time to decannulate the child.

Feeding

Feeding problems associated with clefts of the lip alone are unusual. Mothers should be encouraged to attempt breast-feeding as an adequate lip seal over the nipple can be achieved. Clefts of the palate, and especially the secondary palate, result in an inability to generate sufficient oropharyngeal negative pressure and tongue compression against the palate. Milk reflux into the nasal cavity and associated problems such as respiratory difficulties and fatigue, as well as frustration on the part of the mother, compound the problems. Historically, feeding with spoons and cups have been advocated to allow gravity-assisted presentation of the feed into the oropharynx, as the ability to swallow is not affected by palatal clefts.

A wide variety of proprietary teats with compressible reservoirs and feeding devices have also been designed to facilitate feeding by minimising the need to suck or by attempting to obturate the palatal cleft. Feeding plates comprising an acrylic palatal coverage constructed on a dental cast and secured with ribbon attached to extraoral flanges improve sucking ability, but there is less need for these nowadays with improvements in other feeding techniques, and they are now not generally recommended. In many instances, a normal teat with an enlarged hole to permit a steady, gravity-assisted delivery of milk into the oropharynx is adequate and the mother should be encouraged to identify, by a process of trial and error, the best method suited to mother and baby. However, it is crucial that this process is undertaken under the supervision of a cleft nurse specialist or other member of the cleft team with a specific interest and knowledge of feeding problems in babies with clefts.

Feeding may be seriously compromised by associated respiratory or other problems and it may be necessary to resort to nasogastric tube feeding if adequate nutrition cannot be delivered by oral feeds. However, resident nasogastric tubes are associated with significant morbidity, such as increased risk of respiratory infections, pulmonary aspiration and gastro-oesophageal reflux. In extreme cases, percutaneous gastrostomy might have to be considered. Careful and regular monitoring of weight gain and development is essential to ensure that nutritional requirements are being met.

Surgical treatment

The fundamental objectives of surgical treatment for clefts of the lip and palate are listed in Table 16.5. A wide range of procedures and protocols for surgical management of this deformity has been described and controversies exist regarding the optimum modalities of treatment. Rather than becoming immersed in this debate, it is advisable to grasp the underlying rationale of treatment (Table 16.6).

Surgical procedures

The evolution of surgical procedures for the treatment of cleft deformities has only been possible because of advances in the field of anaesthesia, and especially paediatric anaesthesia. The earliest repairs of clefts of the lip consisted of hastily paring the edges of the cleft deformity without the benefit of anaesthesia and attempting to suture or appose the edges in an effort to seal the gap. Palatal clefts were treated with simple obturators or crude surgical attempts to repair the cleft

Table 16.5 Objectives of surgical treatment of clefts
The restoration of normal facial appearance and facial symmetry Normal speech Normal occlusion Normal hearing

Table 16.6 Treatment of the cleft deformity components
Correction of the surface geometry of the affected tissues Restitution of the underlying structural and functional anatomy Modulation of growth and development of the jaws and dentition Development of normal speech and hearing

Table 16.7	Rule of 10s
Age: 10 weeks	
Weight: 10 lb	
Haemoglobin: 10 g/dL	

Table 16.8	Stages of cleft repair
Primary surgery	
Secondary surgery	
Revision surgery	

defect. As repair of palatal clefts under such conditions was associated with risks of considerable blood loss or other complications, they were often undertaken in adults and, until the 1970s, repair of palatal clefts was not recommended before the age of 18 months. Repair of lip clefts was advocated by the rule of 10s (Table 16.7). These classic recommendations for the timing of surgery are still widely applied today in several leading cleft centres in the world.

Repair of the cleft deformity can be divided into three categories (Table 16.8).

Primary surgery

The objective of primary repair is to close the cleft gap, restore the symmetry or dimensions of the lip by addressing the geometric deformity and restore the underlying structural and functional anatomy of the affected tissues.

The lip

The timing of cleft lip repair ranges from neonatal repair to delaying surgery to between 6 and 9 months of age. The advantages and disadvantages of neonatal repair are listed in Table 16.9.

Lip adhesion

Lip adhesion involves merely approximating the skin without muscle repair. Although it is routine practice in some leading centres to employ lip adhesion as a primary procedure at varying times, there is no evidence to suggest that the procedure confers any long-term benefit and it has the disadvantage of increasing the total number of operative procedures if palatal repair is not undertaken at the time of the definitive lip repair.

Proponents of primary lip adhesion argue that it serves the same function as preoperative orthopaedics to mould the component tissues into a more favourable position without the considerable inconvenience and cumbersome nature of the process. Lip adhesion may have a role in wide bilateral clefts or in wide unilateral clefts if preoperative orthopaedics have failed to narrow the cleft gap or the risks of breakdown of a definitive repair are likely to be high.

Table 16.9	Advantages and disadvantages of neonatal repair of cleft lip	
Advantages	*Disadvantages*	
Theoretical advantage of scarless fetal wound healing	Tissues are more friable and delicate	
Reduction of psychological trauma period for parents and possibly better maternal bonding because of restoration of facial aesthetics	Need for postoperative intensive care, which may adversely affect maternal bonding and compound psychological stress factors	
Higher levels of circulating maternal immunoglobulins conferring improved resistance to infection	Underlying cardiac or other abnormalities may not be manifest at this age. Risk of producing a patent ductus	
Higher haemoglobin level with possibly better wound healing	Neonatal jaundice and risks associated with neonatal anaesthesia	
Dimensions of lip and nose are only slightly smaller than at 3 months. Surgical planning is not compromised	Primary rhinoplasty with alar cartilage dissection is difficult. Functional restoration of muscle anatomy is difficult. Anatomical landmarks are not clearly defined	
Parents take home a baby with a repaired lip cleft	The period of psychological adaptation to an unrepaired cleft may reduce long-term unrealistic expectations	
Underlying alveolus is more malleable and moulded after repair	Repair is more difficult in wide or bilateral clefts with no opportunity to utilise preoperative orthopaedics	

Lip repair at 3 months

This is the traditional recommended timing for lip repair. The anatomical landmarks are well developed at this stage permitting accurate planning and restoration of the geometric anatomy of the soft tissues. The nasal tissues and alar cartilages are also sufficiently developed to permit dissection for a primary rhinoplasty.

Lip repair at 6 months or later

It is easier to repair the palate and undertake a more comprehensive palatal repair, especially of the primary palate and the nasal floor, using the 'working forward from the back' approach. Some proponents advocate a one-stage repair of the entire deformity at this age. 'Functional' repair of the muscles of the lip, nose and palate are believed by advocates of the Delaire functional repair philosophy to be possible at this stage, when the component muscles of the orbicularis oris and perinasal muscle ring can be more readily recognised.

The correction of the vertical dimensions of the vermilion itself is equally important and the value of identifying the 'dry' vermilion and restoring the vertical height of the dry vermilion – and avoiding any use of 'wet' vermilion as a substitute – is being increasingly recognised.

The importance of the restoration of the muscular anatomy of the orbicularis oris in maintaining the proportions of the lip, and especially the symmetry of the face during dynamic movements, is crucial. Meticulous attention needs to be directed to the careful detachment of the abnormal insertions of the muscles into the soft tissues and bony structures adjacent to the cleft as well as reconstruction of the superficial and deep components of the muscle. Some authorities propose that the accurate reconstruction of the superficial part of the orbicularis oris, which arises from the muscles of facial expression, requires radical subperiosteal mobilisation of the facial soft tissue mask to adequately reposition the muscles of facial expression and reconstitute the anatomy of the lip.

Reconstruction of the anterior nasal floor and any associated cleft of the primary palate is desirable at the time of the primary lip repair as the access to these areas is considerably facilitated at this time.

The nose

Primary correction of the cleft nasal deformity is now widely accepted as an essential procedure for the resto-ration of the symmetry of the nose. Several techniques have been described. Those utilising extensive incisions of the nasal lining should be avoided as the risk of stenosis of the nasal airways is high.

The restoration of the nasal architecture, form and symmetry can be properly achieved only by utilising the tissues of the nose. The alar cartilage on the cleft side, or both alar cartilages in a bilateral cleft, may be mobilised quite radically through the cleft lip incisions, avoiding the need for any incisions in the nasal lining. The growth and development of the nose is very dependent on the normal flow dynamics of the nasal airways and the temptation to use the lining of the inferior turbinates or similar structures, which result in gross distortion of the airway architecture, should be avoided.

The alveolus

Primary repair of the alveolus has been attempted by many authorities in an attempt to stimulate normal development of the alveolar arch form. Primary bone grafting, with cancellous bone at the time of lip repair, has been largely abandoned because of long-term facial growth problems that result. There is at present some renewed interest in gingivoperiosteoplasty, which consists of initial orthodontic manipulation to produce abutment of the gingival cleft edges prior to the lip repair and a simple restoration of the gingival continuity with minimal dissection at the time of the lip repair.

Alveolar closure undertaken in the mixed dentition, just prior to the descent of the canine, is often referred to as a secondary alveolar bone grafting procedure to distinguish it from alveolar closure undertaken at the time of lip repair. This is a planned procedure in terms of the timing of surgery and is undertaken at the age when sufficient permanent teeth have erupted to allow preoperative orthodontics with expansion of any collapse at the site of the cleft and alignment of the alveolar segments.

Resorption of the alveolar bone graft is likely to occur if canine descent does not follow soon after the procedure, and the bone grafting is therefore timed to coincide as closely as possible with the time of expected canine eruption at the site of the cleft. At the time of alveolar bone grafting, it is common practice to augment the bony foundation of the alar base on the cleft side with cancellous bone chips or corticocancellous bone block to improve the projection and symmetry of the nose. Revision surgery might be indicated also for the lip and the nose to minimise the total number of surgical interventions.

The primary palate

Closure of the primary palate at the time of the lip repair is recommended as access to this area is extremely difficult after lip closure. The repair may be a single layer repair using the mucoperiosteal lining of the vomer. Two-layer closures have been described if the gap is narrow or using buccal mucosal flaps for the oral lining.

The secondary hard palate

The cleft of the bony secondary palate is often quite wide and attempts to achieve closure may require extensive lateral releasing incisions. Studies evaluating facial growth in patients with unrepaired clefts of the palate or delayed repairs clearly suggest that surgery of the palate may be directly implicated in the subsequent restriction of facial growth.

Some authorities undertake repair of the palate in two stages by initially repairing the soft palate, which encourages descent of the hard palatal shelves and narrowing of the cleft gap, allowing closure at a second stage with minimal dissection.

The soft palate

Early observations that the anteroposterior length of the palate was deficient led to the design of passive push back techniques aimed at lengthening the palate to allow velopharyngeal contact. Detachment of the abnormal insertions of the muscle elements into the soft tissues and posterior edge of the bony hard palate and restoration of the muscular anatomy of the soft palate is essential to achieve effective velopharyngeal closure.

Secondary surgery

Secondary procedures in the management of cleft lip and palate may be grouped chronologically, as listed in Table 16.10.

Fistula closure

Fistula closure following palatal cleft repairs is often undertaken early if it is felt that the fistula may cause functional problems with speech, swallowing or nasal regurgitation of ingested foodstuffs. The presence of a

Table 16.10 Secondary surgical procedures
Fistula closure
Surgery for speech – pharyngoplasty
Rhinoplasty
Orthognathic surgery

fistula does not warrant closure if there is no demonstrable or predicted functional problems likely to be associated with the fistula.

Surgery for speech

As speech develops, the regular and expert assessment of a cleft speech therapist is essential to detect and rectify problems of articulation or other speech problems. Velopharyngeal incompetence resulting from ineffective closure of the velopharyngeal aperture is often not correctable by conservative treatment and early surgical intervention may be warranted.

Pharyngoplasties are designed to reduce the dimensions of the velopharyngeal aperture to facilitate closure or simply increase the resistance of the airway to minimise nasal air escape. They are broadly classified as dynamic – procedures (e.g. orticochea pharyngoplasty), which are designed to mobilise the palatopharyngeus muscle bundles in the posterior tonsillar pillars and attach them to the posterior pharyngeal wall – or passive – procedures that simply narrow the velopharyngeal aperture or augment the posterior pharyngeal wall using implanted materials.

Rhinoplasty

The preschool age is also a common time for parents to request secondary corrective procedures for the asymmetry of the nose by a rhinoplasty procedure. If an adequate primary rhinoplasty was undertaken and the degree of asymmetry is within expected limits, every additional procedure undoubtedly confers additional scars within the nasal tissues, which may compromise the final result. Secondary rhinoplasty at this age, or in the preteen age group, should be undertaken only for gross or obvious deformities causing problems of significant psychological or functional distress.

Secondary rhinoplasty at or nearing the end of the growth phase is common. If orthognathic surgery is planned, it is often preferable to undertake the surgery following the orthognathic procedures to restore the symmetry and aesthetic balance of the face, and especially the bony foundations of the nose. The procedure can be combined with the orthognathic operation, if preferred, to minimise the number of operative interventions.

Orthognathic surgery

With improvements in primary surgical techniques and the recognition of the potentially harmful effects of surgery on facial growth and symmetry, it is anticipated that a smaller proportion of patients will eventually require orthognathic procedures.

In those patients with gross occlusal problems caused by restriction of midfacial growth or other facial skeletal problems, Le Fort osteotomies, bimaxillary surgery, distraction osteogenesis, on-lay bone grafts or other procedures may be indicated. Fixed orthodontic appliances are required to achieve the optimal occlusal outcome in conjunction with surgery. The use of osseointegrated implants and facial reconstruction is becoming more common in the management of patients with clefts.

Philosophy

The management of the patient with a facial cleft deformity is a lifelong project. The long-term consequences of each procedure undertaken must be analysed carefully to weigh-up the potential advantages and disadvantages with the full involvement of, initially, the parents or carers and subsequently the patient. All members of the cleft team should share equal responsibility in the decision-making process. It is essential that the care of cleft patients is undertaken by dedicated cleft teams with adequate centralisation of resources and patient referrals. Continuous and intercentre audit of the outcome of established protocols of care, which are strictly enforced, is essential to monitor outcome and refine techniques. It will also help to identify factors for poor outcome. The search for the optimum protocol of care is currently a subject of considerable interest and speculation.

17 Management of orofacial malignancy

Introduction

Oral cancer is the eighth most common malignancy worldwide, although the prevalence varies from country to country. In countries such as India, oral malignancy accounts for 40% of the total, whereas in the UK around 4000 new cases present every year, accounting for around 3% of all new malignancies. Around 50% of these patients will die from their disease and overall survival rates have not improved over the last three decades, despite advances in surgical and oncological techniques.

The incidence of oral cancer has been rising steadily over recent years; the reasons for which are unclear. Oral cancer generally appears from the sixth decade and increases in incidence in subsequent decades. It should be appreciated, however, that oral cancer can occur at any age and the recent rise in incidence has been more apparent in the younger age groups.

Oral cancer is almost exclusively squamous cell carcinoma, which accounts for 90% of the total; the remaining 10% is made up by salivary gland tumours (8%) (see Ch. 14) and oral lymphoma (2%).

Over the past 30 years, social deprivation has become strongly linked with oral cancer. In the early 1970s, oral cancer was spread relatively evenly over all social classes. When the detrimental effects of smoking became clear, the better educated tended to reduce their cigarette consumption, but those living in deprived areas have continued to smoke to a much greater degree. The aetiology of oral cancer is, however, complex. The high-risk population is that least likely to attend the dentist and therefore most likely to present with advanced disease.

In the UK, the majority of patients tend to present with advanced disease and, by definition, a poor prognosis. In many European countries, more than 70% of patients present with early disease, increasing the chance of cure and reducing the need for radical treatment. Despite the fact that treatment for oral cancer has advanced considerably over the last 30 years, survival has not improved. This is due to the lack of understanding of tumour biology. Research into tumour biology is coming to the fore, hopefully allowing the development of new treatments.

Various aspects of the diagnosis and treatment of oral cancer are discussed here (Table 17.1).

Aetiology of oral cancer

The aetiology of oral squamous cancer is complex. The main factors associated with this disease are tobacco and alcohol consumption. Each of these factors increases the likelihood of oral cancer and both show a strong dose-related increase in incidence. It would seem that heavy smoking and heavy drinking have a synergistic effect, leading to an exponential rise in relative risk (Fig. 17.1).

Tobacco is the main aetiological agent associated with oral cancer. The risk of oral cancer is related to the number of cigarettes per day and the length of time the

Table 17.1 The diagnosis and management of oral malignancy

Aetiology
Morbidity
Premalignancy
Signs and symptoms
Staging of disease
Clinical investigation
Multidisciplinary treatment
Treatment planning
Treatment of the neck
Reconstruction
Quality of life issues

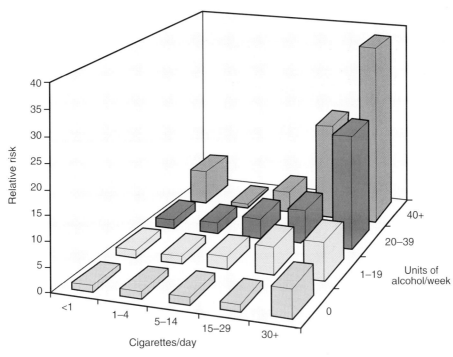

Fig. 17.1   The risk of oral cancer by alcohol/tobacco consumption.

patient has smoked, giving rise to the concept of pack years, where a pack is equivalent to 20 cigarettes:

$$\text{Pack years} = \frac{\text{Number of cigarettes per day} \times \text{number of years smoked}}{20}$$

This formulation allows a calculation of the relative risk of each patient. The relative risk returns to that of a non-smoker 10 years after the cessation of smoking. Topical tobacco, particularly, when mixed with areca nut, slaked lime, and betel and placed as a quid in the buccal sulcus, is a potent carcinogen. On the Indian subcontinent, where the practice of chewing tobacco is common, oral cancer makes up 40% of the total incidence of all carcinomas; it is also prevalent in Asian communities in the UK.

Alcohol *per se* does not appear to be a potent carcinogen but seems to potentiate the effects of tobacco. Someone who smokes 30 or more cigarettes per week has a relative risk of seven-fold that of a non-smoker. A person who drinks 40 or more units of alcohol per week has a relative risk of six-fold; if these factors are combined then the relative risk of oral cancer increases by a factor of 38.

Recent research suggests that genetic factors play a significant part in the promotion of oral cancer. Cancer is prevalent in some families and this can include oral cancer. There is a cohort of patients who develop oral cancer in the third or fourth decade. This group, mainly women, develop aggressive cancers with a poor prognosis.

Cellular biology investigations show that disturbances in the regulators of cell growth and cell death (apoptosis) lead to the development of oral cancer. This is a rapidly expanding field and it is likely that new prognostic indicators and cancer treatments will come from this research.

Other agents that may be implicated in oral cancer pathogenesis include malnutrition, poor dental hygiene, infective agents and sunlight in lip cancer.

Oral cancer morbidity

The number of deaths from oral cancer has been rising over the last 30 years. The death to registration ratio is 0.4, which is higher than many other cancers and similar to cancer of the uterine cervix and breast. The site in the mouth is an important prognostic indicator, with the tongue having the poorest prognosis and highest mortality (Table 17.2).

Table 17.2 Registration and deaths by site in Scotland 1991–1996		
Site	Registrations (%)	Deaths (%)
Tongue	25.0	29.9
Unspecified mouth	19.2	19.5
Floor of mouth	17.6	12.9
Lip	14.5	2.4
Oropharynx	12.5	14.5
Ill-defined sites	6.3	16.5
Gum	4.7	4.2
Cancer surveillance group 1998		

Survival rates have not improved over the past 50 years, mainly due to late presentation of patients with the disease. It has been shown that the delay in presentation correlates well with social deprivation. Education programmes are required to target the at-risk groups, and only when lifestyle begins to change is there a likelihood of an improvement in survival.

Premalignant lesions

The vast majority of oral malignancies arise from previously normal epithelium. A small number of new malignancies may develop from abnormal mucosa.

White or red patches may precede the development of cancer and allow the opportunity of early biopsy. This will determine whether a lesion is premalignant. The site and colour of these lesions can give some idea of their malignant potential. A speckled or red lesion is more likely to be premalignant than a homogeneous white lesion. A lesion situated in the floor of mouth or lateral border of the tongue, irrespective of colour, has a higher chance of being premalignant. Biopsy is helpful in determining the malignant potential of any lesion. A lesion that persists for more that 2 weeks following removal of chronic trauma should be referred for biopsy. Many of these lesions are likely to be asymptomatic.

Signs and symptoms of oral cancer

Tumours can be very advanced before patients develop symptoms that cause them to present to their doctor or dentist. Early warning signs include soreness in the mouth, a lump or thickening, a red or white patch or a non-healing ulcer. Later symptoms include interference with speech or swallowing, weight loss, trismus, an infected ulcer, pain referred to the ear, sensory disturbances and the appearance of a neck lump. Tumours may be of considerable size before the latter symptoms become apparent.

On examination, oral tumours have a variable appearance. They may present as a white or red patch, with or without an ulcer or erosion or as a lump or thickening with intact mucosa. Classically, the squamous cell carcinoma presents as an ulcer with a rolled margin with induration around it. There may be fixation to surrounding tissue and the ulcer may bleed readily after minor trauma. Tumours of the oropharynx and tongue base may first present as a neck lump. To make a diagnosis a biopsy is mandatory.

Staging of the disease

Cancer is staged using the TNM classification, where T measures the primary tumour size, N the draining lymph nodes, and M distant metastasis (Table 17.3). Using this classification, these can be further stratified to stages (Table 17.4). Using this universal language to identify the extent of disease helps provide a prognosis, which is dependent on stage. It also helps in defining treatment protocols and in the analysis of management and survival data. Knowing the extent of the disease is of prime importance for clinicians working in multidisciplinary teams so that the true extent of the disease is known.

Table 17.3 TNM staging	
Tx	Tumour cannot be assessed
T0	No evidence of primary tumour
T1	Tumour ≤2 cm in greatest dimension
T2	Tumour ≥2 cm but ≤4 cm
T3	Tumour >4 cm
T4	Tumour invading adjacent structures (e.g. skin, cortical bone, deep muscles of tongue)
Nx	Regional lymph nodes cannot be assessed
N0	No regional lymph nodes palpable
N1	Single ipsilateral lymph node ≤3 cm
N2a	Single ipsilateral node >3 cm but ≤6 cm
N2b	Multiple ipsilateral nodes ≤6 cm
N2c	Bilateral or contralateral ≤6 cm
N3	Any node >6 cm
Mx	Distant metastases cannot be assessed
M0	No evidence of distant metastases
M1	Distant metastases present

Table 17.4 American Joint Committee on Cancer Staging guidelines on clinical staging

Stage 0	Tis N0 M0
Stage 1	T1 N0 M0
Stage 2	T2 N0 M0
Stage 3	T3 N0 M0
	T1–3 N1 M0
Stage 4a	T4 N0–1 M0
Stage 4b	T1–4 N2–3 M0
Stage 4c	T1–4 N1–3 M1

The extent of the disease will determine the prognosis. The prognosis for stage 1 and 2 disease is good, with reported 5-year survivals rates of 85% and 70%, respectively. The outlook for stage 3 and 4 disease is much poorer, with survival rates of around 45% and 25%, respectively. The presence of lymph node metastases can reduce survival by 50% and lymph nodes displaying extra capsular spread reduces the 5-year survival to as low as 17%.

Initially, disease is staged clinically. However, clinical examination is a poor indicator of the actual extent of disease. Palpation of the neck is only sensitive and specific in around 66% of cases and detection of lymph nodes smaller than 2 cm is difficult, even under general anaesthetic.

Clinical investigation

Clinical examination

When a patient presents with oral cancer, the suspicion needs to be proven histologically. This is straightforward if the lesion is in the anterior part of the oral cavity and a biopsy can be harvested under a local anaesthetic. If this is not possible then it is performed during an examination under general anaesthetic. The examination under anaesthetic allows the surgeon to examine the oral cavity, oropharynx, nasopharynx, hypopharynx and larynx for second primary tumours and, as previously mentioned, the neck is also examined while the patient is relaxed. Fine-needle aspiration of any neck lumps can be carried out at this stage.

With oral cancer, almost 70% of second primaries occur elsewhere in the oral cavity or oropharynx. The major causes of tobacco and alcohol affect the whole of the aerodigestive tract. This suggests that the whole tract is at risk from cancer and more than one area can be affected at any one time. The term 'field change' was coined to describe situations where large areas of the upper aerodigestive tract are affected with malignant or premalignant change. For this reason, some units carry out bronchoscopy and oesophagoscopy at this time. However, these procedures show low pick-up rates for second primaries and tend to be used only when the patient has symptoms.

A tumour found initially is known as the index primary. If a second distinct primary tumour is found at the same time this is known as a simultaneous primary whereas a second tumour found within 6 months of the index tumour is known as a synchronous primary. Any second primary found after the initial 6-month period is described as a metachronous primary.

Most patients with oral cancer are likely to be heavy smokers and drinkers. It is important that all investigations necessary for deciding whether the patient is physically and mentally fit for treatment are carried out. Particular attention should be paid to the cardiovascular and respiratory systems, the nutritional status of the patient, and his or her social circumstances. A psychological assessment can also be of value. This is to allow an informed decision to be made on any further treatment.

Imaging

A plain chest radiograph provides useful information because many patients suffer from chronic obstructive airways disease and some even have a second tumour. An orthopantomogram with other views of the mandible (e.g. occlusal views) provides information on the condition and thickness of the mandible and the state of dentition, and is an essential part in planning treatment for oral cancer. Sophisticated techniques such as computerised tomography (CT) scans or magnetic resonance imaging (MRI) are used for assessment of both the primary and metastatic disease. Many centres favour a CT scan from the diaphragm to the base of the skull to identify evidence of second primaries in the aerodigestive tract, the state of the lungs, and the extent of the primary disease and metastasis in the neck. An MRI scan is slightly more sensitive and specific than a CT scan for soft tissue imaging, with sensitivity up to 83% and specificity of around 85%. Positron emission tomography (PET) scanning is emerging as a useful method for detecting tumours, and also recurrence in previously treated areas, with sensitivities and specificities reported as slightly more than 90%. It is poor at anatomically defining tumours but images can be combined and superimposed on CT or MRI scans to help determine resection margins.

The use of lymphoscintigraphy techniques in determining nodal involvement and directing sentinel node biopsy (see below) is showing significant promise in determining malignant lymph nodes.

The multidisciplinary approach to treatment

The multidisciplinary approach to the treatment of oral and oropharyngeal cancer is now fundamental and all units treating this disease should have a team of specialists. The surgical disciplines of otolaryngology, plastic surgery and maxillofacial surgery should all be involved. A clinical or radiation oncologist with a specialist interest in head and neck malignancy is also mandatory. A specialist nurse, speech and language therapist and nutritionist should also be present and a cytopathologist should be on hand to give the result of any fine-needle aspirates while the patient waits in the clinic. A psychologist and social worker are also helpful in pre-treatment assessment and post-treatment rehabilitation.

This multidisciplinary clinic is where all new patients are assessed. In this environment, the patient's disease can be discussed and a treatment plan formed and put to the patient, based on all the information gleaned from the examination and special investigations. Family and social problems that might impact on treatment or quality of life following treatment should also be discussed. Patients who have been treated are also followed-up at this clinic and problems with ongoing care can be identified and treated.

Treatment planning

Although there have been advances in treatment, the survival rates have not really improved. However, techniques have helped to improve the quality of life for many cancer patients even if survival has not been prolonged.

Treatment comprises surgery, radiotherapy or combined treatment (particularly for larger or more aggressive tumours). These treatments have been the mainstay of oral cancer treatment for the last 50 years. Radiotherapy is given in divided doses, usually over a period of 6 weeks.

One local regime is to give 66 Gy in 33 fractions over a period of $6\frac{1}{2}$ weeks. Other forms of hyperfractionation can be given to reduce the length of treatment and increase the concentration of the radiotherapy effects.

Chemotherapy has a small role to play but, as new drugs are developed and the biology of the disease becomes more understood, its role may increase. Chemotherapy seems to be most effective when it is combined with radiotherapy concomitantly. Currently, the most effective drugs are platinum-based in combination with 5-fluorouracil. Synchronous chemoradiotherapy seems to show some survival advantages as well as improved function in large posterior tumours.

Brachytherapy, or implanted radiotherapy elements, to the local site may be used to deliver a high dose of radiotherapy to the index primary tumour while sparing the surrounding tissues (e.g. the salivary glands). Plastic tubes are looped through the tumour from the neck and, after volumetric planning has been carried out, can be loaded with radioactive wires. If the wires are too far apart then insufficient radiotherapy levels will be delivered to the tumour. Conversely, if the wires are too close then tissue necrosis will ensue. Brachytherapy is an important option for treating the tongue, particularly the posterior tongue, because it allows function to be preserved. The most common side-effect from brachytherapy treatment is pain at the tumour site.

The positive neck is usually treated surgically with the addition of postoperative radiotherapy dependent on the extent of neck disease.

In the UK, if combined therapy is required then the surgery is carried out first in most cases.

When dealing with oral and oropharyngeal tumours, it is critical that surgical margins should be clear of tumour by more that 5 mm on the pathological specimen, because this will have a considerable bearing on the outcome. It has been shown that survival rates are reduced by 10% on similar tumours, despite all other remedial treatment, if the tumour is not completely excised. Many factors seen on the pathological specimen will affect the outcome and a specialist pathology service is therefore mandatory. Tumour thickness, perineural invasion, vascular invasion, lymphatic invasion, differentiation of the tumour cells and whether the invasive front is cohesive are important in deciding further treatment. Tumour thickness has a bearing on the prognosis, with tumours less than 2 mm thick having a much better prognosis than those with a tumour thickness greater than 4 mm. If the invasive front is cohesive then the prognosis is better than that with a non-cohesive front, while perineural invasion has been associated with local recurrence. Not surprisingly, lymphatic invasion is associated with spread to the lymph nodes whereas vascular invasion increases the likelihood of distant metastases. When surgery is performed then the decision to give postoperative radiotherapy may not be made until the final pathology is reviewed.

Treatment of the neck

Treatment of the neck in oral and oropharyngeal malignancy has raised a lot of debate in recent years. The neck is divided into seven levels to describe the position of the regional lymph node basin (Fig. 17.2). Only levels I to V need to be considered when discussing oral malignancy; levels VI and VII tend to be associated with thyroid and parathyroid tumours.

Some definitions need to be discussed when referring to neck dissections. A therapeutic neck dissection takes place when disease is obviously present in the neck and the dissection is undertaken to ablate the disease. An elective neck dissection is used to describe a neck dissection that is undertaken when there is no obvious disease in the neck but there is a high chance of occult disease being present or where the neck is opened for access. This type of neck dissection has become more common since the advent of free tissue transfer, during which the neck needs to be opened to facilitate microvascular reconstruction of the oropharyngeal defect. Many terms have been used to describe neck dissections, such as 'functional', 'supraomohyoid', 'lateral', 'radical', 'extended radical' and 'modified radical'. These terms are confusing and can mean different things to different people. It is now proposed that two terms are used to describe neck dissections:

- If five levels have been removed then this should be described as a comprehensive neck dissection.
- Anything less than five levels should be termed a selective dissection.

As with all neck dissections, the preserved structures should be described and the dissected levels should be named in selective dissections. This system tends to remove any ambiguity when describing the dissection carried out. In comprehensive neck dissections, the accessory nerve should be saved if possible, but not at the expense of good oncological resection, as sacrifice of this nerve leads to poor shoulder function and pain. Other structures, such as the internal jugular vein and sternocleidomastoid, should also be spared if possible.

Surgery is usually the initial treatment for the overtly positive neck with the possible exception of advanced neck disease (N_3) where preoperative radiotherapy or chemotherapy can be used to shrink the mass prior to surgical intervention. For positive disease, most surgeons favour some form of comprehensive neck dissection, attempting to save vital structures wherever possible, without compromising the oncological resection. Management of the N_0 neck and the role of elective neck dissection has been subject to considerable debate. There is some evidence that elective neck dissection confers a survival advantage over monitoring the patient and carrying out a subsequent therapeutic neck dissection when overt disease develops. Many centres adopt the protocol where, if the likelihood of metastatic disease is higher than 20%, elective neck dissection should be considered.

In the clinically N_0 neck, it is perfectly acceptable to carry out some form of selective neck dissection and, for oral cancer, most surgeons dissect only levels I to IV because metastasis in level V in a clinically negative neck is exceptionally rare. All vital structures should be spared to maintain as near normal function as possible but it is important to realise that neck dissection is likely to incur some morbidity no matter how carefully the dissection is carried out.

Sentinel node biopsy is currently under investigation but offers a promising way forward for dealing with the

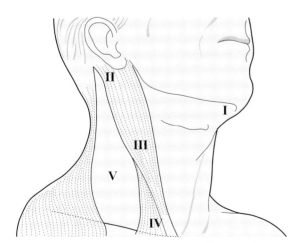

Fig. 17.2 The seven levels of the neck. Showing the position of the regional lymph node basin (level VI is deep and level VII is lower midline; not shown).

clinically N_0 neck. The basis of sentinel node biopsy is that tumour will migrate to the regional nodes and will first collect in a node called the sentinel node. The sentinel node can be identified by using a triple diagnostic approach of lymphoscintigraphy, injection of blue dye and a hand-held gamma probe for localisation at the time of surgery. This offers a relatively easy way of harvesting the sentinel node for histological analysis. If the node turns out to be positive for metastatic tumour, the patient goes on to have a neck dissection.

Reconstruction in the head and neck region

The main aim of reconstruction around the head and neck is to maintain form and function. Many techniques have evolved over the years, resulting in improvements in function and cosmesis and allowing larger and more complex defects to be reconstructed. Despite this, survival rates have not improved, although quality of life is much better. Depending on the defect, a reconstruction ladder can be used, starting with the simplest and leading to the most complex techniques.

A basic principle of reconstruction is to replace like tissue with like. Unfortunately, this is rarely possible in replacing oral mucosal lining, which is very specific. The oral mucosa is moist, sensate, and has specialised receptors for taste. It is sometimes fixed to bone, as in the gingiva and hard palate, or is elastic and freely mobile, as in the buccal area, ventral surface of tongue and floor of mouth. As there is no ideal replacement for oral mucosa, most techniques rely on importing skin. The disadvantage of this is that skin is dry, often insensate, and has no specialised receptors for taste. Often, the best that can be achieved is to restore the anatomy of the oral cavity in an effort to maintain form and function.

Primary closure

Primary closure is the simplest form of reconstruction and is particularly helpful in lip reconstruction. It is possible to resect up to one-third to one-half of the lip without using any flap reconstruction. Primary closure is also used after resection of small tumours of the mobile tongue, floor of mouth and buccal mucosa. Superficial tumours can be excised using a carbon dioxide or KTP laser (see Ch. 38). The use of a laser allows the excision or ablation of tumours without reconstruction, the

wound healing by a mixture of contacture and re-epithelialisation. One problem with laser excision is that any resection specimen will have thermal damage and pathological examination of margins will be impossible. In theory, scarring is less and, if selection of the tumour is correct, then function will be minimally affected. Re-epithelialisation is most effective where there is no possibility of contracture. Raw surfaces can be left in the hard palate, for example, which will re-epithelialise over a period of time.

Skin grafts

It is perhaps surprising that skin grafts can take successfully within the contaminated and wet environment of the oral cavity. They are best used as split thickness grafts and in situations where there is a well-vascularised graft bed such as the muscle of the tongue. The grafts are fixed by sutures, using a quilting technique to avoid shearing during movement of the oral cavity. Grafts are also useful for increasing the height of the labial sulci as in vestibuloplasty where they can be held in position by fixed splints.

Other methods of reconstruction, including local and distant flaps, are discussed in Chapter 15.

Quality of life issues

As mentioned previously, survival has not improved significantly over the past 20 years and one of the main treatment goals is to improve the quality of life for oral cancer patients. The problem is how to measure quality of life. This is now being resolved with questionnaires to try to assess this aspect of treatment. These questionnaires look at psychological and social aspects of patients' lives as well as functional performance. The two questionnaires usually used are The European Organisation for Recognition and Treatment of Cancer (EORTC) and The University of Washington Quality of Life Questionnaire (UW-QOL). The EORTC contains general questionnaires for all cancers and a head and neck module specifically for cancer in that region, whereas the UW-QOL is a head-and-neck-specific questionnaire. With the use of these questionnaires it is becoming easier to recognise which treatments help or adversely affect quality of life. This area of cancer management is still in its infancy, but will generate a lot of interest and will help define the best treatments in the future.

18 Otorhinolaryngology (ENT) surgery

Introduction

Otorhinolaryngology, more commonly known as ear, nose and throat (ENT) surgery, deals with conditions affecting the head and neck, upper aerodigestive tract and organs of special sense. The range of conditions managed by ENT surgeons is vast and includes conditions as diverse as neonatal airway obstruction, cerebellopontine angle tumours and cosmetic rhinoplasty. The scope of ENT reviewed in this chapter has been limited to that which may be encountered in dental and oral surgical practice. Relevant conditions include those affecting the pharynx, nose, paranasal sinuses and neck. Special attention is given to management of airway obstruction and aspects of head and neck malignancy (Table 18.1).

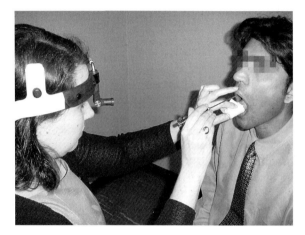

Fig. 18.1 Examination of the larynx and pharynx using traditional headlight indirect laryngoscopy.

Techniques of examination in ENT

Like dental surgeons, ENT practitioners can see most of the organs and areas of interest. Even areas that are not easily or directly visualised, such as the larynx and paranasal sinuses, can be examined indirectly using specialised instrumentation such as mirrors and endo-scopes. The special techniques of physical examination in ENT are difficult to master and trainees in the specialty spend many months acquiring the basic skills needed to view the larynx, nasopharynx and posterior nasal cavity. Traditionally, the pharynx and larynx have been examined using mirrors and headlight illumination (Fig. 18.1), but recently fibreoptic and rigid endoscopes have superseded these techniques (Fig. 18.2).

After an initial review of emergency airway management we will consider some of the more common and relevant ENT conditions. For reasons of relevance and brevity, otology has been excluded.

Table 18.1   ENT conditions encountered in dental practice

Airway obstruction
Diseases of:
   pharynx
   nose
   paranasal sinuses
Neck
Epistaxis
Head and neck malignancy

Emergency management of upper airway obstruction

Perhaps the most challenging clinical situation is a patient with sudden, severe airway obstruction. Although

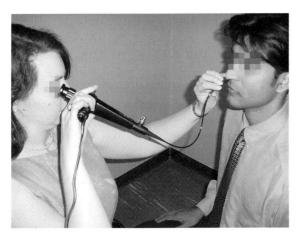

Fig. 18.2 Modern flexible fibreoptic nasopharyngolaryngoscopy.

this scenario is fortunately rare, it is important that clinicians operating in the oral cavity and pharynx have an awareness of the possible causes of acute airway compromise and have the necessary equipment and skill to deal with it. The laryngeal airway is a narrow and functionally complex system whose most important role is to separate and protect the airway from the digestive tract. The diameter of the space between the vocal cords (glottis) is such that even small foreign bodies can cause severe and life-threatening airway obstruction. This risk of airway obstruction is greater in children due to the relatively small dimensions of the juvenile larynx and the natural tendency for children to put toys, beads, pen-lids, etc. into their mouths. Other causes of acute airway obstruction are shown in Table 18.2.

Table 18.2 Causes of airway obstruction
Foreign bodies
food bolus
part of a toy, pen top
tooth
Infection
acute epiglottitis
Trauma
laryngotracheal trauma
orofacial trauma
Caustic inhalation/ingestion
Laryngeal tumour
carcinoma
papilloma

Acute airway obstruction

Sudden complete laryngeal obstruction is easily diagnosed, as severe respiratory distress is rapidly followed by cyanosis and collapse. More often, however, laryngeal obstruction is incomplete and is signified by a less dramatic increase in respiratory effort, difficulty speaking and stridor. Stridor is a coarse inspiratory noise produced as the patient attempts to inhale forcibly through a narrowing at the level of the larynx. Stridor is easily distinguished from stertor, which is a rattling gurgling noise produced by soft tissue obstruction or retained secretions at the level of the oropharynx.

Immediate management of laryngeal obstruction

Emergency management depends on the degree of obstruction and the level of expertise and equipment available to deal with it. Mild stridor requires urgent management but allows time for specialist help to be summoned, whereas acute severe respiratory collapse demands immediate on-the-spot treatment. It is important that all practitioners have a rehearsed plan and the necessary instrumentation available for dealing with catastrophic airway obstruction, even though most will never encounter such a case.

The options for treating are shown in Table 18.3. Of these techniques, only the Heimlich manoeuvre and laryngotomy are appropriate to non-specialist settings. Endotracheal intubation and tracheostomy require advanced skills and instrumentation.

Heimlich manoeuvre

The Heimlich manoeuvre is a technique for relieving airway obstruction caused by an impacted foreign body. If the patient can cough or speak, then the airway obstruction is incomplete and the Heimlich manoeuvre is not appropriate. Stand behind the patient with the arms encircling the patient's abdomen and crossed at the level of the patient's umbilicus. A forceable thrust upwards

Table 18.3 Treatment of laryngeal obstruction
Heimlich manoeuvre
Aspiration and endotracheal intubation
Laryngotomy (cricothyrotomy)
Tracheostomy

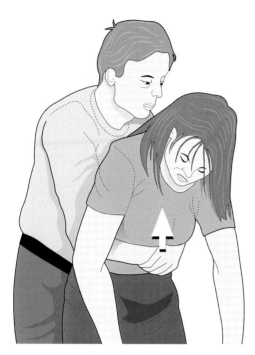

Fig. 18.3 The Heimlich manoeuvre.

and backwards is used to compress the patient's abdomen in an attempt to push the diaphragm upwards and expel the lodged foreign body (Fig. 18.3).

Laryngotomy

If all else fails and the patient is in extremis, an emergency surgical opening into the airway below the level of the vocal cords (most likely level of obstructing lesion) has to be created. The cricothyroid membrane provides an anatomical window for gaining access to the airway. Anaesthesia may not be appropriate as, by the time a decision is made to perform a laryngotomy, the patient is usually semiconscious.

For laryngotomy, full extension of the neck is essential. If the subject is a child, lay the patient across the knee of an assistant with the neck hyperextended and firmly palpate the midline structures of the neck. Starting from the prominence of the thyroid cartilage, run a finger down the midline until the prominent ring of the cricoid cartilage is palpated. Above the cricoid ring and below the lower border of the thyroid cartilage lies the cricothyroid membrane. With the neck sufficiently extended, there are no intervening structures between the cricothyroid membrane and the skin. As a first step, a wide-bore

needle or cannula can be inserted through the membrane into the airway and this may be sufficient to temporarily relieve the obstruction. A horizontal stab incision is then made using a knife or scalpel and, without withdrawing, the blade is turned through 90° to open the incision. Once the cricothyrotomy has been performed it can be held open using a small tube and, in some extreme situations, the outer cylinder of a pen has been used with success!

Specialised cricothyrotomy sets, which include a small-bore endotracheal tube and a specially designed scalpel, are commercially available. General dental practitioners and others carrying out procedures in the oropharynx in non-hospital settings would be well advised to purchase a cricothyrotomy kit and keep a small emergency tray set up in their surgery to deal with such an unlikely emergency.

The pharynx

Anatomy and physiology of the pharynx

The pharynx is a fibromuscular tube that constitutes the upper aerodigestive tract. It is formed by the buccopharyngeal fascia and the overlapping pharyngeal constrictor muscles, which extend from the level of the base of the skull to a lower limit at the sixth cervical vertebra (C6). At C6 the cricopharyngeus fibres of the inferior constrictor form the upper oesophageal sphincter. The pharynx is usually divided into three regions: the nasopharynx, oropharynx and hypopharynx.

The nasopharynx extends from the skull base to the level of the hard palate. It is lined by transitional respiratory epithelium and contains abundant lymphoid tissue. The main structures of clinical note in the nasopharynx are the nasopharyngeal tonsil, or adenoid, and the eustachian (pharyngotympanic) tubes, which communicate between the middle ear and the nasopharynx.

The oropharynx extends from the level of the hard palate to the hyoid bone and is lined by stratified squamous epithelium. Anteriorly, the oropharynx communicates with the oral cavity at the palatoglossal folds. Lymphoid tissue is abundant and, in the oropharynx, the most prominent aggregations of lymphoid tissue are the palatine tonsils and the lingual tonsils.

The hypopharynx extends from the level of the hyoid bone to the upper oesophageal sphincter (cricopharyngeus fibres of the inferior constrictor). It is lined by stratified squamous epithelium and communicates anteriorly with the larynx.

Benign conditions of the pharynx

Nasopharynx

The nasopharynx is often involved in upper respiratory tract infections, and the common cold is usually associated with nasopharyngitis. Symptoms of nasopharyngitis consist of discomfort and pain associated with swelling of the lymphoid tissue, which leads to nasal obstruction and seromucinous secretion more commonly referred to as catarrh. Nasopharyngitis is usually a self-limiting condition but, in some patients, chronic low-grade inflammation can occur, leading to nasal obstruction and chronic catarrh.

In children, the nasopharyngeal tonsil, or adenoid, can occupy almost all of the nasopharyngeal space. Acute respiratory infections can cause acute adenoiditis with mucopurulent postnasal discharge, nasal obstruction and fever. Such episodes of acute infective adenoiditis are common in childhood and may lead to chronic adenoidal hypertrophy, mouth breathing, nasal obstruction and chronic mucopurulent postnasal discharge. The juxtaposition of the eustachian tubes to hypertrophied and inflamed adenoids is thought to be important in the causation of middle-ear effusions. The adenoid may therefore be important in the most common cause of hearing impairment in childhood – otitis media with effusion, more frequently known as 'glue ear'. Children with enlarged and inflamed adenoids often have difficulty eating because they are obligate mouth breathers. Symptoms include disturbed sleep, nocturnal cough and middle-ear effusions. Adenoidectomy offers an effective treatment in such children.

The adenoid gradually atrophies with age and becomes relatively less important as the nasopharynx grows, thus adenoid problems in adults are rare. Symptoms suggestive of adenoidal hypertrophy in the adult should raise the suspicion of a nasopharyngeal tumour (see below).

Oropharynx

Acute infective oropharyngitis presents as a sore throat, pain on swallowing and fever. The cause is usually viral and the condition is self-limiting, responding to symptomatic measures such as paracetamol, saline gargles and a high fluid intake. Throat swabs seldom yield any significant growth. Severe, non-resolving pharyngitis should raise the possibility of glandular fever.

Chronic pharyngitis presents as persistent, dry, sore throat and irritation and discomfort on swallowing. Often the cause cannot be ascertained, but there appears to be an association with nasal disease. The treatment of chronic pharyngitis involves identification of the cause, treatment of any nasal disease, increased fluid intake and avoidance of antibiotics, as these can sometimes lead to secondary candidiasis. In some cases, topical nasal steroid sprays can help reduce the inflammation.

Tonsillitis

Acute tonsillitis is a common cause of a sore throat. Although the initial organism may be viral, super-infection with a beta-haemolytic *Streptococcus* usually ensues. Acute tonsillitis can also be a complication of glandular fever. The symptoms are sore throat, pain on swallowing (odynophagia), systemic malaise, headache and fever. Because of pain on swallowing, patients tend to avoid eating and drinking and, therefore, can become significantly dehydrated and debilitated. Diagnosis is usually obvious with trismus, tonsillar hypertrophy, and pus visible in the tonsillar crypts; there will be associated cervical adenitis. Treatment involves high fluid intake, analgesics and penicillin. In severe cases the patient may be unable to swallow oral antibiotics, thus, a short course of intravenous benzyl penicillin may be indicated (Fig. 18.4). Complications of tonsillitis include a peritonsillar abscess (quinsy).

Tonsillectomy

Tonsillectomy used to be an extremely common operation and was often used incorrectly as a treatment for non-specific sore throat (pharyngitis).

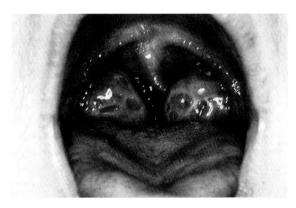

Fig. 18.4 Acute tonsillitis.

Tonsillectomy is carried out by dissecting the tonsils from their fossae and ligating any bleeding points encountered. The most frequent major complication is postoperative haemorrhage, which occurs in approximately 2% of cases. Minor secondary tonsillar haemorrhage can also occur up to 2 weeks after the operation and is usually managed conservatively using antibiotics and saline gargles.

Indicatons for tonsillectomy

Current indications for tonsillectomy include: a clear history suggesting that the sore throats are due to tonsillitis on five or more occasions per year over a period of at least 1 year, or evidence that these episodes of sore throat are disabling and preventing normal function at school or work.

Patients often complain of white or yellow lesions on their tonsils. These are foul tasting and may be associated with halitosis. Examination shows numerous white granules occupying the tonsillar crypts; these are often diagnosed incorrectly as food debris. In fact, the most frequent cause of this is actinomycotic colonies within the tonsillar crypts. Actinomycetes are normal oral commensals but in some patients they 'overgrow' and form so-called 'sulphur' granules within the tonsillar crypts. Patients often use antiseptic mouthwashes to try and cure the problem, but this may well be the cause rather than the cure! Treatment includes reassurance and the avoidance of antiseptic mouthwashes. Some patients, however, are significantly debilitated by this problem and this may be seen as a rare indication for tonsillectomy.

Tonsillectomy can also be used in the surgical treatment of snoring. Significant debilitating snoring, which can lead to extreme social distress, is related to obesity and, in some cases, tonsillar hypertrophy. Most surgical procedures for snoring involve modification and stiffening of the soft palate. The uvulopalatopharyngoplasty (UPPP) operation involves palatal shortening and tonsillectomy. However, there is no good evidence that snoring surgery is beneficial, as results are often poor and snoring recurs within 2 years of successful surgery in 60% of patients. Snoring alone is not an indication for tonsillectomy.

Prions have been demonstrated in tonsillar tissue from patients with new variant Creutzfeldt–Jakob disease (vCJD; see Ch. 7). Because of the potential risk of transmission of prion disease, disposable instruments are now recommended for all tonsillectomies.

Hypopharynx

Benign hypopharyngeal disease often presents as a feeling of something in the throat with or without dysphagia. An accurate history needs to be taken from all patients complaining of pharyngeal discomfort and dysphagia. Warning signs and symptoms are, weight loss, pain referred to the ear and dysphonia (hoarseness).

A common benign cause of 'a feeling of something in the throat' is the globus pharyngeus syndrome, which used to be referred to as globus hystericus. This condition is thought to be due to neurological incoordination of the cricopharyngeus muscle. It is more common in females and is not associated with pain, referred otalgia or weight loss. It is important to note that globus pharyngeus is a diagnosis of exclusion that is made only after normal endoscopy and/or normal barium swallow investigations.

A pharyngeal pouch is a diverticulum at the lower part of the pharynx. Cricopharyngeal spasm is implicated in its causation. Patients present with intermittent dysphagia and regurgitation of partially digested foodstuffs. A characteristic appearance is seen on a barium swallow (Fig. 18.5) and the diagnosis is confirmed at rigid endoscopy. Treatment of pharyngeal pouch can be carried out by open (excision) or endoscopic means (drainage of pouch into oesophagus).

Tumours of the pharynx

Tumours of the pharynx will be considered under benign and malignant lesions affecting the nasopharynx, the oropharynx and the hypopharynx in turn.

Nasopharynx

Benign tumours of the nasopharynx

Tumours of the nasopharynx present with symptoms that can be confused with adenoid enlargement or nasal obstruction. Thus, a high index of suspicion is required and all cases should undergo pernasal endoscopic examination.

Juvenile nasopharyngeal angiofibroma (JNA) is a benign vascular tumour that occurs in adolescent males. It presents with unilateral nasal obstruction and epistaxis.

diagnosis and treatment involves embolisation prior to resection.

Malignant tumours of the nasopharynx

Malignant tumours of the nasopharynx are, fortunately, uncommon. Symptoms include nasal obstruction, epistaxis and, in some patients, deafness due to a middle-ear effusion secondary to eustachian tube obstruction. In advanced cases, nasopharyngeal malignancy will invade the skull base and give rise to cranial nerve palsies. Nasopharyngeal cancer is usually squamous but poorly differentiated or anaplastic variants are not uncommon. Salivary gland tumours (adenoid cystic carcinoma) and non-Hodgkin's lymphoma also occur.

Nasopharygeal carcinoma is much more common in parts of Asia than in the UK. In Hong Kong, nasopharyngeal carcinoma is one of the most common head and neck malignancies, and its aetiology is thought to involve an interaction between infection with the Epstein–Barr virus and racial/genetic predisposition. Malignancy in the nasopharynx often metastasises early to upper deep cervical lymph nodes. Presentation is usually late and curative surgical treatment is seldom possible. Radical radiotherapy (with or without chemo-therapy) can give good results in those patients who are diagnosed in the early stages.

Oropharynx

Benign tumours of the oropharynx

Benign tumours of the oropharynx are relatively uncommon. Tonsillar inclusion cysts, which present as smooth, rounded swellings associated with the upper pole of the tonsil are commonly mistaken for tumours.

Viral papillomata can be found on the faucial pillars, tonsil and posterior pharyngeal wall. Their presence raises the possibility of coexisting laryngeal and genital papillomatosis. Treatment includes excision or laser ablation.

A lingual thyroid presents as a smooth swelling in the midline of the posterior one-third of the tongue. It is due to a thyroid developmental abnormality that results in persistence of thyroid tissue in the region of the foramen caecum.

Tumours of the minor salivary glands may also present in the oropharynx. Numerically they are most likely to be pleomorphic salivary adenomas, but low-grade

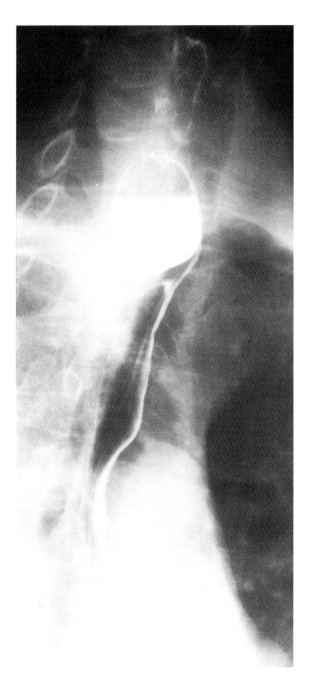

Fig. 18.5 Contrast radiograph of a pharyngeal pouch.

JNA is of unknown aetiology but hormonal influences associated with puberty are thought to be implicated. If a tumour is identified in a young male it is important to consider the possibility of a JNA because biopsy could prove catastrophic! MRI and angiography confirm the

mucoepidermoid tumours should also be considered (see Ch. 14).

Malignant tumours of the oropharynx

Malignant oropharyngeal tumours most commonly involve the tonsils. Squamous cell carcinoma is the most frequent histology and aetiological factors include alcohol and smoking. Tonsillar carcinoma often presents late with spread into the adjacent structures of the soft palate, tongue base and mandible. There is a high incidence of nodal spread to the deep cervical chain at the time of diagnosis. Early tonsillar carcinomas can be treated by radical radiotherapy. More advanced cases need major surgical resection, which involves mandibular splitting for surgical access. Excision of the tumour and adjacent involved structures (mandible, pharyngeal wall, tongue) and comprehensive neck dissection (Ch.17) is followed by reconstruction using radial artery free grafts or pectoralis major myocutaneous flaps (Ch. 15).

The oropharynx may also be the site of non-Hodgkin's and Hodgkin's lymphomas arising in the lingual and palatine tonsils. Treatment of lymphoma includes radiotherapy and chemotherapy.

Hypopharynx

Benign tumours of the hypopharynx

The hypopharynx consists of the piriform fossae, the posterior wall and the postcricoid region. Benign tumours of the hypopharynx are extremely unusual and present with symptoms similar to the globus sensation. Fibromas, schwannomas, papillomata and benign salivary tumours can all occur.

Malignant tumours of the hypopharynx

Although any hypopharyngeal site can be involved, the most common lesions affect the piriform fossa and postcricoid regions.

Piriform fossa tumours are predominantly squamous cell carcinomas. They present with vague symptoms of a feeling of 'something in the throat' and intermittent, variable dysphagia. As the tumour enlarges and invades adjacent structures the patient will present with otalgia due to referred pain. Dysphagia increases and weight loss and aspiration of secretions ensues. In a high proportion, the presenting feature is cervical lymphadenopathy due to nodal metastases. The symptoms of piriform fossa tumours are often relatively minor and it is therefore essential that a high index of suspicion is maintained. In particular, patients should not be diagnosed as suffering from globus pharyngeus unless a full endoscopic examination has been carried out. Piriform fossa tumours can be treated using radiotherapy (if diagnosed early enough), but advanced disease requires laryngectomy, partial pharyngectomy and reconstruction. Adjuvant radiotherapy is usually required and comprehensive neck dissection is used to treat nodal disease.

Postcricoid carcinoma has a presentation similar to other hypopharyngeal conditions. Dysphagia is severe and progressive, with weight loss in advanced cases. Clinical examination reveals pooling of secretions in the hypopharynx and patients will often have cervical adenopathy. Examination under anaesthesia and biopsy through rigid hypopharyngoscopes establishes the diagnosis. Staging relies on the findings at examination under anaesthesia and computerised tomography (CT) or magnetic resonance imaging (MRI) results (see Ch. 17). Early-stage disease can be treated using radical external beam radiotherapy but more advanced cases require surgery. Due to a high incidence of synchronous oesophageal malignancy (skip lesions) concomitant resection of the oesophagus and gastric or free jejunal interposition is the surgical treatment of choice.

Larynx

Benign and malignant disease of the larynx will be considered after a review of its anatomy and functions.

Anatomy and physiology of the larynx

The larynx occupies the junction between the common aerodigestive and respiratory tracts. The basic framework of the larynx consists of the thyroid cartilage articulating superiorly with the hyoid bone and inferiorly with the cricoid bone. Superiorly, the epiglottis and aryepiglottic folds form the laryngeal inlet region, which leads down to the middle section of the larynx consisting of the false and true vocal cords. The false vocal cords, or vestibular folds, lie above and parallel to the true vocal cords and are separated from them by the shallow gutter of the laryngeal ventricle. The principal nerve supply to the larynx comes from the recurrent laryngeal branch of the vagus nerve, which reaches the larynx after looping round the arch of the aorta on the left, and round the subclavian artery on the right. The blood supply is derived from branches of the superior and inferior thyroid arteries, lymphatic drainage is to the upper deep cervical nodes superiorly, lower deep cervical nodes inferiorly, and pre-thyroid nodes anteriorly.

The functions of the larynx are phonation and protection of the lower airway.

Disorders of the larynx may impair the ability of the vocal cords to adduct, resulting in aspiration and weakness of the voice. Inability to abduct the vocal cords to produce a satisfactory laryngeal airway may result in airway compromise which will present as stridor and shortness of breath. Lesions of or on the vocal cords will alter vocal cord tension and resonance leading to hoarseness (dysphonia) as the presenting symptom.

Examination of the larynx

Traditional indirect laryngoscopy used headlight illumination and an angled mirror. The technique is difficult and some patients are unable to tolerate the examination. It is more common today to examine the larynx using a fibreoptic laryngoscope passed via the nasal cavity (see Fig. 18.2). This produces an excellent view of the vocal cords and allows function to be assessed under direct vision.

Benign laryngeal disease

Acute laryngitis

Acute laryngitis is common and often accompanies upper respiratory tract infections, especially if associated with simultaneous voice abuse and ingestion of irritants. Alcohol, cigarettes and voice abuse (shouting or singing) can cause acute inflammation of the vocal cords, as can mechanical and chemical irritation. The patient complains of hoarseness and a mild sore throat, sometimes with pain on swallowing. In the absence of bacterial superinfection, acute irritant laryngitis usually settles with voice rest, a high fluid intake and simple analgesics. If associated with an upper respiratory tract infection, acute laryngitis may progress to bacterial infection, which will present with more severe symptoms and fever. Diagnosis is made on fibreoptic endoscopy. Treatment involves broad-spectrum antibiotics. Failure to respond within 2 weeks is an indication for referral to an ENT department.

Chronic laryngitis

Chronic, painless dysphonia is more common in people who smoke and in those who use their voice to excess such as, amateur singers, teachers and lecturers. In its simplest form, chronic laryngitis is associated with non-specific, low-grade inflammatory thickening of the vocal cords. This produces an alteration in voice quality that responds slowly to conservative measures. Severe cases can progress to Reinke's oedema of the subepithelial space of the vocal cord. This leads to severe dysphonia and, on examination, swollen oedematous vocal cords are evident. In extreme cases Reinke's oedema can produce severe polypoid swelling of the vocal cords.

Vocal nodules are another feature of chronic laryngitis and appear as small fibrotic thickenings of the central portion of the vocal cord. Excision can be carried out using endoscopic microsurgical techniques, or with endoscopic laser therapy.

Vocal cord papilloma

Viral papillomata of the larynx due to the human papilloma virus can affect all ages but are more common in children and young adults than in older people. The usual presentation is dysphonia but papillomatosis can also cause respiratory distress.

Vocal cord palsy

Vocal cord palsy presents as painless dysphonia and a characteristic 'bovine' cough. It is caused by damage to either recurrent laryngeal nerve. Left recurrent laryngeal nerve damage is more common due to its longer course in the thorax. The most common cause of a left vocal cord palsy is a bronchial cancer and, in all patients presenting with a palsy, a chest radiograph is mandatory. Other causes of vocal cord palsy include inadvertent damage to the recurrent laryngeal nerve during thyroid or cardiothoracic surgery.

Malignant tumours of the larynx

Cancer of the larynx is the most common head and neck malignancy encountered by ENT surgeons. Any of the laryngeal subsites (supraglottis, glottis or subglottis) can be involved but in the UK the glottis is the most common site. Even very small tumours involving the vocal cords produce significant dysphonia. The dysphonia produced by a laryngeal cancer is indistinguishable from that produced by a vocal nodule or chronic laryngitis and, therefore, all patients with hoarseness should be treated seriously and early referral in those who do not resolve should be routine. Laryngeal cancer is more common in heavy smokers than in non-smokers, and alcohol intake appears to be synergistic in supraglottic disease. Patients present with dysphonia and, in advanced cases, with respiratory compromise. Squamous cell carcinoma is the usual histology.

Investigation includes indirect or endoscopic laryngoscopy.

The treatment of laryngeal carcinoma depends on the site and stage of the disease. Early tumours can be effectively treated using courses of radical radiotherapy. More advanced cases of laryngeal carcinoma almost invariably require total laryngectomy followed by adjuvant radical radiotherapy and comprehensive neck dissection to eradicate disease.

Following total laryngectomy, speech rehabilitation is required. The most common technique employs a one-way tracheopharyngeal speaking valve, which is placed between the back wall of the trachea and the reconstructed pharynx. This allows the patient to exhale air from the trachea into the pharynx. The shunted air moves the pharyngeal walls and produces vibrations, which can then be modulated into a form of speech. Most patients following total laryngectomy manage to achieve good voice rehabilitation using these valves.

Nose

Anatomy and physiology of the nose

The nose is divided by the piriform aperture into an anterior (facial) component and a posterior nasal cavity. Both components are subdivided into right and left by the nasal septum. The nasal septum is predominantly bony in the posterior cavity and cartilaginous anteriorly. The external nose is covered by skin, subcutaneous tissue and a musculoaponeurotic layer. The upper 40% of the external nose consists of paired nasal bones, which articulate with each other and with the frontal processes of the maxillae and the maxillary processes of the frontal bones. The lower 60% of the external nose is cartilaginous consisting of the paired upper lateral cartilages and lower lateral cartilages.

Posteriorly, the right and left nasal cavities are separated by the nasal septum, which forms their medial wall. The nasal cavities communicate with the naso-pharynx behind and with the nostrils anteriorly. The lateral nasal walls are formed by the inferior middle and superior turbinates with their associated meatuses. The nasal floor is the hard palate and the roof of the nasal cavity lies in the region of the cribriform plate. The nasal cavity has a particularly rich blood supply that is derived from both the external and internal carotid circulations, a feature that is in part responsible for the frequency of spontaneous nasal bleeding (epistaxis).

The nose has five principal physiological functions (Table 18.4).

Nasal malfunction leads to dry, cold, unfiltered air reaching the nasopharynx with resultant risks of inflammation and secondary infection. Nasal conditions can therefore manifest as rhinorrhoea, nasal airway obstruction, pharyngitis and mouth breathing, and abnormalities of olfaction (hyposmia).

Causes of nasal obstruction

Rhinitis

Rhinitis is defined as inflammation of the lining of the nose characterised by one or more of the following symptoms: nasal congestion, rhinorrhoea or sneezing and itching. There are many different causes of rhinitis but the most prevalent is the common cold (Table 18.5).

Table 18.4 Functions of the nose
Airway
Filter
Humidification
Heat exchange (warming inspired air)
Olfaction

Table 18.5 A simplified classification of rhinitis
Allergic
seasonal and perennial
Infectious
acute and chronic
Other
idiopathic
occupational
medicamentosa
hormonal
vasomotor

The treatment of rhinitis depends on the cause. The common cold is usually self-limiting and responds to the short-term use of topically applied decongestants (ephedrine or xylometazoline), which most patients self prescribe. Most other forms of chronic rhinitis respond to potent topical steroids such as beclomethasone or mometasone, but these drugs should not be used without medical supervision. Persistent nasal obstruction, rhinorrhoea and nasal congestion, especially if unilateral, should be seen as a reason for referral to a specialist.

Septal deviation following nasal trauma

The quadrilateral cartilage of the septum may be fractured, resulting in a septal deviation that can give rise to nasal obstruction. Characteristically, this produces unilateral nasal obstruction and examination reveals a convexity of the septum touching the lateral nasal wall. The unilateral nature of the symptoms helps distinguish this from rhinitis. Treatment consists of the operation of septoplasty, which resects and straightens the quadrilateral cartilage, perpendicular plate of ethmoid and vomer, and thus recentralises the septum.

Nasal polyps

Nasal polyps are inflammatory masses that originate predominantly from the lining of the ethmoid sinuses. Polyps are more common in patients with asthma and, in a proportion of patients, there is an association with aspirin allergy. Symptoms are similar to severe rhinitis, with total nasal obstruction, hyponasal speech, hyposmia and nasal discharge. Diagnosis is usually easy on nasal examination. Polyps should be referred for specialist assessment to exclude tumour. Topical or systemic corticosteroid medication can shrink polyps but surgical removal is often required, followed by topical medication to prevent recurrence.

Foreign bodies

Children often put foreign bodies into their nose. The classic presentation is of unilateral, foul-smelling rhinorrhoea (oezena). Common foreign bodies include pieces of foam rubber mattress or pillow, organic matter such as peas, and parts of toys, beads, etc. Often, by the time of presentation there is a secondary vestibular infection, which makes the nose very tender to touch and makes

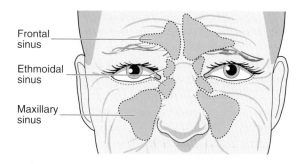

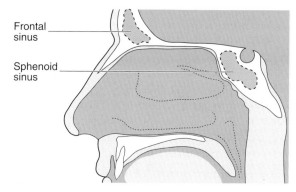

Fig. 18.6   The paranasal sinuses.

instrumental removal difficult. A suspected foreign body is a reason for specialist referral and children will occasionally require general anaesthesia for its removal.

Paranasal sinuses

The nose and paranasal sinuses can be considered to be a single functional unit. There are eight main paranasal sinuses, all of which drain into the nasal cavity. Six major sinuses drain into the narrow middle nasal meatus, which is, therefore, a key area in the causation and treatment of sinus disease. Figure 18.6 shows the general positioning and relationship of the maxillary, ethmoid, frontal and sphenoid sinuses.

Sinusitis

Sinusitis may be acute or chronic, inflammatory or infective.

Acute inflammatory sinusitis is seen in patients with acute seasonal allergic rhinitis, commonly known as hay fever. As such, this condition is seldom diagnosed and the treatment relies on treating the inflammatory rhinitis with topical antihistamines and decongestants. It is only once inflammatory rhinitis becomes chronic and sinus outflow tracts become blocked with oedematous, swollen mucosa that chronic inflammatory sinusitis sets in.

Chronic inflammatory sinusitis occurs in people with allergic nasal conditions (asthma, allergic rhinitis, aspirin sensitivity). It is usually associated with an allergic or inflammatory rhinitis, which is characterised by boggy swelling of the nasal mucosa. Patients present with nasal obstruction, a feeling of congestion, pressure between the eyes and over the nasal bridge and postnasal discharge of mucus. Treatment includes long-term low-dose topical nasal corticosteroids. Antihistamines may be of value in acute flare-ups.

Acute infective sinusitis is an almost universal occurrence during the common cold. This is due to rhinovirus infection and is usually a self-limiting condition needing only general supportive measures in the form of analgesics and nasal decongestants. Topical nasal decongestants (e.g. ephedrine) are preferred over systemic versions. Secondary bacterial infection of ethmoid, maxillary, frontal or, less frequently, sphenoid sinuses can occur following viral infection. Bacterial sinusitis is characterised by pain, which may be severe, and poorly localised (either to the forehead or malar region). There will be a swinging pyrexia with purulent rhinorrhea. Patients often complain of upper dental pain due to involvement of the maxillary sinus. Acute infective sinusitis is a common sequel to an upper respiratory tract infection and should be seen as a potentially serious condition. Treatment with local topical decongestants and systemic antibiotics is required and failure to improve within 3 weeks necessitates specialist referral. Although most cases of infective sinusitis respond to the above measures, some go on to develop complications such as orbital cellulitis, orbital abscess, frontal lobe abscess, meningitis or cavernous sinus thrombosis.

Plain sinus radiographs have little or no role in the investigation of sinusitis, which is mainly a clinical and endoscopic diagnosis. Nasal endoscopy will often reveal oedema and pus in the region of the middle meatus. Failure to respond to conservative measures is an indication for surgical drainage of the infected sinus either via an external or endoscopic intranasal route.

Chronic infective sinusitis may occur in some patients as a result of an anatomical abnormality or an unresolved or inadequately treated infection. Chronic sepsis is most common in ethmoid and maxillary sinuses and less frequently observed in the frontal or sphenoid sinuses.

Bacterial infection results in oedema and secondary development of polypoid mucosa, which ensures that the sinus ostia remain blocked, impeding sinus drainage, which in turn prevents resolution of the infection. Symptoms include nasal obstruction, chronic foul smelling rhinorrhea or postnasal discharge. Specialist referral is required and evaluation will include nasal endoscopy and CT scanning of the sinuses. Surgical treatment of chronic infective sinusitis aims to secure unobstructed mucociliary drainage from the major sinuses. Modern surgical approaches are referred to as functional endoscopic sinus surgery (FESS). FESS aims to remove obstructing hyperplastic tissue from the region of the natural sinus ostia in the middle nasal meatus to enable drainage of purulent secretions.

Paranasal sinus tumours

Fortunately, tumours of the paranasal sinuses are uncommon. The most frequently involved sinus is the maxillary, with the ethmoid being the second most common site.

Maxillary sinus carcinoma

Carcinoma of the maxillary antrum usually presents late as the volume of the sinus allows the tumour to enlarge without causing symptoms. Presentation, therefore, usually occurs only when the tumour invades beyond the margins of the maxillary sinus. Symptoms are due to invasion medially into the nasal cavity, superiorly into the floor of the orbit and laterally into the cheek, and inferiorly, into the upper alveolus. Thus, the patient may present with swelling of the cheek, unilateral epistaxis, unilateral nasal obstruction or diplopia. Histology is typically squamous cell carcinoma, but poorly differentiated or anaplastic variants are common. Diagnosis is made on nasal examination, nasal endoscopy and CT scanning. Treatment includes radical surgical excision in the form of total maxillectomy with or without orbital clearance, followed by radical radiotherapy and treatment of nodal disease.

Ethmoid carcinoma

Ethmoid carcinoma is less common than maxillary sinus carcinoma but, similarly, presents late. Invasion of the medial orbital wall, nasal cavity and anterior skull base leads to the presenting symptoms. Nasal obstruction and epistaxis is universal. There is thought to be an aetiological association with exposure to lignins, which are contained within certain hardwoods. Thus, ethmoidal carcinoma has features of an occupational disease in carpenters. Diagnosis and treatment is similar to maxillary sinus carcinoma.

The prognosis in sinus carcinoma is poor.

Epistaxis

Epistaxis is defined as spontaneous bleeding from the nasal cavity. It is an extremely common condition and most people will at some point in their life suffer from a nosebleed. The range of severity is vast, from the mild self-limiting nosebleed experienced by most people, to severe torrential arterial haemorrhage that carries a significant mortality and morbidity. Epistaxis can be classified into two main groups: childhood and adult.

Childhood epistaxis

Childhood epistaxis is common from age four. It is characteristically minor but none the less alarming. Nosebleeds occur sporadically, with a predilection for nocturnal bleeding. The source of the bleeding is usually on the anterior nasal septum at a rich vascular plexus known as Little's area. This location has led some to believe that nose-picking is the main cause, although there is evidence to suggest other causes may be important. The management of childhood epistaxis includes pinching the nostrils over the soft, lower lateral cartilages, which produces direct pressure over Little's area (the Hippocratic method). Once bleeding has stopped, some antibiotic ointment can be applied to the anterior nares to reduce any associated vestibulitis. Cutting the child's fingernails can also help. Persistent or recurrent nosebleeds in children should be referred for specialist opinion, which will usually lead to the offending blood vessel being identified and cauterised.

Adult epistaxis

Adult epistaxis can be a potentially life-threatening condition, which has a peak age of onset of 60 years. This type of epistaxis is characterised by sudden unilateral severe arterial bleeding. Bleeding in adults often comes from arterial branches of the sphenopalatine artery in the posterior reaches of the nasal cavity. This has led to the term 'posterior epistaxis' being used. Not

surprisingly, this condition does not respond to direct digital pressure over the ala-nasi (Hippocratic method). The management of a severe epistaxis relies on resuscitation of the patient followed by attempts to identify the source of the bleeding. The nose is examined using a headlight, nasal speculum and suction. It is often difficult to identify the bleeding point because of its posterior position. If the source cannot be found, otolaryngologists use endoscopes to examine the posterior nasal cavity and identify the bleeding vessel, which can then be cauterised under direct endoscopic vision. In the absence of specialised equipment, posterior epistaxis is usually managed by some form of tamponade, using either specially designed balloon catheters or nasal packing. Admission to hospital is required and a search for aetiological factors should be undertaken (aspirin use, alcohol excess, thrombocytopenia). Unlike childhood epistaxis, which is recurrent, adult epistaxis tends to be characterised by a single severe episode of bleeding.

The neck

Anatomy

The neck is divided into three zones: an anterior triangle with its apex inferiorly and two posterior triangles with their apices superiorly. The anterior triangle is bounded laterally by the anterior border of the sternomastoid muscles. Superiorly, its base is formed by the mandible and, inferiorly, the apex lies in the region of the sternal notch. The posterior triangles are bounded anteriorly by the posterior border of the sternomastoid muscle, posteriorly by the anterior border of trapezius, inferiorly by the clavicle, and the apices lie posterosuperiorly in the region of the occiput and mastoid processes. Figure 18.7 shows the triangles of the neck with the associated lymph node groups that they contain. Neck swellings are common clinical problems and it is important that a diagnostic strategy is used when dealing with such swellings. The majority of neck swellings are to be found in the anterior triangle and a simple strategy can be used to subclassify into midline: upper or lower, and lateral: upper or lower swellings.

Metastatic nodal disease in the neck

It is important to realise that the lymph node chains of the neck are frequently involved in metastatic spread from

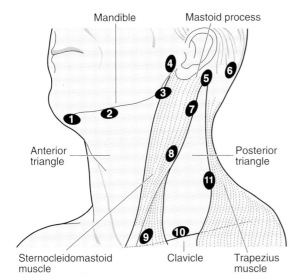

Fig. 18.7 Triangles of the neck and associated lymph nodes. 1, submental nodes; 2, submandibular nodes; 3, jugulodiagastric nodes; 4, parotid/facial nodes; 5, mastoid nodes; 6, occipital nodes; 7, upper deep cervical nodes; 8, mid deep cervical nodes; 9, lower deep cervical nodes; 10, supraclavicular nodes; 11, posterior triangle nodes.

cancers of the upper aerodigestive tract and head and neck. It is, therefore, essential that any patient with an unexplained swelling in the neck is investigated carefully to exclude a carcinoma of the head and neck. Examination of the oral cavity, oropharynx and nasopharynx, and fibreoptic examination of the larynx and hypopharynx are essential when assessing lymph node swellings. Indeed, an isolated lymph node is a common presentation for tumours of the piriform fossa and nasopharynx.

It used to be common practice to biopsy or excise lymph nodes to obtain a diagnosis. The practice of diagnostic excision biopsy of lymph nodes in the head and neck is generally considered obsolete now that highly reliable fine-needle aspiration cytology is available. The procedure of fine-needle aspiration cytology can distinguish between malignant and non-malignant adenopathy in over 90% of cases. If a malignant cytology aspirate is obtained, an examination under anaesthesia is required in combination with detailed imaging of the upper aerodigestive tract, head and neck, and chest. Once a primary has been identified, planned curative treatment can be carried out with nodal disease being treated by radical radiotherapy or neck dissection. Excision of an undiagnosed lymph node, only to later discover that it

contains squamous carcinoma, is highly undesirable as the risks of skin implantation with tumour are significantly increased and further curative resection will be compromised.

Lymphoma involving nodes of the neck is an exception to the above. Once lymphoma has been diagnosed (using fine needle aspiration cytology), node sampling is usually requested in order to histologically type the lymphoma. However, sampling a known lymphomatous node after positive cytology is different from exploratory biopsy of an undiagnosed, possibly carcinomatous, node.

Midline swellings

A midline swelling in the upper neck can represent a submental lymphadenopathy secondary to oral or dental sepsis. However, the possibility of metatastatic nodal spread has to be borne in mind in all patients presenting with a neck lump and, in the upper neck, a thorough examination of the oral cavity is essential.

In children, dermoid cysts can present in the upper midline neck, and these developmental cysts may contain squamous debris, hair and even teeth! A midline swelling in the region of the hyoid bone may represent a thyroglossal cyst. This is a developmental abnormality with cystic thyroid tissue persisting along the thyroglossal duct. A thyroglossal cyst characteristically moves upwards on tongue protrusion due to a continuity of the cyst with the thyroglossal tract leading to the foramen caecum of the tongue. In the lower neck, midline swellings are most frequently related to the thyroid gland. Clinically, it is usually easy to distinguish between swelling *of* the thyroid gland and a swelling *in* the thyroid gland. Swellings of the thyroid gland may be due to simple goitre but thyroid cancer must be excluded. Diagnosis is made by fine-needle aspiration cytology and appropriate use of magnetic resonance imaging and radio-isotope scanning. Occasionally, an early laryngeal cancer presents with metastatic spread to the midline pretracheal or Delphian node.

Lateral neck swellings

Lateral swellings in the upper neck may represent disease of the submandibular salivary gland or inflammatory or metastatic adenopathy of the submandibular, tonsillar and upper deep cervical nodes. Inflammatory or neoplastic disease of the parotid gland can also present as an upper neck lump. In all of these conditions clinical examination of the upper aerodigestive tract and judicious use of fine-needle cytology will elucidate the diagnosis.

A smooth, firm swelling at the anterior border of the sternomastoid near the junction of its upper and middle third is characteristic of a branchial cyst. These are thought to be developmental abnormalities and are, therefore, more common in children and young adults than in older people. Diagnosis is confirmed by fine-needle aspiration, which produces turbid, straw-coloured fluid, the cytology of which reveals cholesterol crystals. Treatment of a branchial cyst is by surgical excision.

In elderly patients, atheromatous or even aneurysmal carotid arteries can present as a pulsatile lateral neck swelling. Auscultation will often reveal a bruit, and ultrasound or MRI can confirm the diagnosis. If a carotid aneurysm is suspected, then fine-needle cytology should not be performed!

The lower lateral neck is a very common site for metastatic adenopathy. Hypopharyngeal tumours often spread to the lower cervical chain first. However, spread from below the clavicles is not uncommon and the Virchow node of gastric cancer and supraclavicular mass of Pancoast's tumour should be borne in mind. Again, clinical examination and cytology will often lead to the diagnosis.

Tuberculous lymphadenopathy seems to show a predilection for the lower lateral (posterior triangle) nodes.

Occasional rarities such as cervical ribs and subclavian artery aneurysms may present as masses in the lower lateral neck.

With almost all of the swellings encountered in the neck, a diagnosis can be made on clinical examination coupled to judicious use of imaging and cytology. As has been stressed, all neck lumps should be considered malignant until proved otherwise, and incisional or excisional biopsy should be avoided.

19 Neurosurgery

Introduction

Neurosurgeons (previously called neurological surgeons) are concerned principally with conditions affecting the central nervous system (CNS), the brain and spinal cord, in which the management of the patient may be aided by surgical means. The boundaries of what constitutes a neurosurgical problem are not clear cut and there are interesting areas of overlap with several other specialties. There is an increasing trend for major operations in such boundary areas to be undertaken by a team of surgeons from two or three specialties, particularly if skin and tissue cover or surgical reconstruction is required, or if the surgical approach to the intracranial lesion is via the maxilla, oral cavity or petrous bone.

Surgery to the spinal column is undertaken by both neurosurgeons and orthopaedic surgeons. Some neurosurgeons distinguish between vertebral surgery, that is surgery to the bones, joints and intervertebral discs of the spine, and spinal surgery, which involves treatment of intradural spinal tumours, arteriovenous malformations of the spinal cord and syringomyelia. Most neurosurgeons and some orthopaedic surgeons handle vertebral surgery, the most common surgical procedures being for prolapsed intervertebral discs and associated spondylitic changes. Generally speaking, only neurosurgeons would tackle spinal surgery.

Neurosurgeons have traditionally had close links with neurologists. The ready availability of sophisticated imaging techniques has rendered much detailed neurological examination redundant. Nevertheless, there are still areas where close cooperation is required between neurosurgeons and their physician colleagues, such as the surgical treatment of epilepsy, movement disorders and trigeminal neuralgia.

This chapter will describe the general neurosurgical approach to problems and outline the common neuro-

Table 19.1 Aspects of neurosurgery
History and examination
Conscious levels
Investigations
Neurosurgical conditions
trauma
intracranial haemorrhage
intracranial neoplasms
intracranial infection
congenital lesions
hydrocephalus
vascular compression syndromes

surgical conditions (Table 19.1). Spinal and vertebral surgery, although forming a large part of the modern neurosurgical workload, will not be discussed other than for the sake of completeness.

Neurosurgical history taking and examination

In neurosurgical patients the history is of major diagnostic value. A patient who is fully conscious will often be able to describe clearly any neurological signs and examination simply confirms the patient's account. The speed of onset of symptoms is usually important. In a patient with a reduced conscious level who is unable to give a history, every attempt must be made to obtain a reliable history from relatives or other witnesses. In cases of trauma, the exact mechanism of injury is often useful.

The details of how to carry out a full neurological examination will be found in any general medicine textbook and will not be repeated here. Unfortunately, students are often taught as if there is such a thing as a routine neurosurgical examination in which all neurological signs and symptoms are tested for. Time constraints alone would preclude such an approach. In practice, neurosurgical history taking and examination is not routine or list based, but more heuristic, that is, goal directed, testing one hypothesis after another. For example, in a patient with a purulent middle ear infection and symptoms of intracranial infection (headaches, neck stiffness, disturbance of conscious level), history taking and examination should be directed initially at detecting signs of a lesion, such as cerebritis or abscess, in the area of brain most likely to be affected. Thus, a middle ear infection can spread superiorly to the temporal lobe, giving rise to a contralateral hemiparesis, visual field defect and, in the dominant hemisphere, dysphasia; or infection can spread posteriorly into the posterior fossa, producing cerebellar signs such as ataxia, nystagmus and ipsilateral incoordination. Therefore these symptoms and signs would be specifically asked and tested for. Such a goal-directed approach does, of course, presume a reasonable basic knowledge of neuroanatomy.

It will be clear in the above example that if such a patient has a limb weakness, detailed testing of individual limb muscle groups and reflexes will add very little to the clinical picture and is therefore unnecessary. By contrast, in a patient with a suspected spinal cord lesion, testing of individual muscle groups and of reflexes may be of great value in determining the level of the lesion and which specific nerve roots may be involved. The examination performed therefore depends on the clinical question to be answered.

Neurosurgical history taking and examination is goal directed, and the goal is in three stages. The first stage is anatomical localisation, the second is to determine general pathology and the third is to determine detailed or special pathology. It is the hallmark of inexperience to try and make a diagnosis of special pathology in the early stages of a patient's presentation. The danger of this is that a patient is labelled with a condition and other possibilities are ignored.

Anatomical localisation

It is usually possible to locate a lesion to one of the three main compartments of the CNS, supratentorial (cerebral hemispheres), infratentorial (brainstem and cerebellum) and spinal.

Certain features always indicate supratentorial pathology. These features are anosmia (inferior frontal lobes),

dysphasia (dominant hemisphere) and seizures (always arise in the cerebral cortex).

Infratentorial (posterior fossa) lesions are characterised by brainstem or cerebellar signs such as ataxia, incoordination, nystagmus, dysarthria and dysphagia. Cranial nerve palsies may often be associated with infratentorial lesions and the presence of a cranial nerve palsy and a contralateral hemiparesis is virtually diagnostic of a brainstem lesion. Mass lesions in the posterior fossa commonly present with signs of raised intracranial pressure from hydrocephalus secondary to obstruction of cerebrospinal fluid (CSF) flow through the aqueduct or the fourth ventricle.

Spinal lesions are characterised first by an absence of the symptoms and signs characteristic of an intracranial lesion, and no disturbance of consciousness. Second, there will often be pain or tenderness at the site of a vertebral lesion. Third, spinal lesions commonly present with bilateral limb symptoms or signs, which is less usual with brain lesions. Fourth, due to the arrangement of the sensory and motor tracts within the spinal cord, there are characteristic syndromes associated with lesions of the spinal cord.

When localising spinal lesions it is important to distinguish between upper motor neuron and lower motor neuron lesions. The lower motor neuron starts at the anterior horn cell of the spinal cord. A lesion involving the anterior horn cell, the nerve root, or the peripheral motor nerve will tend to cause lower motor neuron signs, that is hypotonic weakness, muscle wasting, and reduced or absent reflexes. Lesions of the spinal cord itself will tend to produce upper motor neuron signs – weakness with increased tone, increased reflexes and clonus. A spinal lesion will commonly produce a mixture of upper motor neuron signs (below the level of lesion) and lower motor neuron signs (at the level of the lesion) and thus precise anatomical localisation is often possible.

General pathology

The second stage of the goal of history taking is to determine, as far as possible, which general pathological category the patient's complaints suggest. The general categories are congenital, degenerative, traumatic, infective/inflammatory, vascular and neoplastic. A history of trauma in the recent past will be important. A sudden onset (over a few seconds) of neurological symptoms or signs suggests a vascular origin (if trauma is excluded); an onset over hours or days suggests infection, particularly if there is pyrexia and meningism or evidence of infection elsewhere; and a more gradual onset (weeks or months) would point to a neoplastic process or a chronic subdural haematoma. In younger patients, congenital lesions will be more likely, although congenital lesions can present at any age.

The purpose of anatomical localisation and attempting to define general pathology is to help decide which is the next best investigation to determine special pathology. Modern neuroradiological investigation is sophisticated and accurate but may also be time consuming and expensive. Therefore it is important to be thoughtful about the sequence of investigations most likely to yield useful information.

Special pathology

To make a specific neurosurgical diagnosis usually requires further investigations. For example, a patient with sudden onset of dysphasia and a right hemiparesis has most likely sustained a vascular lesion (general pathology) affecting the left hemisphere. A computerised tomography (CT) scan is required to distinguish the special pathology of an infarct, a haemorrhagic infarct, or an arterial haemorrhage. If a haemorrhage is detected, a cerebral angiogram will usually be needed to display an underlying vascular abnormality such as an aneurysm or arteriovenous malformation.

The range of neurosurgical investigations that may be required to make a precise diagnosis are described later. It is frequently the case, particularly with CNS tumours or infection, that a biopsy will be required to make a definitive diagnosis.

Conscious level and non-localising symptoms

Several common presenting neurosurgical syndromes allow only the vaguest anatomical localisation.

Symptoms and signs of raised intracranial pressure (ICP)

The classic presentation of acute raised ICP is headache, vomiting and papilloedema; with a more chronic build-up of pressure, headache and vomiting may be less marked, even absent. In babies whose skull sutures have not formed raised ICP may simply cause the head circumference to enlarge beyond normal.

Any intracranial lesion can produce raised ICP if it is large enough, or situated in such a position as to obstruct the flow of CSF and cause hydrocephalus.

If unrelieved, raised ICP can lead to herniation of the brain through the tentorial hiatus or foramen magnum (coning). Raised ICP can lead to decreased cerebral perfusion; if ICP rises to equal blood pressure, cerebral perfusion ceases.

Meningism

This refers to the syndrome associated with meningitis, namely headache and neck stiffness, usually accompanied by vomiting. Meningitis means simply inflammation of the meninges. The most common cause in the community is probably viral meningitis, normally a benign, self-limiting condition. Bacterial meningitis is less common but is life threatening. Bleeding (from any cause) into the subarachnoid space also produces meningism. Chemical (non-infective) meningitis is sometimes seen following neurosurgical operations when, for example, cyst contents have escaped into the CSF. All types of meningitis and most cases of CSF or intracranial infection (cerebritis or brain abscess) will give rise to meningism.

Reduced conscious level: the Glasgow Coma Scale

A pathological reduced conscious level can be caused by bilateral cerebral hemisphere lesions, brainstem compression or ischaemia, reduced cerebral perfusion, metabolic disturbance or seizure activity. Most intracranial neurosurgical pathologies can give rise to a reduced conscious level by reason of pressure, direct or indirect, on the brainstem, or by causing raised ICP and reduced cerebral perfusion. Many non-CNS systemic pathologies will also produce a reduced conscious level, for example hypoglycaemia, liver failure, hypoxia (cardiac or respiratory abnormalities) and sepsis. Therefore a reduced conscious level in itself is not an indication of primary intracranial pathology.

Conscious level is universally assessed using the Glasgow Coma Scale (Table 19.2). The three components of consciousness – eye opening, verbal response and motor response – are assessed individually. When assessing each of these components it is important that the examiner starts 'at the top' and works down. Thus, when assessing eye opening, spontaneous eye opening or

Table 19.2 The Glasgow Coma Scale and score		
Feature	*Scale responses*	*Score notation*
Eye opening	Spontaneous	4
	To speech	3
	To pain	2
	None	1
Verbal response	Orientated	5
	Confused conversation	4
	Words (inappropriate)	3
	Sounds (incomprehensible)	2
	None	1
Best motor response	Obeys commands	6
	Localises pain	5
	Flexion – normal	4
	Flexion – abnormal	3
	Extend	2
	None	1
Total Coma score		$^3/_{15}$ to $^{15}/_{15}$

eye opening to speech should be looked for before testing eye opening to pain.

The correct way to test for a motor response often causes some difficulty. If a patient does not obey simple commands, a localising (purposeful) response is tested for. By convention, painful pressure is applied to the supraorbital margin and if the patient brings a hand up to the site of the pain, then the patient is localising. Both arms are tested by holding one arm down at a time.

If the patient does not localise, the other responses are tested by applying pressure to the fingernail bed. A flexion or extension response refers to movement at the elbow. The intermediate response, abnormal (or spastic) flexion is charted if there is either preceding extension movement in arm, or extension in a leg, or two of the following: stereotyped flexion posture, extreme wrist flexion, adduction of arm or fingers flexed over thumb. Because of the difficulty of describing this response, spastic flexion can be omitted from the Coma Scale, but is important to record, if present, as a focal sign (Fig. 19.1). If in doubt, record normal flexion.

When recording conscious level, the 'best' motor response is taken. This means the arm with the best response, not the best response over time. So if a patient is localising pain with the right arm but flexing to pain with the left arm, the conscious level is judged as localising. However, the flexion response in the left arm is an important focal sign, indicating a lesion probably affecting the right hemisphere.

It is common, especially in trauma patients, to be unable to record one or more aspects of the Coma Scale. The patient's eyes might be closed by swelling, or directly injured, making eye opening not possible. The patient may be dysphasic, or have an endotracheal tube or tracheostomy, making verbal response unrecordable. There may be a high spinal injury, brachial plexus lesion, or limb fracture, making motor response unreliable. In all these situations it is important simply to give the reason for not recording the response, rather than to guess at what it might be (see Fig. 19.1).

Coma is defined as not obeying commands, not eye opening even to pain, and not uttering recognisable words. A severe head injury is one where coma, as defined, is present for 6 h or more.

Each component of the Glasgow Coma Scale can be allocated a numerical value, the sum of which can give the Glasgow Coma (GC) Score (see Table 19.2). The GC Score was devised in the 1970s to allow information on large numbers of head-injured patients to be stored and analysed by computer. The GC Score is useful for grouping head-injured patients by severity, for displaying risk factors, and as a form of shorthand used in producing guidelines. Despite widespread practice to the contrary, the GC Score should never be used to describe an individual patient's conscious level in a clinical situation. To do so often results in confusion and significant loss of information. In clinical practice, always use the verbal description of the three components of the GC Scale.

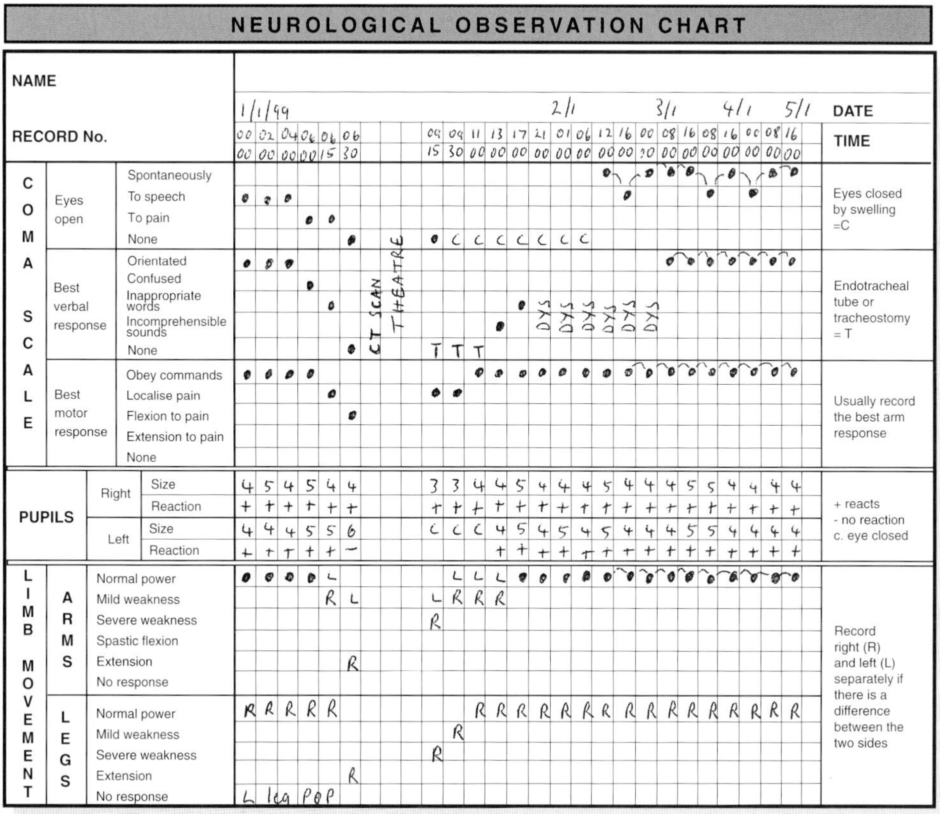

NEUROLOGICAL OBSERVATION CHART

NAME

RECORD No.

DATE: 1/1/99 ... 2/1 3/1 4/1 5/1

TIME: 00 02 04 06 06 06 / 00 00 00 00 15 30 ... 09 09 11 13 17 21 01 06 12 16 00 08 16 08 16 00 08 16 / 15 30 00 00 00 00 00 00 00 00 00 30 00 00 00 00 00 00

C O M A S C A L E		
Eyes open	Spontaneously	
	To speech	
	To pain	
	None	Eyes closed by swelling = C
Best verbal response	Orientated	
	Confused	
	Inappropriate words	
	Incomprehensible sounds	Endotracheal tube or tracheostomy = T
	None	
Best motor response	Obey commands	
	Localise pain	
	Flexion to pain	Usually record the best arm response
	Extension to pain	
	None	

(CT SCAN / THEATRE noted in verbal response columns; DYS = dysphasic; T T T in None row; L leg P&P noted at lower left.)

PUPILS									
Right	Size	4 5 4 5 4 4	3 3 4 4 5 4 4 4 5 4 4 4 5 5 4 4 4					+ reacts	
	Reaction	+ + + + + +	+ + + + + + + + + + + + + + + + +					– no reaction	
Left	Size	4 4 4 5 5 6	C C C 4 5 4 5 4 5 4 4 5 5 4 4 4					c. eye closed	
	Reaction	+ + + + + –	+ + + + + + + + + + + + + + +						

L I M B M O V E M E N T		
ARMS	Normal power	
	Mild weakness	R L / L R R R
	Severe weakness	R
	Spastic flexion	
	Extension	R
	No response	Record right (R) and left (L) separately if there is a difference between the two sides
LEGS	Normal power	R R R R / R R R R R R R R R R R R R R R R R
	Mild weakness	R
	Severe weakness	R
	Extension	R
	No response	L leg P&P

Fig. 19.1 Stylised neurosurgical observation chart of a patient deteriorating with a left-side extradural haematoma who improves following surgical evacuation. The Glasgow Coma Scale (GCS) uses the best motor response but limb asymmetry is also charted; if a response is inaccessible, the reason is given (e.g. C, eyes closed by swelling; DYS, dysphasic). The GC Score is not used for individual patients in a clinical situation.

Neurosurgical investigations and procedures

The purpose of neurosurgical history taking and examination is to determine anatomical localisation and, if possible, general pathology. This in turn guides the investigations that are most likely to assist in further diagnosis (of special pathology) and management.

Lumbar puncture

This is used to diagnose infection of the CSF, in which case the white cell count will be raised. Bleeding into the CSF (from, for example, a ruptured intracranial aneurysm) is diagnosed by frank blood-staining of the CSF and/or xanthochromia in the supernatant. Lumbar puncture (LP) is contraindicated in the presence of an intracranial mass lesion; an LP in this circumstance may lead to a pressure differential and subsequent downward herniation of the brain (coning). This can result in rapid death.

Nerve conduction studies and electromyography

These are tests performed by neurophysiologists and may be very useful in distinguishing nerve root abnormalities from peripheral nerve entrapment or peripheral neuropathy.

Plain radiography

Plain radiographs of the head or spine can be particularly useful in cases of trauma. Radiographs of the skull can show a fracture, a depressed fracture, air in the head or foreign bodies following a penetrating wound. Many head injuries are associated with spinal injury, particularly of the cervical spine, and cervical spine radiograph is almost routine following any significant head injury. Some brain tumours contain calcification or cause bone erosion, which is visible on a skull radiograph. Many pituitary tumours show erosion or expansion of the pituitary fossa on a lateral skull radiograph. In babies or children a skull radiograph can show premature fusion of the sutures (craniosynostosis), and chronic raised ICP gives patchy thinning of the skull vault – the copper-beaten appearance. Some spinal cord tumours or cysts may cause expansion and erosion of adjacent vertebra.

CT scan

This investigation has revolutionised neurosurgery. No longer do neurosurgeons need to rely on careful, detailed neurological examination to identify the exact site of, for example, a brain tumour.

MRI scan

This gives exquisite anatomical images. The two main advantages of the MRI scan over the CT scan are, first, that it is not affected by thick bone and is therefore useful for imaging the posterior fossa and spine. Second, it can image in any plane, and this is particularly informative in sagittal images of the spine.

The disadvantages of the MRI scan is that it is expensive and time consuming. It is contraindicated in patients with pacemakers, implanted stimulators or ferromagnetic implants or foreign bodies. Some claustrophobic patients cannot tolerate lying in the scanner.

Angiography

Carotid and vertebral angiograms are used to visualise intracranial aneurysms, arteriovenous malformations (AVMs), and the vascular supply of tumours. Access is usually via the femoral artery, threading the tracker catheter along the aorta under X-ray control.

Craniotomy

This refers to a flap of bone that is removed with a saw and replaced at the end of the procedure. The craniotomy flap may be of any size but is usually greater than 3 cm diameter. A craniotomy may be an osteoplastic flap,

where the temporalis muscle is left attached to the bone, or a free flap. A craniotomy is the standard neurosurgical procedure to gain access to the intracranial contents.

Neurosurgical conditions

Trauma

> **No head injury is so trivial that it can be ignored, or so serious that it should be despaired of.**

These words are as true today as when written by Hippocrates. Head injuries are common and the majority are minor and do not require investigation or hospital admission. Nevertheless, the potential for complications is always present.

Head injuries can be classified anatomically according to the structure(s) affected (scalp, skull, dura, brain), pathologically, depending on the type of brain damage (primary, secondary, focal, diffuse), or aetiologically, according to the mechanism of injury (blunt, penetrating, acceleration/deceleration, missile).

Isolated scalp injuries are common but not usually serious. Blood loss may look frightening but is rarely enough to cause shock, with the exception sometimes in babies. The history is always important and may alert the examiner to the possibility of a penetrating wound or a depressed fracture, both of which will normally require neurosurgical exploration. First aid treatment of a scalp laceration is to stop the bleeding by direct pressure. Thereafter direct primary suture is usually possible.

A skull fracture may be of the vault or the skull base. A closed (or simple) skull fracture has no overlying scalp laceration. A compound (or open) fracture implies communication of the fracture with the atmosphere. A compound depressed fracture of the skull vault usually requires an operation to debride the wound, elevate the fracture and inspect the underlying dura and brain for lacerations. The main aim of this procedure is to reduce the risk of intracranial infection by removing all foreign material and repairing the dural defect. Penetrating wounds are dealt with in the same way. Simple depressed fractures do not require surgery.

Fractures of the skull base are difficult to see with radiographs but can be diagnosed clinically by the presence of well-defined periorbital haematomas (racoon eyes) and subconjunctival haemorrhage with no posterior

Table 19.3   Risk of an operable intracranial haematoma in head injured patients

GCS (/15)	Risk	Other features	Risk
15	1 in 3615	None	1 in 31 300
		Post-traumatic amnesia (PTA)	1 in 6700
		Skull fracture	1 in 81
		Skull fracture and PTA	1 in 29
9–14	1 in 51	No fracture	1 in 180
		Skull fracture	1 in 5
3–8	1 in 7	No fracture	1 in 27
		Skull fracture	1 in 4

GCS, Glasgow Coma scale
Adapted from Teasdale et al. 1990 British Medical Journal, 300: 363–367

limit (in anterior fossa fractures), or bruising over the mastoid process (Battle's sign) in fractures of the petrous bone. Petrous fractures can damage the middle or inner ear and may have associated bleeding from the external meatus, deafness, dizziness or facial nerve palsy. If the dura underlying a base of skull fracture is torn, there may be a CSF leak through the nose or the ear, or air many enter the subarachnoid space (pneumocephalus). In either event there is a risk of bacterial meningitis. If the dural tear does not heal within 1–2 weeks, surgical repair is usually indicated. Recently published guidelines do not recommend prophylactic antibiotics for a CSF leak.

The main significance of a skull fracture is that it indicates a greatly increased risk of the patient harbouring an intracranial haematoma that requires surgical removal. Table 19.3 illustrates the risks that form the basis for guidelines on the early management of head injuries. Table 19.4 lists the criteria for referral of a head injury to hospital. Further guidelines on the indications for a skull radiograph, admission to hospital, a CT scan, and referral to a neurosurgeon can be found in the Scottish Intercollegiate Guidelines Network (SIGN) publication entitled 'Early management of patients with a head injury (No. 46)', published in August 2000.

Table 19.4   Indications for referral of a head injured patient to hospital

A head injured patient should be referred to hospital if any of the following is present:

Impaired consciousness (GCS <15/15) at any time since injury

Amnesia for the incident or subsequent events

Neurological symptoms, e.g. severe and persistent headache, nausea and vomiting, irritability or altered behaviour, seizure

Clinical evidence of a skull fracture (e.g. CSF leak, periorbital haematoma)

Significant extracranial injuries

A mechanism of injury suggesting:
   a high energy injury (e.g. road traffic accident, fall from height)
   possible penetrating brain injury
   possible non-accidental injury (in a child)

Continuing uncertainty about the diagnosis after first assessment

Medical comorbidity (e.g. anticoagulant use, alcohol abuse)

Adverse social factors (e.g. no-one able to supervise the patient at home).

From Scottish Intercollegiate Guidelines Network (SIGN) Publication Number 46 'Early management of patients with a head injury', August 2000.

Brain damage

Brain damage or dysfunction is the subject of most concern following a head injury. Concussion, seizure activity, mechanical compression and ischaemia, may all render part of the brain dysfunctional, that is, the axons do not conduct or the synapses do not transmit. Such dysfunction may be reversible with appropriate treatment over time. 'Brain damage' is the term used to indicate irreversible

dysfunction, which generally equates with disruption of the structural integrity of the neurons.

Primary brain damage is that which occurs at the time (or very soon after) a head injury. By definition, no treatment will reverse this. The aim of management is to prevent further damage, the causes of which are listed in Table 19.5.

Table 19.5   Causes of secondary brain damage
Ischaemia
hypoxaemia
airway obstruction
chest injury
hypotension
extracranial injuries
other causes of shock
Intracranial haematoma
Brain swelling/oedema
Seizures
Infection (meningitis, abscess)
Metabolic/electrolyte disturbance

Hypoxaemia and hypotension are two of the most common causes of secondary brain damage that can be treated (or prevented) by a non-specialist. Hence the emphasis in all guidelines regarding the management of head injuries on the 'ABC' of resuscitation – the airway and breathing (i.e. adequate blood gases) always take priority, followed by treatment of circulatory disturbances. Treatment of an obstructed airway, or a tension pneumothorax, or bleeding from a ruptured spleen always takes precedence over a possible intracranial haematoma.

Intracranial haematomas

An intracranial haematoma is the complication that most people associate with a head injury, but haematomas requiring surgical treatment are in fact uncommon. The clinical characteristics of such a lesion are severe headache and vomiting, decreased conscious level, contralateral hemiparesis and (a late sign) an ipsilateral unreactive dilated pupil (see Fig. 19.1). Treatment of a significant haematoma will usually be surgical evacuation via a craniotomy. An extradural haematoma (i.e. between the skull bone and the dura) generally carries a better prognosis because it is less often associated with contusions or lacerations of the brain substance. An intradural haematoma is commonly a mixture of subdural blood, brain contusions or intracerebral haematoma, although pure subdural or intracerebral haematomas do occur.

Chronic subdural haematoma (CSDH)

CSDH is a relatively common but poorly understood condition. The typical history is of a minor head injury in an elderly patient, followed weeks or months later by a gradual onset of signs of a cerebral hemisphere lesion. Classically the conscious level fluctuates. Confusion alone is a common presentation and may often be put down to other causes, such as dementia or stroke. Often there is no history of a head injury. An overdraining ventriculo-peritoneal shunt can also result in a CSDH.

Intracranial haemorrhage

Intracranial haemorrhage is subdivided into parenchymal (intracerebral) haemorrhage and subarachnoid or intraventricular haemorrhage. Pure intracerebral haemorrhage may present in the same way as a cerebral infarct (with sudden onset of neurological signs) although is five times less common. Hypertension is the commonest cause and surgery is rarely indicated.

Haemorrhage primarily into the subarachnoid space or ventricles, or intraparenchymal haemorrhage that ruptures into the CSF spaces, presents with a very severe sudden headache, sometimes referred to as thunderclap headache. There may be accompanying neurological deficits and/or a decreased conscious level or coma.

Subarachnoid haemorrhage (SAH) is the most common type of intracranial haemorrhage that concerns the neurosurgeon. The usual cause is a ruptured intracranial aneurysm. Other uncommon causes include arteriovenous malformations, tumours and blood dyscrasias. About 12% of all patients with SAH have no cause found. Usually, such patients are relatively well following the bleed, make a full recovery in time and rarely rebleed.

The diagnosis of subarachnoid haemorrhage is made on the history of sudden severe headache. Some patients liken the onset to being hit on the back of the head with a baseball bat. A CT scan will show subarachnoid blood in 90% of cases scanned within 24 h of the haemorrhage. A cerebral angiogram will demonstrate an aneurysm if present (Fig. 19.2).

Treatment is directed towards preventing a rebleed. The aneurysm may be approached through a craniotomy and a small metal clip placed across its neck to exclude it from the circulation. Alternatively, platinum coils may be packed into the aneurysm sac using angiographic techniques. It is unclear which method gives the best long-term results.

Aneurysmal subarachnoid haemorrhage is a serious condition with a high initial mortality and morbidity. In patients who survive the initial haemorrhage, the risk of rebleeding is 25% in the first 2 weeks and 60% within 6 months, with a mortality of 60%. Therefore early referral and assessment of patients with suspected SAH is important. A common cause of litigation concerns

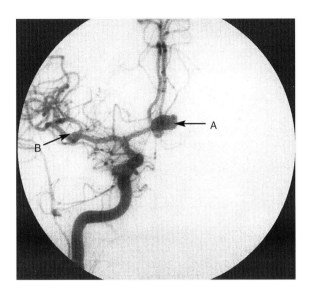

Fig. 19.2 Anteroposterior (AP) view of a right internal carotid angiogram showing an anterior communicating artery aneurysm arising in the midline between the two anterior cerebral arteries (A). A smaller aneurysm can also be seen at the bifurcation of the middle cerebral artery (B).

patients with a minor SAH (who remain relatively well) misdiagnosed as migraine or viral meningitis, only to return a week later with a devastating rebleed.

Intracranial neoplasms

Intracranial tumours form a large part of the neuro-surgical workload. There are many pathological types of tumour and detailed discussion of each is not possible. However, tumours can be grouped broadly into intrinsic tumours (those that arise within the brain substance) and extrinsic lesions. The most common adult intrinsic tumours are gliomas (astrocytomas, oligodendrogliomas, etc.) and metastatic carcinomas. The most common extrinsic tumours are meningiomas, which arise from the arachnoid membrane on the internal aspect of the dura. In children, the most common neoplasms are medullo-blastomas and ependymomas, both intrinsic tumours arising in the posterior fossa.

Depending on their position, size and rate of growth, tumours can present with virtually any neurological symptom or sign. Headache, seizures and confusion are three of the most common. The key feature of neoplastic lesions is that the presenting signs will usually be of gradual onset and progressive. Diagnosis is by CT or MRI scan, although skull radiograph may give a clue in some cases. It is often possible to diagnose with a reason-able degree of certainty the pathological type of tumour based on the CT scan appearance. However, gliomas in particular can have a varied appearance and can some-times look like a metastasis, an abscess, an infarct or a resolving haematoma. Biopsy is often required.

The management of intracranial tumours depends on many factors but the key principle of management is to weigh the likely benefits of the proposed treatment against the possible morbidity or mortality arising from treatment. Factors that tend to increase the risk of surgery are older age, poor clinical condition, location within or close to an 'eloquent' (i.e. functionally important) area of brain, and close involvement of important intracranial arteries or veins.

The usual classification of extracranial tumours into benign or malignant is not so helpful or relevant with intracranial tumours. Most meningiomas, for example, are pathologically 'benign' and have a clear plane of cleavage from normal brain. However meningiomas can invade the dural venous sinuses or bone around the base of the skull, making total removal impractical. Further-more, meningiomas may have 'atypical' features (such as mitotic figures) or be frankly malignant, and in all such situations there is a higher chance of recurrence.

The feature of the majority of gliomas, from low grade to malignant, is that they invade normal brain. It is well established that even if the CT scan shows an apparent clear margin to the tumour, tumour cells extend at least 2 cm beyond the margin into brain substance. Most gliomas respond little to radiotherapy and even less to chemotherapy, and therefore a cure is not possible. The aim of management must be to try and relieve the patient's symptoms and extend the length of good quality life. Attempts at radical resection of the glioma are rarely justified if this means that the patient is to be left even more disabled postoperatively. Conservative manage-ment is often appropriate.

Secondary tumours within the brain are often multiple and most are not referred to a neurosurgeon because they are terminal. Patients with a solitary metastasis in an accessible area and who are generally well may benefit in the short-term from surgical excision.

Intracranial infection

Meningitis

Viral meningitis rarely comes to the attention of the neurosurgeon unless there is suspicion of some other diagnosis such as subarachnoid haemorrhage. Likewise, most cases of bacterial meningitis will be managed perfectly adequately outside a neurosurgical unit. Diagnosis is by lumbar puncture.

Meningitis is seen most often by neurosurgeons as a complication of an open head injury or following intracranial surgery. Treatment is with the appropriate antibiotics. Occasionally, bacterial meningitis, especially tuberculous meningitis, can cause hydrocephalus, which requires ventricular drainage of CSF. Therefore a patient in coma, or who fails to respond to antibiotic treatment, should have a CT scan.

Brain abscess and subdural empyema

A brain abscess (or subdural empyema) may occur as a result of direct spread from infected sinuses, otitis media or a penetrating wound, or by the haematogenous route (Fig. 19.3). Haematogenous brain abscesses are more likely to be multiple and are thought more likely in patients with a cardiac septal defect that allows the normal bacterial filtering action of the lung to be bypassed.

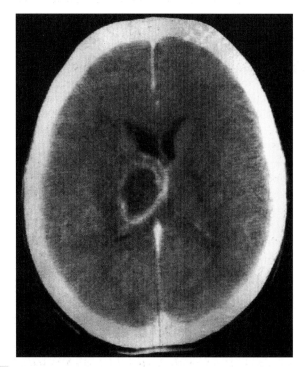

Fig. 19.3 Axial computerised tomography (CT) scan showing an abscess in the region of the thalamus.

Congenital lesions

Congenital lesions of the CNS may occur in isolation or in association with other abnormalities as part of a recognised syndrome. Some lesions are obvious at birth (e.g. spina bifida), and others cause no symptoms and remain unrecognised throughout life (e.g. temporal lobe agenesis). Others, for example, craniosynostosis and aqueduct stenosis, are only diagnosed when they produce symptoms or signs.

Craniosynostosis

This refers to premature fusion of one or more of the skull sutures resulting in abnormalities of the skull shape.

Synostosis may be part of a more generalised abnormality such as Crouzon's or Apert's syndrome, in which case there will be facial, dental and ophthalmic abnormalities to consider, and a multidisciplinary team approach is required.

Surgery consists of resecting the faulty suture line(s) and allowing the skull vault bones to 'spring'. Brain growth will then hopefully mould the skull to a more normal shape and size. Surgery may also be required to the orbits and facial bones.

Spina bifida

This term covers a range of abnormalities from asymptomatic spina bifida occulta to large, open, posterior spinal defects with total loss of cord function. Open defects need to be closed soon after birth. Less major (closed) spina bifida defects may only become apparent as the child grows and develops problems with walking. An MRI scan is the investigation of choice.

Arnold–Chiari malformation

In this condition, the cerebellar tonsils are prolapsed through the foramen magnum. The posterior fossa is often abnormally shallow. In more pronounced forms the lower brain stem will also be herniated.

Mild forms are common and often asymptomatic. Symptoms may range from cough impulse headache to signs of brainstem compression. Chiari malformations may be associated with spina bifida and aqueduct stenosis. Treatment of symptomatic cases is by bony decompression of the foramen magnum.

Aqueduct stenosis

This can give rise to an obstructive hydrocephalus and may present at any age. Ataxia is often an early symptom and headaches are frequently mild or absent even in the presence of papilloedema. Treatment is by insertion of a CSF shunt or by making a fenestration in the floor of the third ventricle.

Hydrocephalus

CSF is actively secreted in the colloid plexus of the lateral third and fourth ventricles at a rate of 20 mL per hour. There is a gentle pressure gradient that causes CSF to flow, in a pulsatile manner, through the aqueduct into the fourth ventricle and then out of the fourth ventricle into the basal subarachnoid space. The flow continues over the cerebral hemispheres to the superior sagittal sinus, where CSF is absorbed through the arachnoid granulations by a passive process dependent on differential pressure between the CSF and the venous sinus. Hydrocephalus refers to the situation where there is an imbalance between CSF production and absorption, causing the ventricles to enlarge. In acute hydrocephalus this causes severe pressure on the brain, decreased cerebral perfusion, herniation through the tentorial hiatus, brain stem pressure and, eventually, death. In more chronic forms there is progressive stretching, ischaemia and destruction of white matter tracts around the enlarging ventricles.

Hydrocephalus occurs as a result of a congenital abnormality (e.g. aqueduct stenosis) or as a complication of some other intracranial pathology. Almost any intracranial pathology can cause or be associated with hydrocephalus and it is one of the commonest problems in neurosurgery.

The term 'active hydrocephalus' implies a continuing imbalance between CSF production and absorption, leading to ongoing raised ICP. Compensated or arrested hydrocephalus refers to the condition of large ventricles (ventriculomegaly), suggestive of previous active hydrocephalus but with no continuing raised pressure. Arrested hydrocephalus is common in the community and although such individuals may have no neurological deficits they might have large heads and enormous ventricles on CT scan. It is important to treat the patient and not the CT scan.

Active hydrocephalus usually requires surgical treatment. The best management in obstructive hydrocephalus is to remove the cause of the obstruction if possible. As a temporary or holding measure a ventricular drain may be inserted to drain CSF into an external reservoir. A shunt consists of a silastic ventricular catheter connected to a subcutaneous valve and reservoir, in turn connected to a tube into the peritoneal cavity (ventriculoperitoneal shunt) or atrium (ventriculoatrial shunt).

The disadvantages and complications of shunts are legion and include blockage, infection and over drainage. Each significant shunt complication requires further surgery; such patients can become very dependent on hospital services.

Vascular compression syndromes

Paroxysmal trigeminal neuralgia (PTN)

This is a relatively common condition characterised by very severe episodes (paroxysms) of shooting pains affecting one side of the face. The diagnosis is made on the history alone and the characteristics are listed in Table 19.6.

In most so-called idiopathic cases of PTN the cause is a blood vessel compressing the trigeminal nerve at the position where it enters the pons. There is evidence that the vessel leads to focal demyelination and ephaptic transmission. MRI scanning will usually demonstrate the compressing vessel.

Treatment is by carbamazepine or other anticonvulsant drugs in the first instance. If the patient still experiences pain on the maximum tolerated dose of anticonvulsants, it is possible to explore the trigeminal root entry zone via a small posterior fossa craniectomy. Separating the compressing vessel from the nerve usually (80% of cases) cures the pain. However, there are cases where no compressing vessel is evident or, if present, decompression does not alleviate the symptoms. Clearly there are other possible causes.

Table 19.6   Features of trigeminal neuralgia
Gradual worsening of severity and frequency of attacks over the years
Periods of remission
No neurological deficits or sensory disturbance
Often aggravated by chewing
A trigger spot where light touch or cold sets off the pain
Responds to carbamazepine

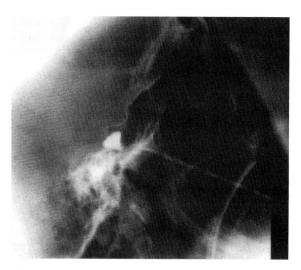

Fig. 19.4 Treatment for trigeminal neuralgia. The lateral skull X-ray shows a needle entering the foramen ovale and a Fogarty balloon inflated with contrast in the trigeminal cistern.

In patients not suitable for the above procedure (i.e. the elderly or unfit) a destructive procedure can be carried out to the nerve. This may be a peripheral nerve block using alcohol or a cryoprobe (usually carried out by oral physicians), or an injection into the trigeminal ganglion via the foramen ovale under X-ray control. The ganglion may be partially denervated by heat (thermocoagulation), chemical (glycerol) or mechanically (balloon compression; Fig. 19.4). The initial success rate of these destructive procedures is high, but so is the recurrence rate.

Patients with multiple sclerosis commonly develop an identical syndrome to idiopathic trigeminal neuralgia. Presumably the origin is a demyelinating plaque somewhere on the course of the nerve root. Vascular decompression procedures will not help but ganglion injection procedures are effective.

Occasionally, a tumour in the cerebellar pontine angle, such as an acoustic neuroma, petrous meningioma or epidermoid cyst may present with PTN. Removal of the tumour is usually curative.

Glossopharyngeal neuralgia (GPN)

This is a similar syndrome to PTN except the pain is in the distribution of the glossopharyngeal nerve that is the posterior tongue and pharynx on one side. Typically, the pain of GPN occurs on swallowing and that of PTN on chewing. Open surgical treatment is highly effective and there is usually a compressing vessel at the glossopharyngeal root entry zone into the brainstem. If there is no vessel, or the vessel is technically difficult to separate, unilateral section of the glossopharyngeal nerve and the upper roots of the vagus is curative and produces hardly any neurological deficit.

Hemifacial spasm

This is the third of the curious cranial nerve vascular compression syndromes. Most people have seen someone with involuntary contractions of muscles on one side of the face. The syndrome usually starts with blepharospasm but tends to progress over the years to involve the whole of the side of the face in dystonic contractions. The patient may effectively lose the use of one eye and the cosmetic effect is distressing.

Once again there is in most cases a blood vessel compressing the facial nerve at its root entry zone. A posterior fossa craniectomy and decompression of the nerve is usually successful in abolishing the spasm.

20 Temporomandibular joint investigation and surgery

Introduction

The most common condition affecting the temporo-mandibular region is temporomandibular dysfunction, or myofascial pain dysfunction. This may be associated with a clicking of the temporomandibular joint. This is a disorder characterised by pain and masticatory muscle spasm and limited jaw opening, which is treated by conservative measures such as soft diet, analgesics, occlusal splint therapy or physiotherapy. Intransigent cases may respond to psychotropic therapy.

Conditions affecting the temporomandibular joint (TMJ) that might require surgery are listed in Table 20.1. A detailed knowledge of the anatomy of the TMJ is necessary and an overview of this follows, with aspects of the history and examination of the patient and details of the investigations that are a prerequisite to appropriate surgical care. This is followed by a discussion of the procedures available for the surgical management of TMJ disorders (Table 20.2).

Anatomy of the temporomandibular joint (TMJ)

The TMJ is a synovial joint with articular surfaces made up of fibrocartilage. Fibrocartilage is adapted to take shearing forces, rather than the compressive forces that act on the hyaline cartilage in the knee joint. The TMJ has an upper and a lower compartment separated by a cartilaginous meniscus. The non-articular surfaces are lined by a synovial membrane, which produces the synovial fluid that lubricates the joint and nourishes the cartilage (Fig. 20.1).

The only time that the joint is loaded is when eating or clenching. When speaking or relaxed the teeth are

Table 20.1   Surgical conditions of the temporomandibular joint
Internal joint derangement
Recurrent dislocation
Traumatic injury
Arthritic conditions
Ankylosis
Tumours

Table 20.2   Surgical procedures for the temporomandibular joint (TMJ)
Arthrocentesis
TMJ arthroscopy
Meniscal plication
Meniscectomy
Eminectomy
Dautrey procedure
Condylotomy
Condylectomy
TMJ reconstruction

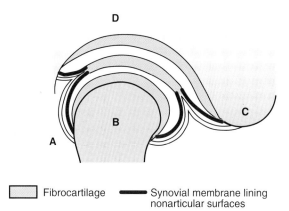

Fibrocartilage ▬▬ Synovial membrane lining nonarticular surfaces

Fig. 20.1   The anatomy of the temporomandibular joint. A, bilaminar zone; B, condylar head; C, mandibular eminence; D, glenoid fossa.

173

apart. When the jaws are closed much of the force is transmitted through the teeth into the facial bones but some of the forces will go into the jaw joints.

The joints are supported by ligaments, which surround the joint capsule. Movement is by the action of the masticatory muscles and information from proprioceptors in the mouth and particularly in the periodontal ligament allow coordination of all components when chewing or speaking. Injury or damage to any of these components affects jaw function.

Investigations

Investigations of the temporomandibular joint include history, examination and special investigations, and these are discussed in turn.

History

The patient's presenting symptoms should be noted. Symptoms might include pain, swelling, clicking, crackling in the preauricular region and limitation of jaw opening. There may also be an accompanying generalised facial ache or a numb sensation over the masseter muscles. When asked about pain, if a patient points to the preauricular region then the pain is likely to be in the TMJ, but if the patient puts a hand over the side of the face as the area of pain then it is likely to be muscular pain. There is often a combination of both in arthromyalgia. TMJ symptoms must be distinguished from other conditions in the orofacial regions.

Previous symptoms, duration and potential causes of the symptoms such as trauma should be elicited from the patient. Any activity that exacerbates or relieves the condition should be noted. Chewing, yawning or parafunctional habits can aggravate TMJ disease.

A full medical and drug history should be taken, as well as a family and social history. Of particular relevance are traumatic life events such as bereavement, a house or job move or a divorce. Stress is a common factor in TM dysfunction.

Examination

A general examination of the head and neck should be carried out, paying particular attention to tenderness in the sternomastoid and temporal muscles. The angle of the jaw may be tender where the medial pterygoid muscle is attached.

Palpation of the TMJs may cause pain and, on movement, clicking or crepitations may be felt or even heard.

On intraoral examination the patient may have limited opening (normal interincisal opening 40–50 mm). There may be deviation of the jaw to one side when asked to open widely due to limitation of movement from that side (normal lateral movement 10 mm to each side).

Palpation of the masseter muscles and the pterygoid muscles should be carried out. To palpate the pterygoid muscles the patient should be asked to deviate the jaw to the side being examined to allow a finger to be passed along the upper buccal sulcus backwards between the ramus of the mandible and the tuberosity of the maxilla. Behind the tuberosity are the pterygoid plates – the origin of the pterygoid muscles. This site is often tender in TM dysfunction, due to muscle spasm and fatigue.

Special investigations

The special investigations which may be considered are listed in Table 20.3.

Plain radiographs include an orthopantomogram, and transcranial and transpharyngeal views of the TMJ. These images give information about the bone structure. Open and closed views will give some indication about jaw mobility.

Arthrography is an invasive investigation using a radiopaque dye, which is injected into the upper joint compartment, the lower joint compartment or a combination of both. This technique can provide information about the internal structures of the joint. The cartilaginous meniscus is outlined. The procedure is usually carried out under videofluoroscopy so that the joint can be imaged in motion. Disc displacement and perforations can be identified. However, extravasation of dye into surrounding tissues will spoil the investigation. With newer imaging techniques this method is now less frequently used.

Computerised tomography (CT) scanning can give a lot of information about the bony relations and bone

Table 20.3   Investigation of temporomandibular joint pathology
Plain radiographs
Arthrography
CT scan
MRI scan

quality of the TMJs. It gives axial views and computer-generated coronal views; it can also give three-dimensional images. This method is very helpful in providing information about trauma to the joint, bony disease in the joint and ankylosis.

Magnetic resonance imaging (MRI) images the soft tissues and is helpful in identifying disc position. It can demonstrate disc perforation and joint effusions. It may also pick out adhesions within the joint. It does give information about the bone but it is not as good as a CT scan.

Surgical management

Arthrocentesis

Arthrocentesis is a method of flushing out the TMJ by placing a needle into the upper joint compartment using local or general anaesthesia. Ringer's lactate (see Ch. 5) is injected into the joint. This compartment will take up to 5 mL of fluid. By filling under pressure, any minor adhesions are broken down or lysed. A second needle placed into the same joint compartment allows through-flow of fluid to be achieved. This allows thorough washing or lavage of the joint. The process is referred to as 'lysis and lavage' and can produce good therapeutic outcomes. It has a particular roll in cases of acute closed lock. In this situation, the meniscus is usually jammed in front of the condyle, preventing translatory movement. By ballooning-up the joint the potential space becomes real and the meniscus may have room to reduce to its normal position. The lavage will wash-out products of inflammation, creating a better environment for healing. Sodium hyaluronate can be injected at the end of the procedure to improve joint lubrication.

TMJ arthroscopy

TMJ arthroscopy can be used both as a diagnostic tool and as a treatment modality. The synovium, joint and miniscal cartilage can be visualised.

The standard technique for TMJ arthroscopy is via a lateral approach. The upper joint compartment, where most of the translatory movement occurs, is entered with a 21 gauge needle posteriorly. After insufflation of the joint with Ringer's lactate, through-flow of fluid is established via a second 19 gauge needle placed anteriorly in the joint space. A trochar and cannula are then introduced into the space created by the fluid in the

joint. The trochar is removed and replaced by the arthroscope. An outport second cannula may be inserted anteriorly into the joint for instrumentation – the working cannula. The upper joint compartment can then be examined for synovitis, displacement of the meniscus, adhesions between meniscus and the joint fossa and other pathology.

If adhesions are seen they can be divided with very small scissors inserted through the working cannula. It is possible in some cases to reduce a dislocated meniscus, biopsy cartilage or synovium, remove loose bodies (fragments of cartilage floating in the joint) and reduce the joint eminence with rotary instruments. Drugs such as corticosteroids or sodium hyaluronate may be injected into the joint to reduce inflammation and improve lubrication respectively.

Splint therapy, soft diet and analgesics are used as part of the postoperative management. The patient is also instructed in gentle jaw stretching exercises.

Meniscal plication

When conservative management has not caused improvement after a period of 4–6 months, and arthrocentesis or arthroscopy have failed to correct meniscal dislocation, then open arthrotomy should be considered.

The usual approach is via a preauricular incision (Fig. 20.2). Once the joint is exposed, entry is made into the upper joint compartment and the position of the meniscus identified. Any adhesions are released and the meniscus is repositioned and fixed with sutures from the lateral aspect of the cartilage and posteriorly into the temporal muscle and fascia. Some surgeons will also enter the lower joint space to increase the mobilisation of the meniscus and remove a wedge of retrodiscal tissue, stitch or plicate the defect created with retrodiscal sutures, repositioning the meniscus more posteriorly. Sometimes these procedures are combined with an eminectomy to increase joint space.

Postoperative management is similar to that of arthroscopy. Physical therapy is important as there is inevitably a degree of scarring following this surgery.

Meniscectomy

This procedure is not commonly performed in the UK but there have been reports of successful outcomes in patients suffering from internal joint derangement by this

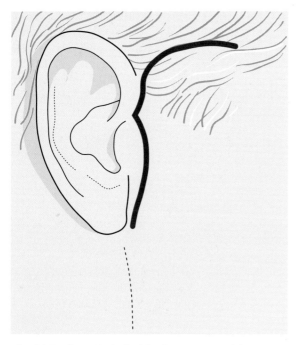

Fig. 20.2 Preauricular incision for exposure of the temporomandibular joint.

method. Essentially, the approach is the same as that for meniscal plication. Once the meniscus is identified the cartilaginous part is excised. There is uncertainty about long-term effects this may have on the joint.

Eminectomy

This procedure is used for recurrent jaw dislocation. The approach is the same as for the plication procedure. The joint eminence, which lies anteriorly to the fossa, has to be well exposed. The eminence is then excised by a combination of bur cuts and a fine osteotome (Fig. 20.3). The

theory is that by taking away this eminence over which the joint head sticks, the joint head has no obstruction to prevent its return into the fossa.

Dautrey procedure

This procedure is another method of stopping TMJ dislocation. The approach is again exposure of the joint via the preauricular incision. The eminence is again exposed but in this procedure the anterior part of the eminence, which is attached to the zygomatic arch, is incised in a more vertical direction (Fig. 20.4). This anterior portion is fractured-off and, still attached anteriorly to the zygomatic arch, is swung downwards and wedged against the remaining eminence to augment the eminence. In theory, because of the increase in eminence height, the condyle is unable to dislocate. Other methods of eminence augmentation have been described, for example bone graft augmentation.

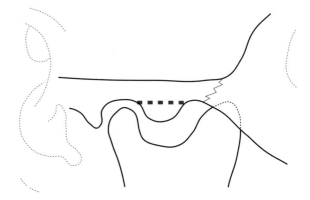

Fig. 20.3 Eminectomy. The hatched line indicates the bony incision line.

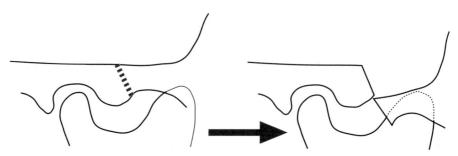

Fig. 20.4 The Dautrey procedure to increase the height of the eminence.

Condylotomy

This technique for treating painful TMJs originally used a blind external approach using a Gigli saw. Nowadays this procedure is carried out via an intraoral approach. The lateral aspect of the ramus of the mandible is exposed and a cut is made below the condyle with an oscillating saw. It may be subcondylar or subsigmoid (Fig. 20.5). This causes reduced pressure on the meniscus and anterior movement of the condylar head, which reduces pain and often allows reduction of the displaced joint meniscus.

Condylectomy

Condylectomy is usually performed when there is either ankylosis or pathology of the TMJ. A preauricular approach is used and, once the condyle is well exposed, it is cut at the neck of the joint and removed. This procedure is generally combined with joint reconstruction.

TMJ reconstruction

On rare occasions the TMJ requires reconstruction. To date no replacement adequately replaces the normal TMJ. Indications for joint reconstruction are listed in Table 20.4.

The goal of treatment is to restore the mandible and TMJ to as near normal an anatomical state. Partial or total TMJ reconstruction may be required; partial reconstruction may be indicated. There are fossa prostheses but these are usually used in conjunction with condylar replacement.

Various synthetic materials or alloplasts have been used for meniscus replacement (e.g. Teflon®). These materials can cause a foreign body giant cell reaction, which is relentless in its destruction of surrounding tissues. For this reason, these materials are now rarely used. Autogenous grafts such as auricular cartilage and dermis are sometimes used. Potential complications from these grafts are disruption or displacement, cyst formation with the dermal graft and fibrous ankylosis.

Ankylosis may be treated with a temporalis muscle flap, gap arthroplasty or total joint reconstruction.

The usual method in gap arthroplasty is by parallel cuts approximately 1 cm apart from the sigmoid notch to the posterior ramus (Fig. 20.6). Interpositional material can be placed to reduce union. Alloplasts such as Silastic® or a chrome–cobalt cap prosthesis have been used.

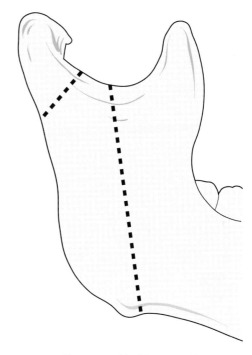

■ ■ ■ ■ Two types of incision on vertical ramus of the mandible for condylotomy

Fig. 20.5 Two types of incision (subcondylar and subsigmoid) on the vertical ramus of the mandible for condylotomy.

Table 20.4 Indications for temporomandibular joint reconstruction
Ankylosis
Joint destruction
Trauma
Infection
Tumours
Previous surgery
Radiation
Developmental deformity

Suturing medial pterygoid and masseter muscles together above the ramus stump is a biological interpositional graft.

Most surgery for ankylosis is carried out through the preauricular approach but when joint replacement is required a submandibular incision is used for access to the ramus for a combined approach. A method of biological reconstruction of the TMJ is the use of an inferiorly based temporalis muscle flap, which is rotated anteriorly beneath the zygomatic arch as an interpositional material (Fig. 20.7).

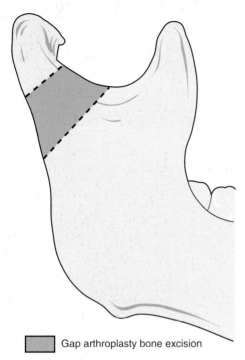

Gap arthroplasty bone excision

Fig. 20.6 Gap arthroplasty. The hatched area is the bony excision.

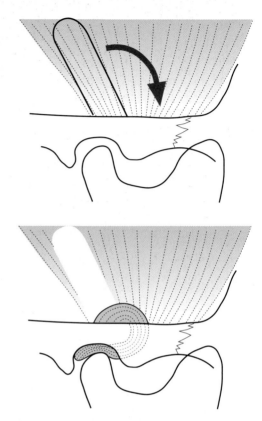

Fig. 20.7 Finger flap of the temporalis muscle rotated anteriorly under the arch of the zygoma into the glenoid fossa.

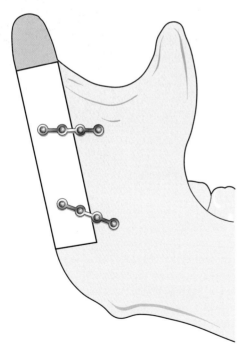

Fig. 20.8 A costochondral rib graft fixed with mini bone plates.

Total joint reconstruction is required where there is no functional joint plus loss of ramus height. This may be necessary where there has been severe trauma, ankylosis, tumour resection or a developmental abnormality such as hemifacial microsomia. Costochondral grafts or vascularised free bone grafts such as the second metatarsal bone from the foot could be used in combination with an interpositional temporalis muscle graft. The most satisfactory method of total joint reconstruction is the combination of the temporalis muscle flap and an autogenous costochondral rib graft (Fig. 20.8).

Several prosthetic joint replacement systems have been devised to replace both glenoid fossa and condyle. Some have had problems from chronic foreign body giant cell reactions to the synthetic materials.

Surgery is not the endpoint of treatment. The postoperative phase, as in all surgery, is very important and neglect in this area is often a reason for failure. Analgesic and anti-inflammatory medications are usually indicated and physical therapy is essential, with jaw opening exercises plus lateral and protrusive movement exercises.

PART II
ORAL SURGERY

21 Introduction

The oral surgery section of this text focuses on those areas of surgical practice that are routinely encountered in general dental practice. Certain procedures, such as uncomplicated extraction of teeth, will fall within the area of competence of every dental practitioner whereas other procedures, such as removal of cysts and certain wisdom teeth, might be performed only by those who have an interest in surgical dentistry and who have developed the necessary competence, through training, to perform those more complex procedures. Regardless, all dental practitioners must have a detailed knowledge of the subject areas covered within the 'oral surgery' sections of this book because they will encounter patients routinely who present with signs and symptoms that require a comprehensive knowledge to diagnose them. Thus, even if referral to a specialist is the management of choice, a dentist must be equipped with the knowledge to make a competent referral and to fully inform the patient of the nature of the problem, the scope of the treatment and the likely prognosis.

This section therefore covers those areas where practical knowledge is core information, whereas the preceding section – 'special surgical principles' – was concerned with areas where theoretical rather than practical information is more important.

References to Part I of this book are extensive, thus minimising duplication of core information relating to basic principles such as homeostasis, surgical sepsis and cross infection control.

The subsequent chapter details the process of history taking and examination and also importantly covers the issue of the patient consent. Further chapters describe specific areas of oral surgical interest.

22 History and examination

Introduction

In oral surgical practice, the same approach to history taking and examination should be adopted as for general history taking and examination. The process should be more focused, however, to the oral region and, for example, a full systemic history and examination is not usually required.

History taking

The elements of the clinical history are shown in Table 22.1.

Introduction to the patient

Introduction to the patient is a most important moment, as discussed in detail in Chapter 2. This allows a rapport to develop with the patient that will facilitate the rest of the interview and enhance the possibility of achieving an appropriate diagnosis and treatment plan. Patient contact at a social level is an important prerequisite to obtaining the rest of the history and is important before examining the patient. Premature physical examination of a lesion may not only reduce the patient's confidence but also unnerve the surgeon if the diagnosis is not immediately apparent with visual examination.

As discussed subsequently, consent to history taking and examination is usually implicit, but nothing should be taken for granted and all of one's questions and examinations should be fully explained.

The presenting complaint

The patient should be allowed to describe the complaint in his or her own words, and then a full history of the presenting complaint should be established. This should be carried out using searching questions that do not lead

Table 22.1   Elements of the clinical history

History of the presenting complaint
Past medical history including drug history
Family history
Dental history
Social history

the patient into giving false information. Patients wishing to avail themselves of the best medical attention will usually wish to please and will therefore tend to agree, using a positive response, to any direct question asked. This problem can be overcome by providing the patient with alternatives: 'Is the pain constant?' is more likely to be answered accurately if the patient is asked 'Is the pain constant or not?'. Several features of the presenting problem should then be elicited:

- When was the problem first noted?
- What is the location?
- Are the symptoms continuous or intermittent?
- Does anything make the problem better or worse?
- Is the problem getting better or worse?

A common presenting symptom in oral surgical practice is that of pain, which requires further specific interrogation to establish its full nature and extent. Key elements to be ascertained are shown on Table 22.2.

Past medical history including drug history

The importance of obtaining a medical history is paramount not only because it allows the surgeon to enquire about other general aspects of the patient's wellbeing that are associated with the presenting complaint but also because it allows the surgeon to ascertain information relating to the patient's medical status that might have an influence on the treatment planning.

Table 22.2   Key features in a history of pain
Principle site affected
Radiation
Character
Severity
Duration
Frequency and periodicity
Precipitating and aggravating factors
Relieving factors
Associated features

A number of systemic diseases have a bearing on surgical practice and these will be discussed below. In addition, however, a number of standard questions should be asked relating to the patient's past medical history. The use of a preprinted questionnaire for this purpose is helpful because patients are likely to produce truthful responses when filling in 'their own' questionnaire, and also because it also provides written confirmation that these questions have been considered (Fig. 22.1). However, the questionnaire should always be verified by the clinician and this information should always be included in the written history that is recorded in the patient's case record.

Cardiovascular system

The cardiovascular status of the patient is particularly important when general anaesthesia is required. A myocardial infarction within the previous 6 months is a contraindication to general anaesthesia and surgery, unless this is vital (see Ch. 35).

Similarly, patients at risk of endocarditis should receive antibiotic prophylaxis and it should also be remembered that many at-risk patients are also on warfarin; their management must take this into account (see Ch. 35).

The respiratory system

An upper respiratory tract infection is a relative contra-indication to surgery and treatment should be deferred until the infection has been cleared. Patients with chronic lung disease may need special care. The history of a productive cough should be elicited, together with sputum production, which may suggest a current pulmonary infection that requires active treatment before general anaesthesia and surgery.

A history of smoking should alert the clinician to the possibility of chronic lung disease and the patient should be advised to stop prior to any surgical treatment under general anaesthesia.

Gastrointestinal system

A past history of liver disease, with or without jaundice, should alert the clinician to the possibility of hepatitis. Such patients also frequently have problems with coagulation, which may require investigation.

Locomotive system

A history of arthritis, especially rheumatoid disease, is important. Such patients tend to have problems with the cervical spine and this may be important, not only for the anaesthetist if the patient requires intubation but also for the oral surgeon treating the patient within a dental chair. Particular care should be taken in patients with Down syndrome because of their tendency to have atlantoaxial dislocation.

Neurological system

Neurological symptoms are important to elicit particularly if there is a history of trauma and these are discussed fully in Chapter 19.

Drug history

It is crucial to know about the drugs ingested by the patient, including over the counter medication, before contemplating any surgery. A history of corticosteroid medication and anticoagulant therapy is particularly important (see Ch. 35). Care should be taken to ensure that the patient's medication will not adversely interact with any medication given to or prescribed for the patient.

Family history

The family history provides information regarding genetic disease, such as haemophilia, and also provides an insight into disease susceptibility by enquiring about concurrent family disease and causes of death in deceased relatives such as heart disease, stroke or cancer.

Social history

This provides information regarding home support for patients postoperatively and should also include questions about smoking and alcohol consumption, as these

TITLE: MR/MRS/MISS/MS (delete as appropriate)   HOSPITAL NUMBER _____

NAME _____   BUSINESS TEL.NO_____

ADDRESS_____   HOME TEL.NO._____

_____   EMERGENCY CONTACT NO._____

_____   OCCUPATION_____

DATE OF BIRTH _____

		YES	NO	DETAILS
1.	Are you an expectant or nursing mother?	☐	☐	....
2.	Have you had rheumatic fever or St Vitus Dance (chorea)?	☐	☐	....
3.	Have you had hepatitis, jaundice or tuberculosis?	☐	☐	....
4.	Have you had any heart complaints, such as heart attack, high blood pressure, angina, heart murmur or a replacement heart valve?	☐	☐	....
5.	Do you suffer from bronchitis, asthma or other chest condition?	☐	☐	....
6.	Do you have diabetes?	☐	☐	....
7.	Do you have arthritis?	☐	☐	....
8.	(a) Are you receiving any tablets, creams, ointments from your doctor?	☐	☐	....
	(b) Are you taking or have you taken steroids in the last 2 years?	☐	☐	....
9.	Are you allergic to any medicines, foods or materials?	☐	☐	....
10.	Do you suffer from epilepsy or are you prone to fainting attacks?	☐	☐	....
11.	Have you ever bled excessively (eg following a cut, tooth extraction or operation)?	☐	☐	....
12.	Have you ever been hospitalised? If yes, what for and when?	☐	☐	....
13.	Are you attending any other hospital clinics or specialists?	☐	☐	....
14.	Do you suffer from blood disorders such as anaemia?	☐	☐	....
15.	Do you have any other medical condition/special needs or disabilities?	☐	☐	....

Doctor's name and address   Dentist's name and address

_____   _____

_____   _____

Tel.No _____   Tel.No._____

Date: Signature: Parent/Patient   :

Fig. 22.1 Medical history questionnaire.

influence not only disease susceptibility but also will influence postoperative recovery.

Examination

Examination of the patient is subdivided into three areas: first, related to the presenting problem; second, to assess the patient's fitness for the proposed procedure and third, to detect any associated or coincidental disease.

The first is dealt with in appropriate chapters within this book. The last two can be dealt with by a system of examination (Table 22.3).

General assessment

All clinicians should look at their patients at the first encounter to see whether they think the patient looks 'ill'. This may mean the patient looks cachectic, flushed

Table 22.3 System of examination for an oral surgery patient

General assessment
Hands
Face
Neck
Oral cavity

and feverish, exhausted, pale or jaundiced, or that other features are apparent. If the patient looks ill, do not hesitate to ask if he or she feels ill.

When assessing a patient for oral or dental surgery, a quick and easy check can be performed as described below.

Hands

Examination of the nails can demonstrate finger clubbing (suggestive of chronic lung disease or even lung cancer), koilonychia or nail spooning (may suggest iron deficiency anaemia), white nails (may suggest liver disease) and cyanosis or bluish discoloration (may suggest heart or lung disease).

Examination of the palms of the hands may show palmar erythema (red and mottled, associated with liver disease), Dupuytren's contracture of the ring and fifth fingers (associated with liver disease and epilepsy), pallor of the palm creases (associated with anaemia) and joint deformity and swelling will indicate arthritis and its nature.

The pulse can now be felt recording the rate and any arrythmia.

Face

Jaundice will be obvious from examination of the colour of the face and conjunctivae. This is a very important sign for the surgeon. Such patients have associated disorders of blood coagulation due to clotting factor deficiencies and are prone to sepsis. If the jaundice is related to viral hepatitis, the patient may be a major risk to the surgeon and the theatre staff.

Examination of the conjunctivae will not only demonstrate jaundice but they may also be very pale, indicating anaemia.

Examination of the eyes may show arcus senilis, a ring of cholesterol deposit around the iris of the eye associated with cardiovascular disease.

Skin rashes may be most obvious on the face associated with allergies, acne, dermatitis, psoriasis, and other disorders. Lichen planus is more typical on the wrists and flexor surfaces of the arms.

Facial paralysis may suggest a previous stroke or a lower motor neuron palsy such as Bell's palsy. A palsy of one side of the face results in the face being pulled to the opposite side because of unopposed muscle action.

Again this examination can take place while talking to the patient and in only a matter of seconds.

Examination of the salivary glands, temporomandibular joints and muscles of mastication should be carried out when indicated.

Neck

Neck inspection is best performed from the front and palpation from behind. It may reveal an obvious goitre especially visible or palpable on swallowing.

Patients receiving treatment for known heart failure may have distension of neck veins, which suggests that the failure is not fully controlled.

Enlarged lymph nodes may be visible and palpable and may be associated with infection, malignancy, or other less common disorders. These usually need to be investigated before any other treatment is instituted.

It is important to remember to inspect the sides of the neck especially in the region of the ears and parotid gland.

Scars in the neck should alert one to previous surgery (e.g. thyroidectomy) and enquiry should be made about this if not mentioned by the patient during the history taking.

Swelling of the neck or elsewhere in the orofacial region is often a presenting feature and should be examined in a rehearsed fashion in order to elicit the important clinical features (Table 22.4).

Oral cavity

The oral/dental surgeon has the great advantage of being able to inspect the oral cavity closely and hence to detect associated diseases that may be apparent here. This is in addition to the presenting problem. The clinical features relating to specific oral disease are detailed in the subsequent chapters.

Table 22.4 Important clinical features of a swelling
Position
Size
Shape
Colour and temperature
Tenderness
Movement
Consistency
Surface texture
Ulceration
Margin
Associated swelling

A full cardiovascular, respiratory, abdominal and neurological examination does not come under the remit of the oral/dental surgeon. Suspicion of underlying disease may be detectable from a clear history and clinical examination as outlined above. Such a history and examination should alert the oral/dental surgeon to an underlying or potential problem and in this situation, specialist advice should be sought before progressing with treatment. The patient's GP will often be aware of the underlying problems and be able to advise on risks and whether further referrals, investigations and management are necessary. If there is any doubt, advice should be sought before any oral surgical or dental treatment is performed.

Conse'nt

The patient must consent to all procedures after full explanation of the options and consequences. Consent to answer questions and to be subjected to routine examination is usually implied. Consent to procedures under local anaesthesia is commonly obtained verbally as patient cooperation is a prerequisite to completing the operation. The consequences, for example, of extraction of an impacted wisdom tooth, may be lip numbness, and it is therefore prudent to fully explain the possible implications and record this in the notes.

Although most dentists will not work on patients under general anaesthesia – most refer patients for general anaesthesia and so hence have the responsibilities of the referring dentist, detailed below – they do have continuing responsibility for their patients postoperatively and so must have detailed knowledge regarding their responsibilities surrounding such referrals.

A detailed discussion about the ethical and legal obligations upon clinicians is not included here but it is important to consider the principles of obtaining consent to treatment.

The use of the term 'informed consent' has led to much confusion amongst healthcare professionals about the nature and extent of the information that should be imparted to a patient. Many clinicians have interpreted this concept of informed consent as a process that has to be undertaken to avoid possible legal actions and, as a result, it is often carried out in a ritualistic way. This approach is most commonly reflected in cursory clinical notes recording, for example, 'warning given regarding possible nerve damage' in association with third molar surgery.

It may be that the term 'informed consent' is a misnomer and that the process of obtaining consent to treatment should, by definition, incorporate all of the information that a patient requires to make an informed decision on whether or not to proceed with the proposed treatment. Rather than thinking in terms of obtaining informed consent, a clinician may benefit from considering the process to be undertaken to obtain valid consent. The concept of obtaining valid consent is one that:

- recognises a patient's right of autonomy
- requires an assessment of the patient's competence to give consent
- imparts information to the patient in a way that is understood
- considers the patient's expectations and aspirations
- obliges the clinician to obtain and assess all information necessary to allow appropriate treatment to be undertaken safely, including sufficient information about the patient's dental condition, the treatment options and the material risks and/or complications arising from the condition itself, or associated with the patient's medical condition
- requires disclosure of the material and relevant risks associated with the treatment options under consideration
- permits discussion about the implications of refusal of treatment by the patient or withholding of treatment by the clinician

Before the process of obtaining consent can be broached with the patient, the clinician must undergo a process of obtaining all relevant clinical information and recording the details in the patient record. The patient record is an invaluable and permanent source of information and it must be possible to rely upon it for accuracy and content at any time in the future. The patient record should also contain the information listed in Table 22.5. The prudent clinician will also record the information listed in Table 22.6.

Following a structured approach to patient assessment and recording, the details in the patient record provide the clinician with all of the information necessary to facilitate meaningful discussions with the patient about the clinical situation. The imparting of all relevant information that the patient needs to make a valid decision on whether or not to proceed with the treatment as proposed is then readily available.

Competence to give consent

The efficient delivery of dental care and/or treatment relies on the fact that the law recognises that consent to every procedure need not be written or even explicitly given. The medical and dental professions rely on the fact that a patient implies consent by cooperating with treatment. However, consenting to treatment is more than simple acceptance or submission. The principles of obtaining or giving consent involve voluntariness, knowledge and competence:

- Voluntariness requires the patient freely to agree to treatment (or not).
- Knowledge requires disclosure of sufficient information in a comprehensible way to allow the patient to make an informed choice.
- Competence means that the patient must have sufficient ability to understand and make an informed decision. Competence to give consent is a prerequisite to obtaining valid consent.

Put simply, the ability to give consent is a function of the patient's age and mental or intellectual capacity. A patient must be able to do the things listed in Table 22.7.

Patients who are not able to make such autonomous decisions are young children (due to their lack of maturity), adults with cognitive difficulties and unconscious patients. These will be considered in turn.

Children

The Family Law Reform Act (1969) in England and the Age of Legal Capacity (Scotland) Act, as amended, confirm that a patient aged 16 years and over could give valid consent to treatment and, by implication, could also

Table 22.5 Essential information contained in the patient record
Patient's personal details
Current medical history
History of presenting complaint or reason for referral
Symptoms experienced
Patient expectations and/or aspirations

Table 22.6 Desirable information included in the patient record
Charting of teeth present
Periodontal assessment and charting
Oral cleanliness
Signs and symptoms noted including extra-oral
Special tests undertaken and results
Assessment of radiographs
Diagnosis and treatment options
Assessment of complications and sequelae
Definitive diagnosis and treatment plan

Table 22.7 Requirements for the ability to give consent
Understand the information
Remember or recall that information
Relate the information to 'self'
Make a judgement on whether or not to proceed
Communicate that decision

withhold consent. Although the law does permit a young person over 16 years to give valid consent, the prudent clinician undertaking a major procedure on a patient between 16 and 18 years should consider involving the parents, but only with the patient's consent.

For young children the consent of the parent or guardian is sufficient and must be obtained.

For older children, the Children Act (1989), the judgement in the Gillick Case and the Age of Legal Capacity (Scotland) Act, as amended, effectively permit a patient under the age of 16 years to give legally valid consent if he/she has sufficient intelligence and maturity to fully understand the nature and consequences of the proposed procedure.

Although the law does permit a child under 16 years to give consent, it is subject to an assessment by the clinician of the patient's level of understanding, and practitioners should always attempt to confer with the parents of patients under 16 years unless the patient declines parental involvement.

Mental capacity

There are varying degrees of mental capacity/understanding that affect a patient's ability to understand the nature and purpose of the treatment and to give valid consent. Where an adult patient is unable to give consent then, in an emergency, the law relies upon the 'principle of necessity'. If emergency treatment is considered necessary to preserve the health and wellbeing of the patient then the clinician can proceed without formal consent. To proceed with treatment on an elective basis for such patients, a clinician would be wise to take advice from his/her defence organisation.

Unconscious patients

In the case of temporary incapacity, such as unconsciousness, it is recognised that treatment can be carried out without consent provided that such treatment is clinically necessary and in the patient's best interests.

General anaesthesia

As a result of guidance issued by the General Dental Council, the availability of general anaesthesia for dental treatment has been removed from the general dental practice setting. There will be a continuing demand, albeit a reducing one, for general anaesthesia in the secondary care sector and an increasing requirement for sedation facilities, and it is therefore important to define the obligations on dental practitioners.

The referring dentist

The General Dental Council places the following obligations on a dentist who refers a patient for treatment under general anaesthesia:

- to assess the patient's ability to cooperate
- to describe the various methods of pain control, including an assessment of the relative risks associated with each
- having decided that the patient requires treatment under general anaesthesia, or by sedation, to provide a written referral specifying the following:
  - the patient's details
  - the relevant medical and dental history
  - details of treatment to be undertaken
  - confirmation that the patient assessment has been undertaken and specification of the reason for referral.

The referring dentist is also required to ensure that the provider to which the patient is referred complies with the General Dental Council guidelines on staff, equipment and facilities for the safe delivery of care.

The operator dentist

Operator dentists are required to ensure that the treatment to be undertaken is not beyond their level of expertise and knowledge and that the facility complies with General Dental Council requirements on anaesthetic and support staff, equipment and drugs and that there is a protocol in place for the care of the collapsed patient. Staff training in monitoring of the patient and in dealing with emergency situations is mandatory and should be undertaken regularly. Before embarking on the provision of care the operator should:

- confirm the identity of the patient
- confirm the nature and extent of the treatment to be undertaken
- assess the need for diagnostic radiographs if not provided
- assess the patient's level of cooperation and reinforce the alternative methods of pain control
- obtain written consent – following an assessment of the patient by the anaesthetist, including an evaluation of the medical history – if general anaesthesia is deemed necessary
- give appropriate advice about postoperative complications or sequelae.

When a patient is referred for treatment under general anaesthesia the consent process is dependent on:

- the patient disclosing all relevant information
- the referring dentist undertaking an assessment of the patient, including the level of cooperation as well as the treatment required
- the operator confirming the need for treatment and the appropriateness of the request for general anaesthesia
- in concert with the anaesthetist, obtaining written consent following an assessment of the patient's fitness for anaesthesia.

Postoperative care

It could be difficult for the patient to find out-of-hours care after a referral for treatment under general anaesthesia, and this is particularly true if the provider is some distance from the referring practice. The referring practitioner retains overall responsibility for the care of the patient and should therefore ensure that the patient, or a responsible person or carer, is informed of the arrangements for the provision of emergency care.

23 Basic oral surgical techniques

Introduction

The majority of oral surgery skills can be learnt by most with good practical training, an awareness of basic principles of surgery (see Part 1), knowledge of the anatomy of the region and careful preparation for the procedure. Whatever surgical operation is being undertaken, the operator must have considered the following points (Table 23.1).

Preoperative considerations

The surgeon must consider if the procedure is necessary. For example, oral surgeons over recent years have looked more critically at the removal of impacted wisdom teeth, given the unpleasant short-term effects and, more importantly, the longer-term possibility of inferior dental or lingual nerve damage. In the light of more careful scrutiny of these aspects, many surgeons are now advising an increasing number of patients not to have these teeth removed unless quite strict criteria are fulfilled (see Ch. 27).

The patient must be made aware of other possible, perhaps non-surgical, treatments. A good example of this is the treatment of periapical infection by surgical means where endodontic alternatives may be considered more appropriate.

The short-term and long-term consequences of the operation must be explained to the patient, particularly in relation to known risks. Many surgeons now prefer to prepare information leaflets on the more common procedures, such as removal of impacted wisdom teeth, so that verbal preoperative warnings are reinforced with written information.

The most appropriate measures for control of pain and anxiety during the procedure must be considered. Practically, there must be a decision on whether local anaesthesia, local anaesthesia with some form of sedation, or general anaesthesia is the preferred method. Patients have an important contribution to make when reaching such a decision but the operator may advise sedation or general anaesthesia where the procedure would take an unacceptably long time, where access might prove difficult in the fully conscious patient, or where postoperative care would benefit from the expertise of skilled nurses.

Patients should be urged to accept local anaesthesia, with or without sedation, for straightforward procedures given that the additional risk of general anaesthesia, although small, should be avoided where possible (see Ch. 10). Only when these issues have been fully addressed with the patient will he or she be in the position of being able to give informed consent to the operation. Several of the points above can be supplemented with preoperative explanatory literature and the patient's signature is finally required for documented consent. This is mandatory

Table 23.1 Preoperative considerations
Equipment for oral surgery
Operative techniques
incision
raising a flap
bone removal
tooth division
elevators
debridement
suturing
types of suture
Postoperative care
postoperative instructions
analgesia
prevention of infection
postoperative bleeding
Follow-up

where sedation or a general anaesthetic is employed but is implied in many centres where local anaesthesia is used alone. Informed consent is discussed fully in Chapter 22.

Equipment for oral surgery

Surgical instruments

Although there may be individual preferences for particular surgical instruments, there is a general consensus on basic items that are commonly used. Figure 23.1 shows a typical oral surgical kit. In oral surgery there is almost invariably a need for a hand-piece and drills and, when soft tissue surgery is being carried out, a bipolar diathermy unit can be invaluable. The use of the various instruments will be discussed later in this chapter and the importance of instrument sterilisation has already been discussed in Chapter 7.

Good lighting is essential to oral surgery and multifocal surgical lamps reduce dark spots and minimise the head or shoulder shadow of the operator or assistant. Dark protective spectacles reduce the patient's discomfort from the glare of a good light, in addition to protecting their eyes from any possible debris or instruments.

Suction

Suction should be low volume and aspirator heads or tips should be narrow bore. This combination allows maximum efficiency without undue soft tissue obstruction of the system.

Radiographic viewing screens

Most oral surgical operations require good radiographs and adequate viewing facilities within the operating room.

Assistance

Competent assistance is extremely valuable in oral surgery. Good assistants realise that they can materially aid the operator's access and vision of the operative site and are aware of the importance of their role in reducing tissue damage by careful retraction. They should be fully aware of the objectives of the surgery being undertaken and operative problems that might be encountered.

Operative techniques

Incision

For most minor oral surgery, a Swann-Morton number 15 blade is the most common choice for incision of the mucoperiosteum (Fig. 23.2). The operator should have a clear picture preoperatively of the access that will be attained, and the incisions will be made appropriate to this need. Scalpel blades should be new for each patient

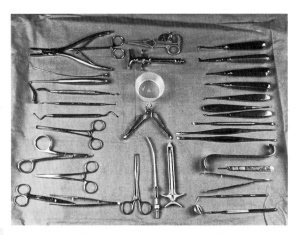

Fig. 23.1 Typical oral surgery kit.

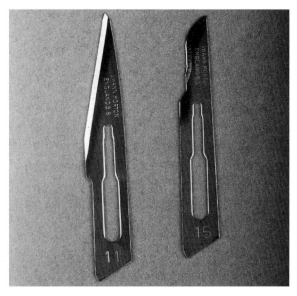

Fig. 23.2 Swann-Morton scalpel blades number 11 (left) and number 15 (right).

and, given that the cutting edge can be rapidly blunted by pressure onto a bony surface, they can and should be renewed as necessary intraoperatively. The cut should be made at right angles to the underlying bone surface such that the epithelium on each side of the incision is not chamfered but each edge should lie as close as possible to 90° to the basement membrane. This will maximise the chance of good healing when the tissues are reapposed. Any laxity in the soft tissue that is a feature of the free rather than the attached gingiva can be tensed and hence be more stable by a finger stretching the sulcus and holding it firmly against the underlying bone. The scalpel should move at uniform speed and with sufficient firmness to cut through not only the mucosal surface but also the periosteum overlying the bone. It should be made, ideally, with one movement, avoiding redefining or chopping actions, which produce ragged margins.

Raising a flap

This is undertaken with periosteal elevators such as the Ash pattern or Howarth elevators. Other instruments that can be used are the small blade end of a Mitchell's osteotrimmer where the tissues are particularly adherent to the bone beneath, or the reverse side of the right or left Warwick James' elevators for careful raising of interdental papillae. The term 'raising a flap' is probably not well chosen, for it implies that the tissues are lifted up actively from the bone surface. In fact, the periosteal elevator should be firmly pushed at approximately 30–45° to the surface of the bone such that the periosteum is stripped from it. It is important to try to raise both mucosa and periosteum in one layer and this does require a considerable force to be applied. Each push of the periosteal elevator should only be designed to achieve a movement of about 5–10 mm, with the emphasis on the sharp edge of the instrument being kept on the actual surface of the bone. Occasionally, a dry, sterile swab can be interposed between the periosteal elevator and the bone, particularly where muscle fibre attachments are very adherent to the periosteum. This measure can more effectively clean the bone surface totally of overlying soft tissue.

Most mucoperiosteal flaps are buccally situated and are designed to have one horizontal and one vertically arranged limb. The vertical cut is often known as the relieving incision. For this reason many refer to this configuration as 'L'-shaped. For virtually all flaps the horizontal arm should extend from the distal forward to the operative site, with the vertical limb anteriorly placed. This ensures that when the flap is taken back and retracted, it is being held away from the operator's line of vision, thus increasing access and visibility. From time to time there may be a need for a distal (posteriorly) placed vertical limb in addition to the anterior one, and this can be an advantage where there is a more marked convexity to the curvature of the arch such as in the lower anterior segment. In general, however, the second vertical cut is avoided because the flap is never as stable when replaced in such circumstances. Palatal flaps do not require any vertical relief whatsoever, as the concave configuration puts no requirement for it whether in the dentate or edentulous mouth.

In the edentulous patient, horizontal incisions are made along the crest of the ridge or where there is any instability due to resorption of the underlying bony alveolus, slightly to the buccal aspect of the crest. Incisions around standing teeth require care to avoid undue damage to the gingival cuff both for buccal or palatal flaps. The vertical incision needs to be carried from the attached into the free gingiva to a varying length, depending on the access needed. It should be angled forwards such that the base of the flap must always be longer than its free margin, thus ensuring adequacy of the blood supply to it. Only the mental nerve is at risk from a vertical cut in the oral cavity. Care should always be taken to avoid the mental foramen with a vertical incision and even the horizontal incision may need to be swung to the lingual side around this area where, in the edentulous patient, there has been gross alveolar bone atrophy and the foramen is lying for practical purposes on the crest of the ridge.

Finally, in the edentulous ridge, it may be possible to increase the length of the horizontal (crestal) limb of the incision such that the need for a vertical relieving cut is obviated. This is sometimes known as an 'envelope' flap and it certainly reduces postoperative discomfort as movement of the lips and cheeks tends not to pull directly on it, and also where a denture is being inserted this can be worn more comfortably. This principle (i.e. increasing the length of the horizontal incision to allow access without any vertical relief) can also be used in dentate patients as, for example, in the removal of wisdom teeth (see Ch. 27).

Buccal retraction can be effected with a variety of designed retractors. Some of these contain a rake edge, containing multiple teeth, which should be held against the bone but which can cause considerable damage to the undersurface of the flap if its teeth are allowed to rotate and tear into the flap. This might happen if the assistant tires later on in the procedure. Many prefer, therefore, to use periosteal elevators, one held by the operator and the other by the assistant. The main objective of good retraction is to protect the soft tissues from damage during the procedure and this includes not only the mucoperiosteal flap but also the lips and cheeks, which are particularly liable to frictional burning from bur shanks if the operator and/or the assistant is not duly vigilant.

Bone removal

Many dentoalveolar procedures require bone to be removed to allow access to a buried root, unerupted tooth, cyst, or whatever pathological condition is being treated. This can be done by a variety of methods.

Thin or weakened bone can often be removed with hand instruments such as osteotrimmers, curettes or even elevators. Under local anaesthesia this may be a less alarming method for the more nervous patients and can in some cases eliminate the use of drills. Bone rongeurs (bone nibblers) can also be used to enlarge existing bone defects, as for example round cysts, in addition to their use for trimming sharp edges on completion of the operation.

A hand-piece and drill is the most frequently used method for bone removal. For most dentoalveolar surgical purposes an engine with a capability of 40 000 revs per minute and with good torque is needed, either air or electrically driven. As oral surgery techniques utilise direct visualisation, a straight hand-piece is inevitably the instrument of choice. High-speed air rotors do not give the same desirable sense of feel to cutting bone and run the risk of air escape into the wound causing air emphysema. Air introduced at pressure can be a most alarming occurrence to both patient and operator as it causes immediate swelling. Palpation of the resultant swelling will elicit characteristic crepitus, a creaking sensation that tends to 'move about', not always being felt at the same point of the swelling.

A variety of different burs are available but round burs and fissure burs are most commonly employed. For most procedures where bone alone is being cut, steel is a good material but where tooth sectioning is likely, tungsten carbide burs have faster cutting potential and can reduce the time spent cutting through enamel, as, for example,

when dividing a tooth. Removal of bone and how much to remove is a skill learned by experience but, in general terms, sufficient bone should be removed to allow adequate further instrumentation to achieve the desired result. Ideally, bone removal is kept to the minimum consistent with the provision of satisfactory access. During the cutting, sterile water or saline should act as a coolant and aid the successful aspiration of any loose bony fragments, thus maintaining maximum visibility.

Chisels can be used as hand instruments or with a hammer. When the latter is employed, the patient would normally be under a general anaesthetic as the procedure would be unduly alarming to the conscious patient. The most common use of the hammer and chisel is in the removal of lower third molars where the lingual plate is split (split bone technique) allowing the tooth to be rotated lingually to effect its removal (see Ch. 27). The bone must not be unduly brittle as this will increase the chance of uncontrolled splitting of the bone and jaw fracture. It is therefore confined to young patients and, although the split of the bone may be less controlled than using a drill and hand-piece, it can be a very quick and remarkably atraumatic technique in skilled hands.

Tooth division

Division of an impacted tooth is usually carried out to reduce the amount of bone removal that would otherwise be required to effect its elevation and delivery. Division of a tooth is normally carried out with a hand-piece and bur, the latter often being a fissure bur. Teeth may be divided in any way appropriate to their position, but most often this involves sectioning of the crown from the root complex. There are instances where, for example, in a mesioangular impacted lower third molar there are two clearly separate roots on radiograph, the tooth may more easily be divided longitudinally to separate the mesial root and its adjacent crown from the distal root and crown. The additional benefit of division of a tooth is the resultant reduction in its resistance to elevation.

Separation of the roots of a multirooted tooth will also reduce the mechanical advantage of its resistance to removal and some teeth do require sectioning of crown from roots, followed by root from root separation. Although this clearly requires more use of the drill, the forces that have to be applied with elevators are consequently reduced and this more than compensates for the alarm that patients might experience as a result of excessive forces being used during elevation.

Elevators

A variety of elevators are available for removing teeth or roots from their sockets: Coupland's chisels (originally designed as hand-held bone chisels), Warwick James' elevators, Cryer's elevators and dental luxators (Fig. 23.3). Dental elevators work either on the principle of 'block and wedge' or 'wheel and axle', and should never be used as crow-bars (Fig. 23.4). Hence, a dental luxator with its sharp edge is pushed between the root of a tooth and its alveolar bone via the periodontal space. This wedging effect should cause the root to be moved from its socket

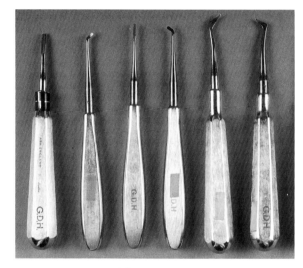

Fig. 23.3 Elevators left to right Coupland's chisel, Warwick James' left, straight and right, Cryer's left and right.

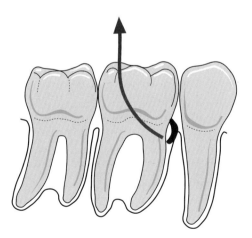

Fig. 23.4 The correct application of an elevator between the bone and the tooth.

as the elevator is advanced. Coupland's chisels can be used in a similar fashion and are more effective in this way if their edge is well maintained and sharp.

The other method is accomplished by rotating the elevator along its long axis such that its edge exerts a displacing force on the tooth or root. The straight Warwick James', Coupland's chisels, and, with their pointed blades, Cryer's elevators are used in this way. Great care should be exercised to avoid using an adjacent tooth as a fulcrum for elevators except where several teeth are to be extracted, when movement of the adjacent tooth will not be a problem and may indeed be desirable.

Elevators should be applied to teeth with an awareness of the most advantageous point of application so that the tooth will move along the line of its least resistance. Hence, as most roots in the lower molar region curve distally, elevation from the mesial aspect is more likely to be successful. Similarly, elevation from buccal rather than lingual is technically more practicable when using the rotation principle.

Debridement

Following the completion of any surgical procedure it is important to ensure that there are no impediments to good healing. These can take the form of loose bone spicules or fragments insufficiently attached to periosteum to maintain an adequate blood supply, dental fragments lying loose or hidden under the flap, or infected soft tissues such as infected follicular tissue around the removed crown of an impacted tooth. Bony or dental fragments should be carefully aspirated with thorough irrigation paying particular attention to spicules hidden under the retracted flap. Soft tissues should be curetted or removed with tissue forceps such as 'mosquito' or Fickling's forceps. Any sharp bony edges can be nibbled with rongeurs or smoothed with a larger 'acrylic' bur.

Suturing

Inserting sutures into a mucoperiosteal flap allows accurate repositioning of the soft tissues to their pre-operational site. In many cases, this will re-establish the anatomical position of the flap but in certain circumstances the flap may be moved for good reason. Such a situation arises where a buccal flap is pulled across an oroantral fistula to be attached to the palatal aspect of the socket. This is known as a buccal advancement flap and, as will be discussed later in Chapter 26, it does require periosteal release by incising the periosteal layer at the base of the flap to allow sufficient elasticity to move the tissues across the defect. In the majority of cases, however, sutures hold the soft tissues in the desired healing position and prevent the wound opening, with the consequent exposure of bone beneath and encourage haemostasis.

Materials required

A suturing kit is shown in Figure 23.5 and involves the following:

Needle holder

These instruments come in a variety of sizes and design and operators tend to choose one that suits them, having tried various forms. In general, they will be either ratchet or non-ratchet designed, the former allowing the needle to be locked into the beaks of the instrument whereas the latter requires the operator to actively hold the needle within the beaks.

Tissue forceps

Sometimes known as dissecting forceps, the important requirement is that they hold the soft tissues atraumatically so avoiding crushing and with little chance of slippage. This is achieved by a rat-toothed design, which, although possibly causing tiny puncture points, is ideal for the purposes of suturing and holding soft tissues generally (Fig. 23.6). The use of non-toothed forceps will result in crushing of the tissues as, to prevent tissue slippage from grasp, the instrument must be held too tightly.

Soft tissue retractor

The relevance of this instrument is obvious but it does indicate that an assistant is necessary during suturing to hold the soft tissues aside to allow access and to use the aspirator.

Needles

These are made of stainless steel and, for oral surgical purposes, are usually a curved shape from three-eighths to one-half the circumference of a circle; on cross-section they are triangular. A full description of suture needles and sutures appears in Chapter 3. The length of the needle varies but between 18 and 26 mm is a reasonable range for intraoral work. The triangular cross-sectional view of the needle either has the apex of the triangle facing inwards (i.e. on the concave side) or outwards. The former (i.e. inward pointing) is known as the cutting needle and the latter as a reverse cutting needle. These designs allow minimal soft tissue trauma during needle insertion as they cut a path through the soft tissues and do not therefore require excessive force on the part of the operator.

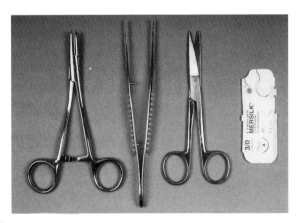

Fig. 23.5 Suturing kit containing a Kilner's needle holder, Gillies toothed tissue forceps, suture scissors and suture.

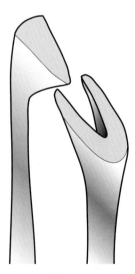

Fig. 23.6 The head of Gillies toothed tissue forceps showing the interdigitating nature of the points.

Suture material

There is a wealth of choice of material for suturing purposes (see Ch. 3) but most commonly in oral surgery materials such as silk, catgut (now in its softgut format) vicryl and nylon are used. Sutures are available either as non-resorbable (e.g. silk and nylon) or resorbable (e.g. catgut or vicryl). The gauge or thickness of the chosen material must be determined and this is denoted by O gradings. As the thickness of the material decreases, the O grading rises. Hence 2/0 is thicker than 3/0, which is thicker than 4/0 and so on. Most intraoral suturing is carried out with 3/0 or 4/0 gauge material but on extraoral skin surfaces, finer gauge is preferred such as 6/0 or even finer. This helps reduce scar visibility.

Types of suture

Different designs of suture usage can be chosen according to the particular needs of the clinical situation (Fig. 23.7). These vary from the simplest, such as the interrupted suture, to more complex mattress designs to continuous sutures placed either over the wound or, particularly with skin surfaces, beneath it. These latter continuous sutures are sometimes known as subcuticular sutures. The vast majority of intraoral sutures will be simple interrupted sutures.

Mattress sutures have particular advantages in certain clinical situations. The horizontal mattress is often helpful in reducing the surface area of a bleeding lower molar socket and exerting pressure on the overlying mucoperostium. It can also be a useful suture in closing an oroantral fistula where it encourages eversion of the margins of the wound, thus ensuring better connective tissue contact and discouraging epithelial contact which would prevent healing by primary intention.

The vertical mattress suture also helps the apposition of connective tissue surfaces and hence trouble free healing. One example of its application is the interdental papilla particularly of an anterior tooth where accurate gingival repositioning of the flap is desired (see Ch. 29).

Suture technique

Flaps are normally 'L'- or inverted 'L'-shaped. Most operators prefer to suture the angle of the 'L' first as this will correctly align the vertical and horizontal limits of the flap. The tissue of the flap should be held firmly by the tissue forceps and the needle passed through the mucoperiosteum about 3 mm from the margin, more if the flap is friable because of chronic infection. The needle is then pushed through the corresponding tissue on the other side of the incision, again about 3 mm from the margin. The suture is pulled through such that there are only a few centimetres from its entry point to the end of the suture. The knot should be tied as in Fig. 23.8 and the ends cut. Where possible, the knots should be drawn to lie to one or other side of the line of incision and the tissue should not be drawn too tightly together (which is usually seen by blanching) as it causes the thread to 'cheese cut' through the flap and produce a painful ulcer.

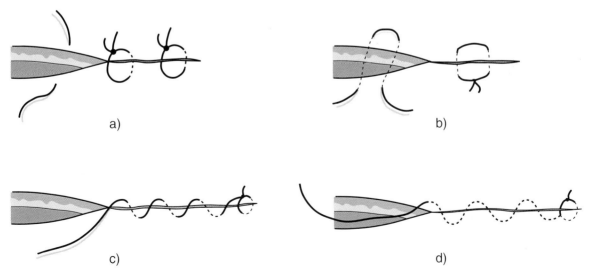

Fig. 23.7 Diagram showing types of suture: (a) interrupted; (b) mattress; (c) continuous; (d) subcutaneous continuous.

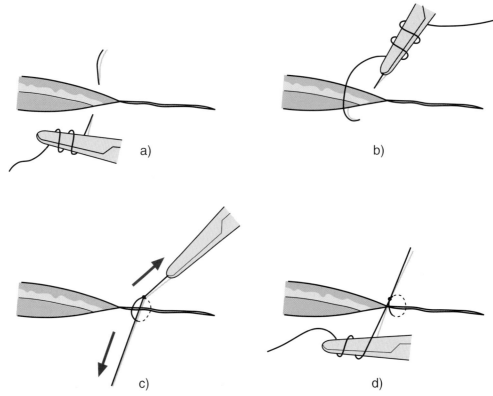

Fig. 23.8 Suture tying: the suture is wound round the needle holder clockwise (a) before pulling the free end through (b) to create the first tie (c); the suture is then wound counter clockwise to complete the knot (d).

Sutures placed intraorally are normally removed 5–7 days postoperatively. Surface anaesthetic can be very helpful if the stitch has become embedded. In the removal of sutures, normal dental tweezers such as college tweezers should grasp the free ends of the thread and the suture should be cut by sharp scissors or a suture blade close to the knot. The suture should then be pulled though in its entirety.

Postoperative care

The responsibility of the surgeon to a patient under treatment does not stop as the last suture is placed. Successful healing can be enhanced by regimes designed to minimise pain, prevent infection and reduce the chance of bleeding. This involves not only necessary prescription of drugs to patients but also appropriate instruction as to the measures patients can follow to encourage fewer postoperative problems.

Postoperative instructions

These can be given orally or by printed instruction sheets; both compliment each other because oral instructions given immediately on completion of treatment are seldom retained fully by patients who have just come through what to most of them has been an ordeal. Figure 23.9 outlines the information that should be given to patients. The list of instructions should not be over-detailed and their design should bear in mind the ability of the patient to understand them. A contact telephone number is useful and instructions on where to get help during 'non-office' hours is reassuring even if not needed.

Analgesia

As far as most patients are concerned, control of post-operative pain is the most important factor during the early phase of healing.

1. **MOUTH CARE**

    a)   Avoid rinsing for the first 6 hours after operation.

    b)   Then use warm to hot salt water (1 teaspoon in 1 tumbler) gently for the first few rinses, then progressively more vigorously at least 6 times per day.

    c)   Do not explore the wound with tongue or fingers.

    d)   Avoid alcohol and also excessive physical exercise for first 24 hours.

    e)   Brush other teeth – but avoid the wound or socket.

    f)   Keep your lips and cheeks moving as much as possible.

2. **PAIN**

    a)   Some discomfort is normal.

    b)   Use painkillers as prescribed or from the chemist but always read the label and do not take more than the suggested dose.

    c)   Start the painkiller before the numbness of the injection wears off.

    d)   If the pain is not reducing after 24 – 48 hours, seek help.

3. **BLEEDING**

    a)   Some staining of saliva with blood is not uncommon on the first day or two after the operation.

    b)   If bleeding is ocurring, then roll up the swabs provided (or a clean handkerchief) into a pad, place it over the socket (or wound) and bite firmly for 10 – 15 minutes without releasing the pressure.

    c)   If still bleeding, this can be repeated.

    d)   If bleeding stops, mouth-rinsing should not be started again for 4 hours.

    e)   If the problem persists, seek help.

4. **SWELLING**

    a)   Swelling after a mouth operation is very common and not a cause for undue anxiety. There may also be bruising.

    b)   Softer food may be necessary for a few days as opening the mouth and chewing may be made difficult by swelling.

    c)   If swelling increases after 48 hours then advice should be obtained.

5. **ANTIBIOTICS**

    a)   If these have been prescribed use them as directed by the surgeon or nurse.

    b)   Antibiotics can reduce the effectiveness of 'the Pill' (oral contraceptive) and additional forms of contraception may therefore be needed during and for 1 week after the completion of the antibiotic course.

CONTACT No. ....

OUT OF HOURS HELP: ....

Fig. 23.9   Postoperative instructions leaflet.

Local anaesthesia

Many operators now administer local anaesthetics to control immediate postsurgical pain. Under local anaesthesia with or without sedation, the necessary injections are given and tested presurgically as a matter of course. Under general anaesthesia local anaesthetic is given perioperatively, normally at the start of the procedure, and many now prefer to use longer-acting agents such as bupivacaine. It is obviously important to inform patients that the area in question will be numb when they first recover consciousness, and this is particularly important when they have been warned preoperatively of the possibility of nerve damage as a consequence of the procedure. Even if longer-acting local anaesthetics are not used, some operators reinforce anaesthesia with the usual agent on completion of the surgery, whether under local or general anaesthesia. It does appear that immediate control of pain for the first few hours postoperatively seems not only to have an early benefit but may also reduce the discomfort throughout the several days following surgery.

Systemic analgesia

The normal agents employed following minor oral surgery are non-steroidal anti-inflammatory drugs or paracetamol. Recourse to narcotics is seldom needed, other than codeine-containing preparations. Opiates may be needed after more extensive surgery but these patients will generally be inpatients under the supervision of skilled nursing personnel. There may be an advantage in prescribing drugs with an anti-inflammatory action as well as an analgesic effect. However, certain groups of patients, such as asthmatics or those with a history of peptic ulceration, are at risk from these drugs and the use of paracetamol with or without codeine is more prudent.

All patients should be prescribed adequate analgesics, and given instructions on their correct usage. There seems little doubt that, whatever drug is prescribed, patients should be instructed to take the analgesic before the local anaesthetic effect has worn off. Some suggest that analgesics are best started preoperatively, to ensure that there is an adequate plasma level of the drug when the local anaesthetic begins to wear off. Many patients have their 'favourite' preparation and in these circumstances should be encouraged to use a drug that has a proven success for them.

Prevention of infection

Antibiotics

Prescription of antibiotics as a prophylactic measure in this context remains a contentious issue. The evidence for their use is far from convincing and it is true to say that most surgeons rely on their clinical experience when making the decision of whether or not to use them. Many operators justify their use based on the presence of infection in the surgical field (see Ch. 8) or the removal of substantial amounts of bone during the procedure. The blood supply in the maxilla is more profuse than in the

mandible and infection is consequently a more uncommon complication and most antibiotics are therefore prescribed for procedures carried out on the mandible.

Arguments against antibiotic use are based on their overprescription resulting in increasing numbers of bacteria that have developed resistance to these drugs, and in some cases multiresistant organisms such as the methicillin-resistant *Staphylococcus aureus* (MRSA) that now poses such serious problems. The possibility of more and more organisms having multiresistance is without question a serious and potentially disastrous scenario of which both the medical and veterinary professions are becoming increasingly aware. There is good cause, therefore, for all clinicians to consider carefully the perceived advantages and disadvantages of antibiotic prescription, particularly where they are being used for prevention of possible infection rather than the actual treatment of existing infection. Many clinicians now reduce the length of time for which antibiotics are prescribed because this measure in itself will reduce the chance of the emergence of resistance in bacterial colonies. Amoxicillin or metronidazole are probably the most commonly prescribed antibiotics when the postoperative risk of infection is considered significant. Their use for patients with a reduced capability of coping with infection, such as those with a reduced immune response (for example, poorly controlled diabetics, HIV-positive patients or those on immunosuppressive drugs) in whom the results of infection can be correspondingly serious, is therefore uncontroversial. A further discussion of the use of antibiotics in surgery is given in Chapter 8.

Mouthwashes

Patients are universally advised on the use of mouthwashes and they undoubtedly play an important role in maintaining wound cleanliness if used frequently.

Chlorhexidine

This is an antiseptic mouthwash which is effective in controlling plaque but may also have positive benefits for wounds. With inability to use toothbrushes in the areas of the surgery, both plaque control and local antiseptic action are needed and this mouthwash is commonly prescribed as a routine post-operatively. Use of chlorhexidine is probably best restricted to 2 or 3 times per day with the intervening periods covered with simple saline rinses. Pre- or perioperative use of a chlorhexidine mouthwash has been shown to reduce the risk of post-operative infection and reduce the incidence of 'dry sockets'.

Saline mouthwashes

These should be made up with approximately one teaspoonful of salt to one tumbler of warm to hot water. They are the mainstay of wound cleanliness and should be encouraged. Their use should initially be gentle rather than vigorous but, as the days progress, a more vigorous use should be encouraged. In addition to increasing the use of mouthwashes after the first 24 h, patients should also be encouraged to keep their mouths moving so that stagnation of saliva does not result, as this can encourage infection. Mouthwashes upwards of six times per day should be discontinued only if bleeding from the wound occurs.

Postoperative bleeding

Bleeding from intraoral wounds is seldom due to a defect in the haemostatic mechanism or in the clotting process (see Ch. 6) but is more commonly due to leakage from small vessels in bone or periosteum. It is more frequently seen within a few hours of surgery and may in some cases be reactive bleeding resultant upon the dilatation of vessels previously constricted by local anaesthetic containing adrenaline (epinephrine). Another contributory factor may be inappropriate exploration of the wound by fingers or tongue and by mouth rinsing too soon after the surgery.

Control of such bleeding is usually affected by use of local haemostatic agents such as regenerated oxidised cellulose, further suturing of the wound and direct masticatory pressure via a suitably placed swab.

Secondary haemorrhage caused by wound infection is characteristically seen around 10 days postoperatively but is very uncommon in dentoalveolar wounds.

Follow-up

Following surgery, most patients will be seen between 5 and 7 days later to ensure that healing is progressing satisfactorily. Sutures are removed when necessary and debris may need to be irrigated from the wound area if the patient's oral hygiene measures have been inadequate. For some patients, results of histological examination of tissue can be explained and, if necessary, further appointments arranged. For many patients, however, there is no further need for follow-up and they can be discharged. For routine removal of wisdom teeth or retained roots, for example, and where resorbable sutures have been used in the surgery, some operators see only those patients who have continuing problems. Where this format of management is used, a full postoperative leaflet is issued, which indicates the particular problems that could occur and might need further consultation. The required contact telephone numbers are a necessary inclusion in such a leaflet.

24 Local anaesthesia

Introduction

Achieving good local anaesthesia is a prerequisite for virtually all dental surgery, and in oral surgery the confidence this gives is mandatory from both the patient's and the operator's point of view. The ability to administer a comfortable local anaesthetic to any patient is a fundamental skill that dental surgeons should strive to achieve. This will allow stress levels in both giver and receiver to be greatly reduced, and technique must be constantly reviewed and revised to this end.

Not only is the actual injection of local anaesthetic important, the operator must give the drug adequate time to block nerve transmission and must have confidence in his or her ability to recognise the subjective changes it will bring about before testing its adequacy. One of the most common faults is testing the effect of local anaesthetic before reasonable time has elapsed, when lack of necessary depth of anaesthesia causes discomfort. This immediately results in loss of confidence by the patient, who becomes more apprehensive and may therefore be far more difficult to convince that adequate anaesthesia, even after further administration, is finally attained.

Patients must be told before the testing of an anaesthetic that all sensation is not, and will not, be lost, and that it is specifically pain that will be abolished. This is particularly true in oral surgery practice, where the procedure may often involve causing a very real feeling of pressure that can be alarming to patients who have not been fully briefed on what the local anaesthetic can and cannot do. If patients are asked to report 'feeling anything' during the testing procedure they might truthfully say that they feel something, and this could lead to further, and possibly unnecessary, administration of local anaesthetic. Finally, awareness that good local anaesthesia is one of the most important criteria by which patients judge their operator makes this subject worth studying and knowing well.

Uses of local anaesthesia

The uses of local anaesthesia are listed in Table 24.1 and these are discussed in turn.

Diagnostic use

Administration of local anaesthetic can be a useful way of finding the source of a patient's pain. An example of this is the pain of a pulpitis, which can be very difficult for both the patient and the dentist to isolate because of its tendency to be referred to other parts of the mouth or face. Particularly useful is the infiltration technique, which achieves a localised action and can discriminate between maxillary and mandibular sources, and even between individual upper teeth provided they are not immediately adjacent. Another example is the patient with myofascial pain who is convinced that an upper tooth is causing the problem. Local anaesthesia may help this patient and the surgeon in this situation to eliminate the tooth as the cause of pain and may thus avoid its unnecessary treatment.

Table 24.1   Uses of local anaesthesia

Diagnostic: to isolate a source of pain
Therapeutic: to reduce or abolish the pain of a pathological condition
Perioperative: to achieve comfort during operative procedures
Postoperative: to reduce postoperative pain

Therapeutic use

Local anaesthetics can, in themselves, constitute part of a treatment regimen for painful surgical conditions. The ability of the dentist to abolish pain for a patient, albeit temporarily, is a therapeutic measure in its own right. The use of a block technique to eliminate the pain of dry socket (localised osteitis) (see Ch. 26) can be immensely helpful to the management of this very painful condition, particularly in the first few days. Inferior dental blocks of long-acting local anaesthetics such as bupivacaine can give total comfort for several hours, allowing patients to catch up on lost sleep and perhaps reduce the use of systemic analgesics to avoid overuse. Moreover, the patient can return for further local anaesthesia if the pain once more becomes too demanding. Although it would be impossible to keep administering local anaesthetic blocks, there is enough, albeit anecdotal, evidence to suggest that when the pain returns after the block wears off, it is not at the same level of intensity.

Blocks of the inferior dental, mental or infraorbital nerves can also be used for the treatment of trigeminal neuralgia when pain breakthrough, despite medication such as carbamazepine, has become unacceptable. Long-acting local anaesthetic in this context seems, in some patients, not only to give comfort during the duration of the anaesthetic but also to break the pattern of break-through in the longer term.

Perioperative use

The provision of pain-free operative surgery is by far the most common use of local anaesthetics, and provides an effective and safe method for almost all outpatient dentoalveolar oral surgical procedures. It can, in con-junction with sedation techniques, allow more difficult or protracted procedures to be carried out without the additional risks of general anaesthesia, and this may be particularly of value in patients with significant cardio-vascular or airway disease (see Ch. 11).

Additionally, however, local anaesthetics are often given to patients undergoing oral or maxillofacial surgery under general anaesthesia. This serves several purposes:

- It reduces the depth of general anaesthesia needed.
- It reduces the arrhythmias, which are noted on electrocardiogram (ECG) during the surgery when significant afferent stimulation is taking place. This can be seen, for example, when a tooth is being elevated.
- It also provides local haemostasis to the operative site and provides immediate postoperative analgesia.

Postoperative use

After surgery with either local or general anaesthesia, the continuing effect of the anaesthetic is a most beneficial way of reducing patient discomfort. It helps to reduce or even eliminate the need for stronger (often narcotic) systemic analgesics, which have their own drawbacks. Many operators now use longer-acting agents, such as bupivacaine, to prolong the immediate postoperative analgesia. There is some evidence to suggest that this measure, allied to early prescription of systemic analgesics, can more effectively control pain and that this early benefit may well be sustained throughout the days following surgery.

Local anaesthetic agents

Table 24.2 shows the commonly used local anaesthetic agents. In oral surgery there is a distinct advantage in using a local anaesthetic with adrenaline (epinephrine), which, by its vasoconstrictive action, improves the visibility of the surgical site by reducing small-vessel bleeding.

Action

Both lidocaine (lignocaine) and prilocaine hydrochloride are good local anaesthetic agents and account for the vast

Table 24.2 Commonly used local anaesthetic agents		
Anaesthetic drug	*Vasoconstrictor*	*Duration (ID block)*
Lidocaine (lignocaine) hydrochloride 2%	Adrenaline (epinephrine) 1:80 000	2.5–3 h
Prilocaine hydrochloride 3%	Felypressin 0.03 international units	2.5–3 h
Bupivacaine hydrochloride 0.5%	Adrenaline (epinephrine) 1:200 000	6–8 h

majority of local anaesthetic administrations in oral surgery. They are both tertiary amines that form hydrochloride salts for use in solution. When injected into the tissues, these agents dissociate into cationic quaternary amides with a positive chemical charge, although some remains in the uncharged base form. It is this uncharged lidocaine (lignocaine) or prilocaine that passes through the nerve membrane to once again dissociate into the cationic form. These intracellular cations of the anaesthetic agents are believed to be primarily responsible for blocking the sodium channels in the membrane, which in turn blocks the rapid sodium inrush to the cell during nerve impulse propagation. Distortion of the axon membrane by uncharged local anaesthetic also appears to have a role in blocking this transmission.

Maximum safe dose

Local anaesthetics such as lidocaine (lignocaine) and prilocaine are extremely safe given their extensive use in both medicine and dentistry. The addition of adrenaline (epinephrine) to lidocaine (lignocaine)and of felypressin to prilocaine reduces the rate of uptake from the site of injection, thus reducing the possible toxic effects of the local anaesthetic agent and increasing, in theory, the volume that can therefore be used. Apart from the actual amounts used, three other considerations should be taken into account: (1) the avoidance of intravascular injection by use of an aspirating syringe; (2) the rate of administration of the local anaesthetic – a slow rate reduces the chance of overload and hence possible toxic effects; and (3) the status of the patient. Extremes of age, physical size and medical background should be determined for each individual patient, all of which may modify what could be considered a safe quantity.

Most authorities do now acknowledge that the toxic effects of the local anaesthetic agents – which mainly arise from central nervous system depression, and in particular respiratory depression – must be balanced against the possible undesirable effects of adrenaline (epinephrine) where that is included in the solution. The action of adrenaline (epinephrine) on the heart (causing increase in myocardial excitability, rate, force of contraction, and stroke volume) is potentially undesirable, particularly in patients with known heart disease. It is in this group of patients that many operators prefer to use adrenaline (epinephrine)-free local anaesthetics. Others argue that lidocaine (lignocaine) and adrenaline (epinephrine) provide a more profound anaesthesia with less chance of

pain breakthrough, and that for oral surgical purposes the relatively bloodless field they produce is a significant advantage.

In general terms, the maximum safe dose can be expressed as 4.5–5.0 mg per kg body weight of lidocaine (lignocaine) with 1:80 000 adrenaline (epinephrine) and 3 mg per kg body weight of prilocaine. When translated into millilitres of 2% lidocaine (lignocaine) with adrenaline (epinephrine) or 3% prilocaine with felypressin in a fit 70-kg adult patient this means that a maximum of six cartridges of lidocaine (lignocaine) (or four of prilocaine), each of 2.2 mL, is well within the safe limit. The preoccupation with volume is misleading as it tends to cause unthinking administration, and not consideration of each patient's individual situation allied to safe technique.

Local anaesthetic technique

There are a variety of techniques used in local anaesthetic administration and these will be discussed in turn (Table 24.3).

Infiltration

This can be used to achieve anaesthesia of upper teeth and lower anteriors. It is achieved by depositing the solution around the apex of a tooth on its buccal aspect in the sulcus. The porosity of the bone allows it to diffuse through the outer plate of bone to affect the apical nerve or nerves. It normally achieves anaesthesia within 1–2 min and has the added surgical advantage (where adrenaline (epinephrine) is in the solution) of small-vessel vasoconstriction, which provides reduction in bleeding and

Table 24.3   Local anaesthetic techniques
Infiltration
Block anaesthesia
inferior dental block
mental nerve block
posterior superior alveolar block
infraorbital block
greater palatine block
nasopalatine block
Other injection techniques
periodontal ligament block
intraosseous injection
intrapulpal injection

increased visibility as a consequence. Administration should be considered as a two-part technique:

1. needle insertion
2. deposition of local anaesthetic.

Needle insertion

To achieve minimal discomfort, topical local anaesthetic should be applied 2–3 min before the injection. The index finger or thumb of the 'free' hand should pull the lip or cheek such that the sulcus tissues are taut, as this will minimise discomfort on introduction of the needle. The tip of the needle needs to be advanced only 3–4 mm into the tissue adjacent to the tooth to be anaesthetised (Fig. 24.1).

Deposition of local anaesthetic solution

The solution should be deposited slowly because the lumen of a dental needle is very fine and undue force of the solution being injected can lead to unwanted pain and tissue damage. This therefore takes time and patience but is essential in reducing discomfort.

For palatal anaesthesia, the greater palatine (or naso-palatine) nerve anteriorly supplies the mucoperiosteum.

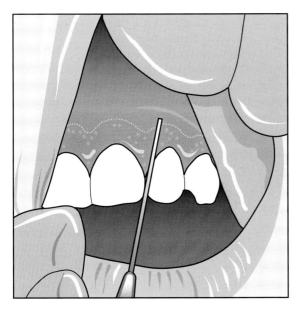

Fig. 24.1 Position of the needle for the infiltration of local anaesthetic to achieve anaesthesia of an upper lateral incisor.

Only a small quantity of local solution should be introduced and use of topical anaesthesia and strong finger-pressure adjacent to the point of entry of the needle can help to reduce this notoriously unpleasant injection. The injection is normally given adjacent to the surgical site but many consider that the area midway between the midline of the palate and the gingival margin of the tooth is less tightly bound down to the underlying bone, and is therefore less uncomfortable.

Another technique is to achieve buccal anaesthesia in the usual way, then pass the needle from buccal to palatal through both the interdental papillae (anterior and posterior) of the tooth under treatment. This does appear to reduce discomfort even if an additional palatal injection is necessary to be quite sure of adequate anaesthesia.

Block anaesthesia

Several block injections of nerve trunks can be used for oral surgical purposes. By far the most common is the inferior dental block, but others include the mental block, the posterior superior dental block and the infraorbital block. The hard palate can be anaesthetised by greater palatine and nasopalatine blocks if more extensive areas of palate require to be anaesthetised.

Inferior dental block

Several techniques have been suggested but only two will be described here, the first being a standard block and the second a closed-mouth technique that can be very useful if restricted opening is a problem.

The nerves affected are: (1) the inferior dental nerve, which provides sensation to the pulps and periodontal membranes of first incisor to third molar, the bone investing the teeth, the buccal gingivae and the sulcus from premolars to incisors, lower lip and chin; and (2) the lingual nerve, which supplies the anterior two-thirds of the tongue, the floor of mouth and the lingual gingiva.

Technique

The precise technique will vary but the following will serve as a guideline for administering an inferior dental block injection.

The patient should be seated with good head and neck support and with the neck slightly extended such that the lower occlusal plane will be approximately horizontal on fully opening the mouth. With the mouth widely opened, the finger or thumb of the 'free' hand should pass along the lower buccal sulcus until it rests posteriorly in the retromolar triangle, which lies between the (external) oblique line of the mandible and the continuation of the mylohyoid ridge or internal oblique line.

The pterygomandibular raphe should then be identified as an almost vertically running soft tissue line. This takes its origin from the pterygoid hamulus and runs downwards to its insertion on the lingual aspect of the mandible in the third molar region. The raphe gives rise to muscle attachments running laterally (buccinator) and medially (superior constrictor).

The syringe should be introduced from the lower premolar teeth of the other side parallel to the lower occlusal plane such that the needle penetrates the tissues lateral to the pterygomandibular raphe and at a level halfway up the finger or thumb lying in the retromolar triangle (Fig. 24.2).

The 'long' dental needle (3.4 cm) should be advanced about 2.5 cm until bone is touched lightly. The needle should then be withdrawn a millimetre or two and aspiration performed. If blood in the form of a smoky red trail is noted in the cartridge, the needle should be withdrawn a millimetre or so before reaspirating.

The local anaesthetic should then be deposited slowly, using most of the 2.2 mL cartridge and with the local anaesthetic being deposited on slow withdrawal to 'catch' the lingual nerve, which lies anteromedial to the inferior dental nerve.

This technique introduces a local anaesthetic solution to the inferior dental nerve as it enters the mandibular foramen on the medial aspect of the ramus. In patients who, for a variety of reasons, have trismus and cannot open sufficiently to allow this technique, a closed technique can sometimes be useful.

The patient should be seated such that the occlusal plane is approximately horizontal. The cheek should be retracted with the index finger or thumb of the 'free' hand and the needle advanced horizontally at about the level of the gingival margins of the upper molar teeth. The needle should penetrate to a depth of 1–1.5 cm before aspiration. Slow deposition of most of the 2.2 mL cartridge is normally required.

This technique leaves the local anaesthetic solution at a level higher than the standard technique, which means that it is deposited above the mandibular foramen but still below the level of the mandibular notch.

Determination of adequate anaesthesia

As mentioned in the introductory paragraph, it is important not to embark on surgery until full anaesthesia is achieved. This is normally done by asking the patient what subjective changes he or she feels in the lower lip and chin of the affected side. A feeling of pins and needles or a tingling sensation denotes early-stage changes, which would normally progress to a numb, swollen, thick or rubbery sensation. At this point the area can be tested objectively with a sharp probe passed between the tooth to be extracted, or operated upon, and the attached gingiva. Patients must be told that the sensations of touch, and especially pressure, will not be totally abolished, although pain should not be felt. Patients should always be advised that, once the surgery begins, they must immediately indicate if there is any pain breakthrough because more local anaesthetic can be given.

Buccal injection

The sulcus region in the lower premolar and molar regions may have innervation from the buccal nerve and this must be covered by a separate injection.

The buccal injection can be given more comfortably by waiting for the inferior dental block to become effective. Rather than a single block given in the cheek at

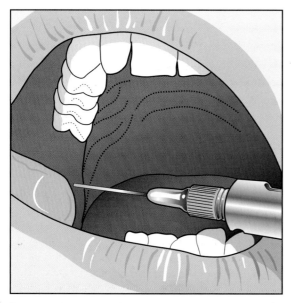

Fig. 24.2 Position of the needle for an inferior dental block.

the level of the crown of the third molar at the anterior border of the ramus, many operators simply infiltrate around the surgical site, for example, in the sulcus of the third molar region where an impacted third molar is being treated since this will have the added benefit of haemostasis of the flap.

Complications of inferior dental block

Systemic complications such as allergy, fainting or inadvertent intravascular injection with cardiac or central nervous system effects are rare, with the exception of fainting, which can usually be averted by placing the patient in the supine position. Specific to this injection, however, are certain local complications and these are listed in Table 24.4.

Facial nerve paralysis (palsy) occurs when the injection is given too far distally and the parotid gland is penetrated, allowing diffusion of the local anaesthetic through the loose glandular tissue, which then affects all five terminal branches of the facial nerve. The effect is seen in the lack of the corrugation of the forehead, inability to close the eye or blink, and inability to raise the corner of the mouth or puff the cheeks. Patients may feel that something is wrong but be unable to identify exactly what the problem is, and it is usually the operator who notices these specific changes. Patients should be informed, reassured as to the transitory nature of the palsy, and the eye should be protected with a loose pad such that the cornea is protected until the protective blink reflex returns. Recovery often occurs in a relatively short time (within an hour), unlike the inferior dental nerve itself, which can take up to 3 h.

Postinjection trismus may also arise. The diagnosis of this distressing complication is normally fairly easy in that the trismus occurs within hours of the injection. It is believed to be due to damage to the medial pterygoid muscle, resulting in its spasm and consequent inability of the muscle to relax and allow opening. It is not painful but many patients are extremely anxious and do need reassurance. In terms of technique, it may be attributed to an injection at too low a level and perhaps using too

much force to deliver the anaesthetic solution. If undue resistance to any injection is felt (as when in a muscle bed) excessive force should be avoided and the needle withdrawn. The free-running of the cartridge plunger should be checked and the needle reinserted at a higher level. Trismus can also occur after the extraction of teeth, unrelated to the anaesthetic technique. This is especially so with mandibular third molar teeth (see Ch. 27).

If the problem does occur, some prescribe a benzo-diazepine to try to alleviate muscle spasm. The mainstay of management, however, is reassurance and encourage-ment to the patient to try to gain further opening. Use of wooden spatulae may be a convenient method for the patient to measure progress. The trismus may last for weeks and even months, and resolution may occur slowly or quite dramatically over a day or two after even a prolonged period of limitation.

Prolonged anaesthesia is a rare and poorly documented complication. It can affect the inferior dental nerve or lingual nerve, and very occasionally both. It may represent physical trauma to the nerve by the needle or an idiosyncratic reaction to the local anaesthetic. Prognosis is difficult to judge as there is little evidence of outcome and resolution appears unpredictable.

Visual impairment is a reported complication but is very rare. Its cause is unknown although vasospasm has been suggested as a possible factor. Any impairment of vision warrants immediate referral to an ophthalmic specialist.

Mental nerve block

This injection will anaesthetise the pulps and periodontal membranes of the lower incisors, canine, first premolar and variably the second premolar. For surgical procedures, it must be remembered that the lingual mucoperiosteum will require separate infiltration as the mental block anaesthetises the teeth through the incisive branch of the inferior dental nerve and the peripheral distribution of the mental nerve.

Technique

In dentate patients, the mental foramen lies below and between the apices of the lower premolar teeth, approxi-mately half way between the cervical margins of the teeth and the lower border of the mandible. The injection is similar in all respects to an infiltration injection, and the objective is to deposit the solution at or near the

Table 24.4	Complications of inferior dental block
Facial nerve paralysis	
Postinjection trismus	
Prolonged anaesthesia	
Visual impairment	

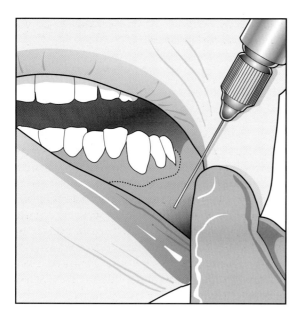

Fig. 24.3 Position of the needle for a mental nerve block.

foramen (Fig. 24.3). No attempt should be made to 'feel' the distally facing foramen because this is totally unnecessary and often causes haematoma formation through damage to the mental blood vessels.

In edentulous patients, the foramen may lie nearer the crest of the ridge as a result of alveolar resorption and due allowance for this should therefore be made before the injection is given.

Posterior superior alveolar (dental) block

This block is intended to anaesthetise the posterior superior dental nerve as it penetrates the posterolateral aspect of the maxillary tuberosity before it pierces bone. As such, a close relationship exists between the site of the injection and pterygoid venous plexus lying laterally and above and which can easily therefore be entered by the needle. This can cause an immediate and alarming haematoma visible both in the sulcus and externally in the face just below the zygomatic arch.

Technique

The technique, which is in effect high infiltration, is seldom, if ever, really necessary as diffusion of anaesthetic from the conventional infiltration is almost always effective. If it is considered necessary, then the

needle should be angled inwards towards the buccal plate as much as possible, given that the opening of the mouth will restrict this. The other angle to remember is the alignment of the needle at approximately 45° to the occlusal plane after entering the sulcus in the second molar region.

Infraorbital block

This injection, although given infrequently, can be a very valuable technique for achieving anaesthesia in the anterior part of the maxilla. The local anaesthetic solution is deposited around the infraorbital foramen, where it can diffuse back along the infraorbital canal to affect the anterior and, where present as a separate nerve, the middle superior dental nerve. Ideally, therefore, in addition to anaesthesia of the soft tissues of the upper lip, side of nose, cheek and lower eyelid, the upper incisors, canine and premolars will be affected together with the adjacent sulcus and gingivae.

For oral surgery purposes this injection can be given to avoid injecting into inflamed tissues in the incisor or canine region, but can also achieve a more dependable and profound anaesthesia for larger lesions such as cysts. Use of a long-acting agent such as bupivacaine to achieve control of trigeminal neuralgic pain breakthrough also makes knowledge of this technique valuable.

Technique

Although several techniques can be used, the most commonly employed, which uses the upper first and second premolar as the key landmark, is described.

The buccal sulcus is tensed with the finger or thumb of the 'free' hand in the premolar region. Some operators suggest that a finger be placed over the infraorbital foramen on the face to 'feel' the local anaesthetic as it is administered and ensure that it is in the correct location. In practice, however, this is often not a realistic measure. The needle is introduced such that it is parallel to the long axis of the premolars; it penetrates the lateral aspect of the sulcus about 1–1.5 cm from the buccal bone surface and it is advanced upwards approximately 1.5 cm into the tissues (Fig. 24.4). After aspiration, the local anaesthetic is slowly introduced to the tissues when 1.5–2.0 mL of the preferred solution is normally sufficient.

Alternative techniques include direct injection through the skin to the foramen. The lower orbital margin rim

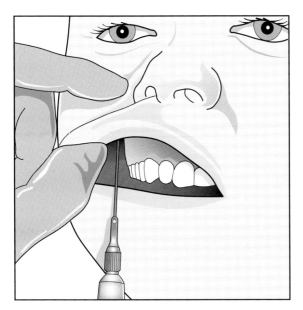

Fig. 24.4 Position of the needle for an infra-orbital block.

should be palpated carefully before injecting about 1 cm below this landmark, and at the midpoint of the infra-orbital bony margin. Administration of local anaesthetic in this way can be alarming to a patient, and careful explanation of what is being done is necessary. The eye should be protected by the fingers of the 'free' hand, with one finger carefully palpating the lower orbital bony margin.

Other injection techniques

Periodontal ligament injection

This technique introduces local anaesthetic directly into the periodontal space and, as the force required is quite substantial, specialised syringes are available to achieve this. In oral surgery, the intraligamentous injection is most frequently used if pain is being felt despite the normal techniques of infiltration or block anaesthesia. This can occur when a tooth is 'hot' through acute pulpitis or apical infection. It may also be of value if limitation of jaw mobility makes block injection difficult or impossible. One of its advantages is the small volume of local solution needed, but it is often uncomfortable to administer and will cause a bacteraemia which should be

prophylactically covered with appropriate antibiotic in an endocarditis at-risk patient.

Intraosseous injection

This technique will achieve excellent anaesthesia limited, however, to the immediate locality of the injection. The local is administered through a trephined hole best prepared with a specially designed bur through the outer cortical plate of bone. Initial infiltration anaesthesia of the area is hence a prerequisite and, after the entry is cut, a short needle is introduced into the medullary space before injecting a small quantity of solution. The diameter of the trephined hole should ideally be matched to the needle to prevent leakage. Again, the advantages of the technique are the small quantity of local anaesthetic used and the ability to achieve a good depth of anaesthesia where access may be limited through trismus.

Intrapulpal injection

This injection is normally used where, despite apparently good anaesthesia by other conventional means, the tooth remains painful on manipulation. This again is a feature of some pulpal or apical infections. In oral surgery, the tooth is normally being extracted and either the pulp canal(s) are already accessible or can be accessed using a small round bur. The technique is imprecise and escape of the solution is almost invariable. It can, however, be remarkably successful if sufficient local can be introduced. Discomfort during its administration is often a reliable indication that it will prove of benefit.

Difficulty in obtaining anaesthesia

The above techniques can all be helpful in achieving sufficient anaesthesia where prior, more conventional, methods have been unsuccessful. One other measure is the use of a stronger local anaesthetic solution, such as 4% prilocaine. The higher concentration appears in some cases to obtain a more profound depth of anaesthesia. If an inferior dental block fails to allow surgical comfort despite all the subjective features of adequacy, it may be useful to consider giving a second block with the stronger anaesthetic solution rather than simply repeating the procedure with the same agent.

Extraction techniques

Introduction

Teeth are extracted for a number of reasons, including caries, trauma, periodontal disease, impactions and orthodontics. Tooth extraction techniques improve with clinical experience. Two aspects of tooth extraction are important in successful completion of the operation: equipment and technique.

Equipment

Most teeth are extracted with dental forceps of which a variety of types are available.

Lower forceps have their blades at 90° to the handles and upper forceps have the blades either angled slightly forwards or straight in relation to their handles (Fig. 25.1). Forcep design has developed over many years and is based around the principle of creating a displacing force on the roots of the tooth, not the crown. When teeth fracture during extraction it is most commonly the result of poor forceps placement. Forceps are therefore designed around the root morphology of the tooth they are intended to remove (Fig. 25.2). The appropriate forceps choice is outlined in Table 25.1.

Root forceps that have smaller beaks for smaller teeth or fractured roots are available. There are other specific forceps with more limited application, such as upper third molar forceps, which have an elongated 'gooseneck' for access to the posterior maxilla.

Elevators may be used as an alternative method of mobilising or extracting teeth, and these are discussed in Chapter 23. There has been a recent increase in the use of instruments known as luxators to assist with extractions. Luxators are designed to help the operator gain space for application of the forceps. They are very sharp-bladed elevators that are used to increase the gap between the tooth and the surrounding bone, thus loosening the tooth and producing more space for forcep application. They can be very helpful but care must be taken due to the potential soft tissue damage. They should be used to 'unscrew' the tooth, not to elevate it.

Technique

Every clinician will develop specific techniques for tooth extraction, but all follow the same basic pattern (listed in Table 25.2), and these will be discussed in turn.

Application

Having chosen the forceps that best fit the root morphology of the tooth to be removed, surgeons must first position themselves and the patient to achieve good access and vision, as well as allowing the surgeon to

Table 25.1 Types of forcep

Forcep	Tooth
Upper universals	Upper incisors and premolars
Upper straights	Upper canines
Upper molars (R/L)	Upper molars (R/L)
Lower universals	Lower incisors, canines and premolars
Lower molars	Lower molars
Cow-horns	Lower first and second molars

Table 25.2 Extraction technique

Application of forceps
Consolidation of grip
Displacement of tooth
Postdelivery care

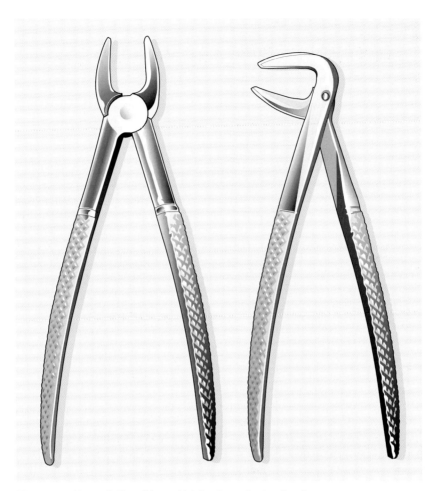

Fig. 25.1 Upper (left) and lower (right) universal extraction forceps.

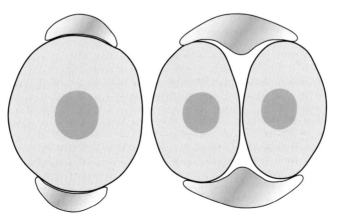

Fig. 25.2 Blades of universal forceps (left) and lower molar forceps (right) applied to the roots of an incisor and lower molar, respectively.

Table 25.3 Operator–patient position for extraction		
Quadrant	Patient	Operator
Upper right and upper left	Supine	In front
Lower left	Upright	In front
Lower right	Upright	Behind

put appropriate force on the tooth. For a right-handed operator this is outlined in Table 25.3. It is usual practice to remove lower teeth before upper teeth, and posterior teeth before anterior teeth, to avoid blood obscuring the operator's view if a number of teeth are to be extracted.

The patient's head should be at the level of the surgeon's elbow. The next stage is to position the surgeon's non-dominant hand. This is important because it improves access by retracting soft tissues and allows the surgeon to place a counterforce on the jaw to assist tooth extraction. For example, when buccally expanding an upper molar it is necessary to have an opposing force provided by the operator's passive hand. It is conventional to place a finger and a thumb on either side of the tooth to be extracted.

Application of the forceps is the most important stage and the basic principle of tooth removal must always be borne in mind: application of the beaks of the forceps to the root rather than the crown of the tooth. It should usually be as easy to remove a tooth fractured at gingival level as a fully intact tooth because the forcep blades are placed on the root face not on the enamel of the tooth.

This application involves the placing of the blades under the gingivae, taking care to minimise soft tissue damage. The forceps should then be pushed apically, completing this stage of the procedure. This may require considerable force.

There are exceptions to these general rules, for example, cow-horn forceps fit into the bifurcation of lower molars and, because of their unique design, produce an upwards force. Their application is therefore different.

Consolidation

To remove the tooth efficiently, the forceps must be pushed together firmly to engage on to the root surface, with the handles of the forceps being gripped with the palm of the hand with an apical force applied at the same time as forcing the handles together. This avoids the beaks of the forceps sliding around the root of the tooth on rotation rather than the efficient transfer of forces from operator to tooth.

Displacement

Displacement depends on root morphology. Teeth can be removed in two ways: by rotational movement or buccal movement (expansion).

Upper incisors and lower premolars can be rotated. All other teeth are best removed by controlled buccal expansion. Upper first premolars are an exception as they often present with two thin roots. The best extraction technique is a combination of gently wiggling the teeth and slight expansion, both bucally and palatally.

Rotational movement involves increasing destruction of the periodontal ligament by a circular movement both clockwise and anticlockwise. Buccal expansion involves the enlargement of the bony socket allowing tooth delivery. This is usually a staged process where the tooth is forced bucally and, with sustained pressure on the buccal alveolar bone, the tooth is extracted.

There are variations of the above basic movements: lower molars can often be removed efficiently by a combination of rotation and buccal expansion (a figure-of-eight movement is often suggested); also lower third molars can be expanded lingually where the lingual plate is thinner than the buccal bone.

Postdelivery

The extraction socket usually heals without incident, even when multiple extractions have produced a large, open wound. Healing can be aided by a number of procedures: sockets that have been expanded should be squeezed to replace the bone to its original position; sharp pieces of bone can be removed and the patient should be instructed to bite on to a damp piece of gauze to aid haemostasis. Once haemostasis has been achieved, postoperative instructions should be given (Ch. 23). Postoperative instructions should include leaving the socket undisturbed for 4–6 h and then gentle rinsing with hot saline mouthwashes after each meal. Patients should also be advised of control measures if bleeding occurs postoperatively and how to contact the appropriate emergency service in case of complications.

Risk assessment in tooth extraction

Teeth should be assessed preoperatively to anticipate potential difficulties with extractions. Preoperative assessment can be carried out using the history, examination and special investigations.

History

A history of difficult extractions or postoperative complications can give an early indication of potential problems. The age of the patient is also important: the bone of older patients is less flexible than that of younger patients, making standard techniques such as buccal expansion more difficult.

Examination

Clinical examination will reveal gross caries, which can make forceps placement very difficult. Imbrication or crowding can make forceps placement and delivery of the tooth difficult. Wear facets, indicating increased occlusal load, increase supporting bone strength making extractions more difficult.

Radiography

Radiographs are helpful in showing the number, shape and relationship of the roots of the tooth. They also reveal whether the roots of a lower molar tooth are convergent or divergent. Radiographs can also indicate areas of hyper-cementosis and bony pathology that may complicate the extraction.

26 Complications of extractions

Introduction

Complications can arise during the procedure of extraction or may manifest themselves some time following the extraction. These will be discussed in turn. Problems of local anaesthesia are discussed in Chapter 24.

Immediate extraction complications

These occur at the time of the extraction and are listed in Table 26.1.

Fracture of the crown of a tooth

This may be unavoidable if the tooth is weakened either by caries or a large restoration. However, the forceps may have been applied improperly to the crown instead of to the root mass, or the long axis of the beaks of the forceps may not have been along that of the tooth. Sometimes, crown fracture arises from the use of forceps whose beaks are too broad (see Ch. 25) or as a result of the operator trying to 'hurry' the operation. The management of this complication is to remove all debris from the oral cavity and review the clinical situation. Surgical extraction of the remaining fragment may then be necessary (see Ch. 23).

Fracture of the root of a tooth

Ideally, it should be possible to ensure that the whole tooth is removed every time an extraction is carried out. However, when a root breaks a decision about management of the retained piece of root has to be made.

Further management depends on the size of the root fragment, whether it is mobile, whether it is infected, how

Table 26.1   Immediate extraction complications

Fracture of tooth:
  crown
  root
Fracture of alveolar plate
Fracture of mandible
Soft tissue damage
Involvement of maxillary antrum:
  oroantral fistula
  fractured tuberosity
  loss of root (or tooth) into antrum
Loss of tooth or root:
  into pharynx
  into soft tissues
Damage to nerves or vessels
Dislocation of temporomandibular joint
Damage to adjacent teeth
Extraction of permanent tooth germ with deciduous
  tooth
Extraction of wrong tooth

close it is to major anatomical structures such as the maxillary antrum or inferior dental canal, patient cooperation and the ability of the surgeon to successfully complete the procedure taking into account the constraints of time, equipment and surgical expertise.

If the decision is made to leave the root then this must be written in the case notes and the patient fully informed. If the procedure is deferred, the root fragment should have the pulp removed and a dressing placed.

If a deciduous tooth is being removed, it must be kept in mind that the roots are usually being resorbed with the roots being pushed towards the surface by the permanent tooth. It is often prudent therefore to leave these fragments, as injudicious use of elevators can cause damage to the underlying permanent tooth.

Fracture of the alveolar plate

This is a common complication and is often seen when extracting canine teeth or molars. If the alveolar plate has little periosteal attachment and is hence liable to lose its blood supply then it should be carefully removed by stripping off any remaining periosteum with a periosteal elevator. If, however, it is still adequately attached to the periosteum, a mattress or simple suture over the socket margin will stabilise the plate and allow its incorporation into the healing process.

Fracture of the mandible

This is an uncommon complication of dental extraction, which is usually heralded by a loud crack. The most important thing is to stop the extraction and reassess the situation. The patient should be informed of the possibility that his or her mandible might be broken and a radiograph should be taken. If a jaw fracture is confirmed then the patient should be referred to a maxillo-facial centre as an emergency. It would be advisable to administer another inferior dental block injection. If this involves a significant delay, then further analgesia should be provided and appropriate antiseptic mouthwashes and antibiotics prescribed.

Soft tissue trauma

Soft tissues must not be crushed. For example, the lower lip is at risk from the handles of the forceps when removing maxillary teeth. It should be ensured that recently sterilised instruments are not too hot and the patient's eyes should be protected from instruments and fingers using safety spectacles. Soft tissue damage is more likely to be encountered when the patient is under a general anaesthetic and cannot communicate. Care should be exercised to avoid application of the beaks of forceps over the gingival soft tissues, especially lingually in the lower molar region where the lingual nerve may be damaged. Protective finger positioning is required when using elevators that may slip and damage the tongue, floor of mouth or the soft tissues of the palate. The soft tissues at the angle of the mouth may also be damaged by excessive lateral movement of forceps particularly when extracting an upper tooth when an ipsilateral inferior dental block has been administered or where the patient is having general anaesthesia.

Involvement of maxillary antrum

Oroantral fistula (OAF)

The roots of the maxillary molar teeth (and occasionally the premolar teeth) lie in close proximity to, or even within, the maxillary antrum. When the tooth is extracted, a communication between the oral cavity and the antrum may be created. The operator may be aware of this possibility from the study of a pre-extraction radiograph (Fig. 26.1) or may suspect the creation of an OAF by inspection of the extracted tooth or the socket. An upper molar may have a saucer-shaped piece of bone attached to the trifurcation of the roots, indicating that the floor of the antrum has been detached. The socket itself may show abnormal architecture such as loss of the interradicular bony septae. To confirm the presence of an OAF the patient can be asked to pinch the nostrils together and blow air gently into the nose. The operator can then hold cotton wool in tweezers under the socket and look for movement of the fibres. Sometimes, the blood in the socket can be observed to bubble or the noise of the air moving through the fistula can be detected. Some operators favour inspection of the socket with good lighting and efficient suction using a blunt probe to explore the integrity of the socket. The noise of the suction often becomes more resonate if a communication exists between socket and sinus.

Once confirmed, an OAF can be treated in two ways: if small, the socket can be sutured and a haemostatic agent such as Surgicel® can be used to encourage clot formation. Strict instructions should be given to avoid nose blowing because this can increase the intrasinus pressure and break-down the early clot that covers the defect. The patient should be prescribed an antibiotic

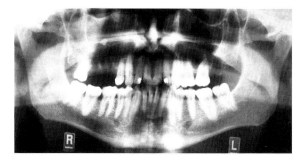

Fig. 26.1 Radiograph of the upper molar region showing the close association of the maxillary antrum to the upper molar roots. On the right side a root apex has been displaced into the maxillary antrum.

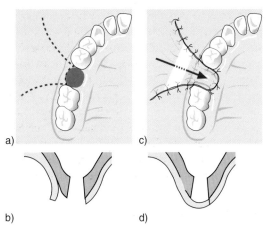

a)

c)

b)

d)

Fig. 26.2 A buccal advancement flap: (a) and (b) show a buccal flap, which is inelastic due to the underlying periosteum; (c) and (d) show the flap advanced to cover the fistula after incising the periosteum.

because of the risk of infection, which would prevent the sinus healing and lead to a chronic oroantral fistula. The patient should be reviewed 1 week later to check progress and then 1 month later to ensure that the socket has healed.

If the OAF is large then it should be closed immediately by means of a surgical flap. Most commonly this is done by means of a buccal advancement flap. This is a U-shaped flap with vertical relieving incisions taken from the mesial and distal margins of the socket. The flap is mucoperiosteal, which means that the periosteum lies on its inner aspect. Periosteum is a thin sheet of osteogenic soft tissue that has no elasticity and must therefore be incised to allow the whole flap to be advanced to the palatal margin of the socket (Fig. 26.2). The incision is made horizontally along the whole length of the base of the flap; it need not be deep because the periosteum is relatively thin. Some surgeons reduce the height of the buccal plate of bone to reduce the length of the advance. Horizontal mattress sutures encourage wound margin eversion and aid primary healing. A prophylactic antibiotic would normally be prescribed and the patient asked to avoid nose-blowing.

Fractured tuberosity

The maxillary tuberosity is the posterior part of the tooth-bearing segment of the maxilla. Occasionally, during extraction of a maxillary molar tooth a segment of bone becomes mobile. As with the fractured mandible,

the operator should stop the extraction and assess the problem, as continuing to extract the tooth will lead to tearing of the soft tissues and displacement of the fractured segment. Assessment can be carried out clinically by palpating the area to gauge the size of the bone fragment. This can be confirmed by taking radiographs including periapicals, oblique occlusals or panoramic films. It must be decided whether to retain the fractured piece of bone or to remove it with the associated tooth, or teeth. The principal consideration is size of the defect that will be left when the segment is removed, as this can complicate future denture provision. If the decision is made to remove the tooth and the bone, then a mucoperiosteal flap should be raised and the segment dissected out carefully. The soft tissues can then be sutured and the wound closed completely. As there is a breach of the maxillary antrum, antibiotics and analgesics should be prescribed for the patient.

The more common management is to retain the tooth and bone in position and allow the fracture to heal. First, the segment must be reduced if it is displaced, and this can normally be done with digital pressure or through forceps on the tooth. The tooth that has been giving rise to pain will have to have appropriate pulp extirpation or obtundent dressing. The next stage is to take an impression for construction of an appropriate splint to hold the fractured segment in position and protect it from trauma from the mandibular teeth. Alternatively, a segment of preformed arch bar can be wired to the buccal aspects of the fragment, extending forwards as far as the canine. Orthodontic wire can be used in much the same way, either using brackets or more simply attached with composite. The patient should be prescribed analgesics and antibiotics. The splint should be kept in place for approximately 4 weeks, after which time healing should be assessed. If the fragment is firm and there is no sign of infection, the tooth should be removed surgically by raising a flap, removing buccal bone and dividing the tooth into separate roots to avoid applying lateral pressure to the relatively weak tuberosity segment.

Loss of the root (or tooth) into the antrum

Another complication involving the antrum is pushing part or all of a tooth into the antral cavity. Normally the operator should arrange for the removal of this root as the patient is again at risk of the development of maxillary sinusitis with or without an oroantral fistula. The patient should have radiographs taken to confirm the presence of the root in the antrum and the operator should then raise a buccal flap from the mesial and distal margins of the socket. Access to the antrum should then be increased by bone removal with bone nibblers and drills. The root can then be removed from the antrum by a variety of techniques including suction, the use of small caries excavators or direct removal by tweezers. If these methods are unsuccessful then the antrum can be flushed-out with sterile saline in an attempt to 'float' the root out, or the antrum can be packed with ribbon gauze, which might dislodge the root when it is removed. Once the root has been removed from the antrum, the resulting defect should be closed with a buccal advancement flap, as in the closure of an oroantral fistula. In the rare circumstances where a whole tooth is dislodged into the maxillary antrum, its removal is often paradoxically easier.

Loss of tooth/root

Occasionally, during removal of a tooth, parts of the tooth can be dislodged and disappear. If this happens, a search should be instituted, using good suction. The patient may be aware of swallowing the tooth, or part of the tooth. If the tooth or root cannot be located then a radiograph, first of the abdomen, should be arranged to check whether the tooth or root has been swallowed, which is most likely. It is important to ensure that the object is not in the patient's airways.

Roots that are elevated incorrectly can occasionally be pushed through a very thin bony plate overlying the socket and disappear – bucally or lingually – into the soft tissues. This is more problematic when a root (often an additional third root) is pushed through the lingual plate in the lower third molar region, because these can be very difficult to recover.

Damage to nerves or vessels

This complication applies more commonly to the surgical removal of teeth rather than simple extractions but one must always be aware of difficulties when operating in the region of the inferior dental, lingual or mental nerves.

Dislocation of the temporomandibular joint

Occasionally, a patient will open the mouth so widely during an extraction that the mandible is dislocated; or the operator might apply force to an unsupported mandible, causing it to dislocate. In this event, the operator

should try, as quickly as possible, to reduce the dislocation by pushing the mandible downwards and backwards. If this is not done relatively quickly, muscle spasm of the powerful elevator muscles of the mandible will ensue and the patient will require sedation, or indeed even a general anaesthetic, to reduce the dislocation. When extracting teeth under general anaesthesia the mandible can dislocate due to the loss of muscular tone. It is important to ensure the mandible is repositioned before the patient recovers from the anaesthesia. Recurrent dislocation of the temporomandibular joint is discussed in Chapter 20.

Damage to adjacent teeth

When extracting teeth, fillings from adjacent teeth may become dislodged and this should be dealt with appropriately. Inexperienced operators sometimes damage teeth in the opposing jaw when the tooth being removed comes out of its socket rather more quickly than expected. It is important to recognise that damage has been caused and to deal with it appropriately.

Extraction of a permanent tooth germ along with the deciduous tooth

When extracting deciduous teeth there is occasionally a significant amount of soft tissue attached to the apex of the deciduous root. It is often difficult to ascertain clinically whether this is a granuloma or abscess, or whether it is the permanent tooth germ attached to the root. If there is concern, the specimen should be sent for histopathological investigation to confirm whether the permanent tooth germ has been removed.

Extraction of the wrong tooth

Extraction should be considered to be an irreversible procedure and therefore extreme vigilance should be employed to ensure that the correct tooth is extracted. The most vulnerable clinical situation is where one is extracting teeth for orthodontic reasons and the teeth have no obvious clinical problem. Extracting the wrong tooth is medicolegally indefensible.

Postextraction complications

Postextraction complications can occur a variable length of time after the extraction. They are listed in Table 26.2 and will be considered in turn.

Table 26.2 Postextraction complications
Haemorrhage
Dry socket
Osteomyelitis
Swelling, pain, echymosis
Sequestra
Trismus
Prolonged anaesthesia
Actinomycosis
Chronic oroantral fistula
Infective endocarditis

Table 26.3 Predisposing factors in dry socket
Infection
Extraction trauma
Blood supply
Site
Smoking
Sex
Systemic factors, e.g. oral contraceptives

Postextraction haemorrhage

Haemorrhage is one of the complications that clinicians worry about most and it can seriously complicate the extraction of teeth. Prevention of haemorrhage is desirable. To achieve this, the patient must be questioned carefully as to any previous history of excessive haemorrhage particularly in relation to previous extractions (see Ch. 6). If a history of postextraction haemorrhage is elicited it is important to try and ascertain for how long the bleeding continued and what measures were used to stop the bleeding on previous occasions. It is also important to discover when the bleeding started in relationship to the time of the extraction. General questions regarding a history of prolonged bleeding after trauma or other operations, or a family history of excessive bleeding or known haemorrhagic conditions may be relevant. It is also important to question the patient about the use of drugs, such as anticoagulant drugs. If there is any doubt regarding the existence of a haemorrhagic abnormality the patient should be investigated as discussed in detail in Chapter 6.

A postextraction haemorrhage is first dealt with by removing any clot from the mouth and establishing from where the bleeding is originating. The patient can then be asked to apply firm pressure by biting on a gauze pack for 10–15 min. It is advantageous to infiltrate local anaesthetic with a vasoconstrictor into the region, as this will make any manipulation of the socket more comfortable and the vasoconstrictor in the local anaesthetic will also aid in reducing the haemorrhage. Suturing is essential in the management of a postextraction haemorrhage and a horizontal mattress or interrupted sutures should be used to tense the mucoperiostem over the underlying bone so that the haemorrhage can be controlled (see Ch. 23). The use of haemostatic agents such as Surgicel® is helpful. Agents like bonewax can help to stop bleeding from the bony walls of the socket. Although postextraction haemorrhage can be dramatic, significant blood loss is unusual. Patients should, however, be assessed for evidence of shock if bleeding appears significant (see Ch. 4).

Dry socket

Dry socket is also known as focal or localised osteitis and manifests clinically as inflammation involving either the whole or part of the condensed bone lining the tooth socket (lamina dura). The features of this are a painful socket that arises 24–72 h after extraction and may last for 7–10 days. Clinically, there is an empty socket with possibly some evidence of broken-down blood clot and food debris within it. An intense odour may be evident and can be confirmed by dipping cotton wool into the socket and passing it under the nose. The overall incidence of dry socket is about 3% but this figure is much higher if the definition of postextraction pain is used as the sole diagnostic criterion.

The aetiology of this condition is incompletely understood but many predisposing factors exist and these are listed in Table 26.3.

Infection

This could occur before, during or after the extraction. However, many abscessed and infected teeth heal without leading to a dry socket. The oral flora in some patients can be shown to be haemolytic and these individuals may be more susceptible to recurrent dry sockets.

Extraction trauma

Excessive force may be associated with an increase in the incidence of dry socket. This is not always the case and it may occur after very easy extractions. The difficulty of extraction may be important, as the bony wall of the socket may be burnished during the extraction, crushing small bony blood vessels and so impairing the repair process.

Blood supply

Vasoconstrictors in local anaesthetics may predispose to a dry socket by interfering with the blood supply to the bone and dry sockets certainly occur more frequently after extractions with local anaesthetic than after those using general anaesthetic.

Dry sockets are much more common in the mandible than in the maxilla. The relatively poor blood supply of the mandible predisposes to the development of this problem and food debris also tends to gather in the lower sockets more readily.

Site

The incidence of dry sockets increases further back in the mouth with the highest incidence in the mandibular molar region. The most common tooth involved is the lower third molar, where the incidence may be significantly more than 3% (see Ch. 27).

Smoking

Tobacco use of any kind is associated with an increase in dry socket. This may occur, in part, due to the significant vasoconstrictor effect of nicotine on small vessels that occurs in smokers.

Sex

Dry sockets are significantly more common among females.

Systemic factors

It has been suggested that systemic factors are involved, although these have not been elucidated. Oral contraceptive use is associated with an increased incidence of dry sockets.

In an attempt to reduce the incidence of this painful condition, the teeth to be extracted should be scaled to remove any debris and preoperative flushing with 0.2% chlorhexidine may reduce the incidence. The operator should use a minimum amount of local anaesthetic and the teeth should be removed as atraumatically as possible. Where patients have a consistent history of this problem, some clinicians advise prophylactic use of metronidazole.

Management

Management of a dry socket firstly involves the relief of pain and secondly resolution of the condition. The socket should be anaesthetised and irrigated gently and all degenerating blood clot and food debris should be removed. A dressing should be inserted into the socket to protect it from further irritation by food debris. The most appropriate dressing is a matter of personal choice but Whitehead's varnish pack, a zinc oxide pack or the use of proprietary agents such as Alvogyl® are commonly used. Analgesics are an essential part of the management, as is the use of regular mouthwashes to keep the area clean. It is important that the patient is reviewed regularly to ensure that healing is progressing. When pain is intolerable, long-acting local anaesthesia such as bupivacaine blocks may afford relief and allow patients to sleep.

Osteomyelitis

This rare complication is often a result of an immune-comprised state or a reduction in the blood supply, usually of the mandible following radiotherapy. The patient is usually systemically unwell: there is an increase in temperature and severe pain. Often the mandible, which is more commonly involved, is tender on extraoral palpation. The onset of disturbance of labial sensation after an extraction is characteristic of acute osteomyelitis. The patient will often be admitted to hospital for management of this condition. The principles of treatment are the drainage of pus, the use of antibiotics and the later removal of sequestra once the acute infection has been controlled. Prevention is best achieved, in a predisposed patient, by ensuring primary closure of the socket by bone trimming and suturing (see Ch. 33).

Swelling, pain, echymosis

Some swelling, pain or bruising can be expected after any surgical interference and it is important for the operator to realise that if the soft tissues are not handled carefully these features can be exacerbated. The use of blunt instruments, excessive retraction or burs becoming entangled in the soft tissue all predispose to increased swelling and discomfort. If sutures are tied too tightly, postoperative swelling due to inflammatory oedema or haemotoma formation can cause the sutures to cheese-cut through the soft tissues, causing unnecessary pain. It is helpful for the patient to bathe the area with hot saline mouthwashes in an attempt to reduce debris around the wound. Surgeons must be aware of the possibility of wound infection and be prepared to institute drainage and consider antibiotic therapy.

Sequestra

There will be occasions when small pieces of bone become detached and cause interruption to the healing process. The patient will return, complaining of something sharp in the area of the socket and may feel that the operator has left a root fragment behind. These sequestra can be dealt with either by reassuring the patient and await shedding of the piece of bone or by administering some local anaesthesia and removing the piece of loose bone with tweezers. In some cases, granulation tissue may be apparent with pus discharging especially on probing the socket. This will respond well to a curettage of the socket, thus removing the sequestrum in the curettings.

Trismus

Trismus is a common feature after the removal of wisdom teeth (see Ch. 27) and may be associated with other extractions. It can also be related to the use of inferior dental block local anaesthesia (see Ch. 24). It is important to ascertain the cause of the trismus and then to manage it appropriately. On most occasions the trismus will resolve gradually over a period of time, which will vary depending on whether the condition is due to inflammatory oedema or perhaps direct damage to the muscles following local anaesthesia. The management is discussed in Chapter 24.

Prolonged anaesthesia

This is usually a feature of the removal of difficult or impacted teeth, particularly wisdom teeth, and is considered in detail in Chapter 27.

Actinomycosis

This is an uncommon chronic suppurative infection caused by *Actinomyces israelii* and classically characterised by swelling in the neck with multiple sinus formation and widespread fibrosis. The common site of presentation following extraction is the region around the angle of the mandible. Extraction wounds from lower teeth or fracture of the mandible provide pathways for the entry of the organisms. A detailed consideration of cervicofacial actinomycosis is given in Chapter 33.

Chronic oroantral fistula

This complication arises when a communication between the socket of an upper molar (or more rarely premolar)

and the maxillary air sinus has not been noted at the time of extraction and infection both in the socket and the air sinus occurs. The patient may present with a variety of symptoms and signs either within a week or two following the extraction or many months (and even years) later. Common to all, however, is failure of the normal healing process and persistence of the socket. As infection of the air sinus becomes acute, symptoms of diffuse unilateral maxillary pain, nasal stuffiness, bad taste and intraoral pus discharge may occur; these can be intermittent in character.

On examination, the socket can appear empty or be filled with granulation tissue. Occasionally, distinctly polypoidal tissue can grow down from the opening, reflecting the sinus origin of the tissue. In other cases, the socket can appear almost totally closed, with only a very small opening into the sinus. Diagnosis by careful probing is normally straightforward and an occipito-mental radiograph will show the extent of infection within the sinus.

The management involves two stages. First, the acute infection must be controlled, then the opening should be closed surgically. Initially, any accumulation of pus in the sinus should be drained. This often requires excision of the infected granulation tissue and polyps from the socket to allow free drainage and also to ensure histologically that the formation of the fistula is not related to downgrowth of an antral neoplasm. Nasal decongestants and antibiotics also help to control more acute infections.

Once the acute phase is controlled, most fistulae can be closed using the buccal flap advancement. The margins of the opening must be freshened by excising a rim of soft tissue, because epithelium will often have grown-up into the opening and, if not removed, will prevent healing. Where infection is limited to the immediate vicinity of the fistula, a limited curettage is carried out. However, where the whole sinus is filled with polypoidal granulation tissue, a more thorough exploration of the sinus may be required, and this often is performed under general anaesthesia.

Infective endocarditis

Infective endocarditis may arise in susceptible patients with cardiac lesions who are not given appropriate antibiotic prophylaxis. A detailed consideration of antibiotic prophylaxis for dental procedures is given in Chapter 35.

27 Wisdom teeth

Introduction

Third molars are the last teeth to erupt in the human dentition and are popularly known as wisdom teeth. They frequently give rise to problems when they are erupting and the management of these problems has become colloquially known as the 'bread and butter' aspect of the speciality of oral surgery. Through evolution, the human jaws are occasionally no longer large enough to accommodate all of the permanent dentition and therefore the last ones to erupt are short of space. Most of the problems associated with wisdom teeth occur between the ages of 18 and 25 but adults of any age can have problems.

A consideration of the criteria for removing wisdom teeth will be followed by discussion of pericoronitis. The clinical assessment and management of impacted wisdom teeth will then be outlined, including preoperative assessment, the procedures used to remove wisdom teeth, postoperative care and – finally – complications of surgery (Table 27.1).

Criteria for removal of wisdom teeth

Over recent years there has been debate over the advisability of removing symptom-free wisdom teeth or leaving them in place. The trend in recent years has been to be conservative in the management of these teeth and this has been driven, to some extent, by the incidence of complications associated with their surgical removal, and particularly the small, but measurable, risk of damage to the inferior dental nerve or the lingual nerve.

The controversy surrounding wisdom teeth has led to the publication of guidelines, the most recent of which are 'Management of unerupted and impacted third molar teeth' a National Clinical Guideline from the Scottish

Intercollegiate Guidelines Network (SIGN) and 'Removal of wisdom teeth' guidance from the National Institute for Clinical Excellence (NICE). These guidelines inform the decision on whether to remove wisdom teeth.

Surgical removal of impacted third molars, it is recommended, should be limited to patients with evidence of pathology. These are listed in Table 27.2 and will be discussed in turn. Further possible indications to be considered are listed in Table 27.3.

Table 27.1 Management of impacted third molars
Criteria for removal of wisdom teeth
Pericoronitis
spread of infection from pericoronitis
treatment of pericoronitis
Clinical assessment
Radiographic assessment
Clinical management
preoperative information
techniques
lower third molars
upper third molars
Postoperative care
Complications of surgery

Table 27.2 Indications for removal of wisdom teeth
Infection
pericoronitis
untreatable caries
untreatable pulpal or periapical pathology
periodontal disease
Cystic change
External or internal resorption
Wisdom tooth in tumour resection

219

Table 27.3   Further possible indications for removal of third molars
Transplantation
Fractured mandible
Atrophic mandible
Denture or implant design
Access to dental care
Medical condition
Orthodontic considerations
Orthognathic surgery or reconstructive surgery
Use of general anaesthesia
Age of patient

Infection

Pericoronitis

The most common reason for recommending removal of wisdom teeth is that patients have experienced significant infection associated with them. This usually manifests itself as pericoronitis and a discussion of the clinical features and management of this will follow. Pericoronitis is only an indication for extraction if the first episode is very acute or there has been more than one episode.

Untreatable caries, pulpal or periapical pathology

Another common indication for removal of wisdom teeth is the development of caries either in the wisdom tooth itself or in the adjacent second molar. This occurs because the patient is unable to clean the distal aspect of the second molar or the area around the wisdom tooth, which is often partially erupted. This leads to the accumulation of food debris and plaque and then caries of the adjacent tooth surfaces. This may lead to untreatable pulpal or periapical pathology.

Periodontal disease

As a result of the unsatisfactory relationship between the second and third molars, the area is prone to periodontal disease, which may compromise the second molar. This can be improved by the removal of the third molar.

Cystic change

When third molars are unerupted they may be the source of a dentigerous cyst, which can enlarge considerably before giving rise to symptoms. The risk of developing these cysts is low but is also unpredictable and gives rise to a clinical dilemma of how often radiographic assessment of unerupted third molars is necessary to diagnose a cyst before its size makes the management more complicated.

External or internal resorption

A less common reason for removal of third molars is external resorption of the second molar due to pressure from the unerupted third molar. As with the formation of the dentigerous cyst, this resorption can be extensive before the patient experiences symptoms. Internal resorption within the wisdom tooth is also an indication for removal.

Wisdom teeth in tumour resection

If an impacted wisdom tooth is associated with a tumour at the angle of the mandible, or is within the tumour resection margins, it should be removed.

Transplantation

When a patient presents with a heavily restored or carious first molar tooth and a partially erupted third molar tooth it is possible to transplant the third molar into the socket of the first molar. This procedure is complicated by the difficulty of removing the third molar without damage and also because the root morphology of these teeth is different, which causes problems accommodating the third molar in its new site. Once transplanted, the tooth will often require to be splinted for a period and, with a low success rate, this procedure is rarely carried out.

Fracture of mandible

If a fracture of the mandible through the angle occurs, an opportunity may arise to remove the third molar when surgical access is being made to treat the fracture itself. Some authorities consider that unerupted third molars should be removed in those individuals who participate in contact sports like rugby and boxing, in whom the risk of mandibular fracture is increased.

Atrophic mandible

It has been argued that an unerupted third molar in an already atrophic mandible might be a potential site for fracture and consideration should be given to removing it in a controlled manner before a fracture occurs.

Denture or implant design

Restorative dentists can request the removal of unerupted third molar teeth to facilitate denture design or the accurate placement of implants.

Access to dental care

Where patients are in a situation where they do not have easy access to dental care, it is appropriate to consider the removal of potentially troublesome third molar teeth. This could for example, include submariners or occupations that involve working in isolated areas where dental help may be difficult to find. With modern means of travel and communication, this reason for removing third molar teeth has assumed less significance.

Medical conditions

Removal of third molars may be indicated in certain medical conditions, such as prior to cardiac surgery or in those scheduled to have radiotherapy of the jaw. Removal of third molars following radiotherapy increases the likelihood of the development of osteoradionecrosis, and is therefore better carried out before such treatment (see Ch. 36).

Orthodontic considerations

Orthodontic treatment plans may include the removal of impacted lower and upper third molars in an attempt to prevent or reduce imbrication of the incisor teeth. There is no evidence, however, that third molars contribute to this problem (see Ch. 31).

Orthognathic or reconstructive surgery

Third molars may also need removed when orthognathic surgery is being planned, particularly with procedures such as sagittal split osteotomy (see Ch. 13).

General anaesthesia

More rigorous criteria for removal of lower third molars can lead to further difficulties in determining whether symptom-free third molar teeth on the other side of the mouth should be removed when general anaesthesia or sedation is being used for the removal of a symptomatic third molar tooth. The fact that the tooth is present is not sufficient reason to remove it while the patient is anaesthetised. However, as in all situations regarding third molars, all four teeth should be subject to a risk–benefit analysis.

Age of patient

Finally, removing third molars in young fit patients and not leaving them until an older age when the bone is denser and more difficult to manage, and when the patient may have medical problems related to older age groups, is still a common point of view. Contrary to this argument is the view that the small but significant morbidity following removal of wisdom teeth supports a more conservative approach, and so removal for this reason alone can no longer be condoned. The more conservative approach is now more commonly adopted but many oral surgeons are mindful that they may be storing up difficulties for later years, both for their patients and for their surgical successors. Time alone will answer this question

Pericoronitis

This condition is characterised by inflammation around the crown of a tooth and only occurs when there is communication between the tooth and the oral cavity. The tooth is normally partially erupted, and hence visible, but occasionally there may be little evidence of communication between it and the oral cavity and careful probing of the gingiva immediately distal to the second molar may be necessary to demonstrate some communication, however small.

The patient's main complaint will be pain, which initially may be of low intensity. As the condition develops the pain increases in intensity. Swelling over the affected site may develop and this will cause further discomfort when the patient occludes with the opposing teeth. As the swelling increases, the pain on occluding becomes more severe and the patient will be discouraged from bringing the teeth together. The 'lid' of gum over the involved tooth is known as the operculum and this may show evidence of trauma from the cusps of the opposing maxillary teeth. There may be pus formation and a bad taste. There will be marked inflammation in the tissue adjacent to the affected tooth and this can lead to trismus and difficulty in swallowing. The patient may be generally unwell, with lymphadenitis and pyrexia. There will often be marked halitosis.

Spread of infection from pericoronitis

On occasion, pus associated with an impacted lower wisdom tooth will track buccally forwards above the buccinator attachment forming a sinus in the region of the first permanent molar. This may lead to some confusion as to the source of the infection and can lead to unnecessary removal of the first permanent molar. This condition is referred to as a migratory abscess. Pericoronitis can also be associated with acute ulcerative gingivitis causing marked halitosis and gingival sloughing and ulceration. Spread of infection can occur in various directions (Table 27.4), including laterally into cheek, or distobuccally under the masseter muscle to give rise to a submasseteric abscess characterised by profound trismus. It can also spread to the sublingual or submandibular region and also into the area around the tonsils and parapharyngeal space (see Ch. 33). Less commonly, it can ascend through the anterior pillar of fauces into soft palate causing marked dysphagia. Early and competent management of acute pericoronitis will hopefully limit this spread.

Treatment of pericoronitis

The management of pericoronitis is similar to the management of any acute oral infection. It is essential to provide drainage for any pus. Once drainage is adequate it is important to clean the area beneath the operculum.

Table 27.4 Spread of pericoronal third molar infection	
Region	*Direction of spread*
Migratory abscess of sulcus	Forwards, bucally above buccinator
Soft tissue of cheek	Laterally
Submasseteric	Distally and bucally
Sublingual space	Lingually above mylohyoid
Submandibular space	Lingually below mylohyoid
Parapharyngeal space	Distally and lingually
Soft palate	Upwards through anterior fauces

This can be carried out mechanically by irrigation with warm chlorhexidine or saline solution. This should remove any accumulated food debris and plaque. Application of antiseptic or mildly caustic solutions underneath the operculum may be beneficial. Examples include Talbot's iodine and trichloracetic acid. These agents are astringents and will cause soft tissue damage, and must therefore be used with caution. If the maxillary third molar has overerupted and is causing trauma to the operculum, the single most effective treatment is its removal. This can be carried out easily, even in the presence of some degree of trismus, and often leads to resolution. The patient's general condition needs to be assessed and a decision made regarding the prescription of an antibiotic (see Ch. 33). The patient should be encouraged to use regular hot saline mouthwashes and discouraged from applying heat to the cheek area extraorally. Arrangements should be made for early review of the patient's condition (within 2–3 days), when some resolution should have occurred.

Clinical assessment

Once the symptoms of pericoronitis have settled the patient needs to be assessed fully regarding the future management of the wisdom teeth. It is important to consider all four third molars as a unit and to make a decision on each of them. A general assessment of the mouth should be made, including caries activity and the level of periodontal disease. The patient's oral hygiene should be checked with particular reference to the accumulation of debris around the third molars. The eruption status of each of the four third molars is made using three categories – unerupted, partially erupted or fully erupted. Note should be taken of the patient's age because the management of third molars can be significantly influenced by this factor. It is also important to assess the surgical access to the third molar region by asking the patient to open widely and to note the space available between the distal aspect of the second molar and the vertical anterior border of the ascending ramus. This is particularly important when removal of these teeth under local anaesthesia is being contemplated.

Radiographic assessment

Radiographs are an essential part of the assessment of a patient's wisdom teeth. When removal is contemplated it is important that the entire tooth and the surrounding bone can be seen clearly using a panoramic view of the oral cavity. A periapical radiograph may be helpful if lack of detail in the panoramic view compromises assessment of the root morphology or its proximity to the inferior dental canal.

Table 27.5 lists the information which should be available from the radiographs.

Most operators initially assess the depth and the position of the impacted tooth. The simplest method of depth assessment can be made by looking at the position of the crown of the impacted tooth relative to the second molar (Fig. 27.1). A crown-to-crown relationship indicates a superficial impaction, crown-to-crown-and-root of the second molar indicates intermediate depth and crown of wisdom tooth to the roots only of the second molar implies a deep position. The angulation should be assessed by comparing a line joining the mesial and distal images of the cusps of the wisdom tooth with the curve of Spee formed by joining the cusps of the pre-molar and molar teeth. If the lines are parallel then the wisdom tooth is vertical in position. However, if the wisdom tooth line, when extended posteriorly, would meet the Spee line then the tooth is mesio-obliquely impacted (Fig. 27.2). Conversely, if the wisdom tooth line when extended posteriorly would never meet the curve of Spee, then it is disto-oblique in position. The most common position is mesio-oblique and the most difficult to remove is the deep disto-angular impaction, because its path of removal impacts into the ramus of the mandible and there is often little space to elevate the tooth from its mesial aspect.

The crown may show evidence of distal bone loss or follicular enlargement, which is indicative of chronic pericoronal infection and often facilitates removal of the tooth.

The crown of the impacted tooth should also be examined for evidence of caries, as caries will tend to weaken it and make fracture more likely on elevation. Paradoxically, a carious crown is also more difficult to section and split than an intact crown. The size, number and shape of the roots, and how they relate to each other, is fundamental to the assessment of difficulty in removal. Fused roots tapering to the apex present little difficulty in elevation and removal compared to converging or diverging roots with apical dilacerations.

The relationship of the roots to the image of the inferior dental canal should be scrutinised carefully (Fig. 27.3). Features likely to indicate close proximity

Table 27.5 Information obtained from radiographs of wisdom teeth

Angulation of the wisdom tooth (for example mesioangular, distoangular, vertical or horizontal)
Depth of the wisdom tooth
The relationship to the inferior dental canal
Crown features
The root morphology
The texture of the surrounding bone
Any associated pathology (e.g. dentigerous cyst)
Surgical access
The state of the second permanent molars (including root morphology, presence of caries or extensive restoration)

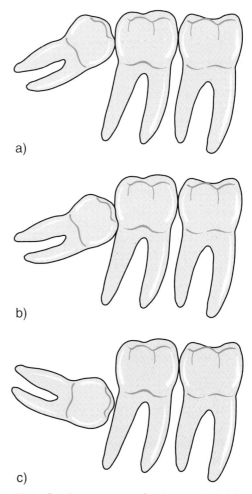

a)

b)

c)

Fig. 27.1 Depth assessment of an impacted wisdom tooth on a radiograph: (a) superficial impaction; (b) intermediate depth; (c) deep position.

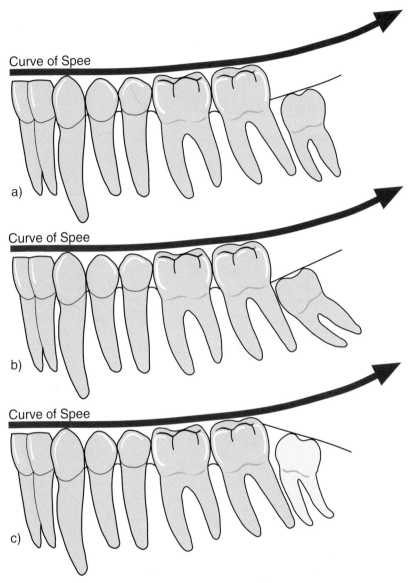

Fig. 27.2 Angulation of a wisdom tooth on a radiograph: (a) vertical: the intercuspal line of the wisdom tooth is parallel to the line of Spee; (b) mesio-oblique: the intercuspal line of the wisdom tooth is converging with the line of Spee; (c) disto-oblique: the intercuspal line of the wisdom tooth is diverging from the line of Spee.

include narrowing of the canal as it passes across the outline of the root, loss of continuity of the radio-opaque roof of the canal or deflection of the normal arc of the canal as it passes across the root(s). Additionally, the apices of the roots may show severe dilacerations as they approach the outline of the canal. Although less reliable, any radiograph that shows the root image crossing that of

the canal may indicate anatomical closeness. Conversely, it is important to understand that separation of the images of roots and the inferior dental (ID) canal with interposed bone on any radiographic view indicates lack of close approximation because, if the root(s) were anatomically close, such a separation could not be shown radiographically, regardless of angulation.

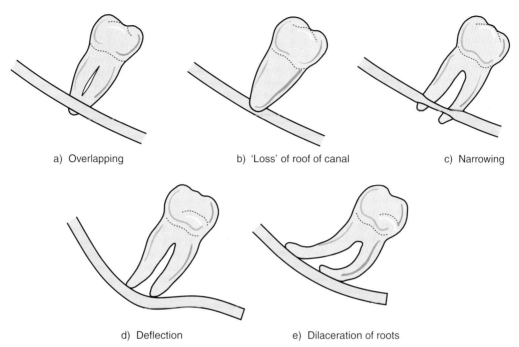

a) Overlapping   b) 'Loss' of roof of canal   c) Narrowing

d) Deflection   e) Dilaceration of roots

Fig. 27.3 Radiographic features likely to denote close proximity between root(s) and inferior dental canal.

Finally, the morphology of the roots and distal restorations present in the second molar should be noted as forces carelessly applied to the third molar may cause movement to this tooth or risk dislodging the restoration.

Clinical management

Once the decision has been made to remove a patient's wisdom tooth, the options for anaesthesia should then be considered. Consideration of either local anaesthesia and sedation or general anaesthesia may be indicated. Decisions regarding the form of anaesthesia used will depend upon the patient's anxiety about the procedure, the number and the degree of difficulty of removal of the wisdom teeth and the availability of patient-care options.

Preoperative information

Before treatment commences, the patient should be given information regarding the possible complications of the removal of wisdom teeth. This is best done not only verbally on a one-to-one basis with the clinician but also by the use of written information, which the patient can study and discuss with the surgeon before the procedure. The information provided to the patient should include a description of the discomfort that follows removal of these teeth and the associated swelling and difficulty in opening the mouth for a short period. Bruising of the face at the angle of the jaw can cause alarm. Dry socket is more frequently experienced when lower wisdom teeth are removed than other teeth (see Ch. 26). The most serious complication is numbness of the tissues supplied by the inferior dental or lingual nerves. It is mandatory that the patient is advised of this possible complication prior to their procedure. Around 15% of patients who have lower wisdom teeth removed will experience some temporary alteration in sensation along the distribution of the lingual or inferior dental nerves but permanent numbness occurs in under 1%. It is important that the case record is fully documented with the information that has been given to the patient regarding the possible complications and also to indicate whether written information has been given to the patient.

Techniques

Lower third molars

Access to the tooth is gained by lifting a buccal mucoperiosteal flap (Figs 27.4 and 27.5). Raising the flap lingually can lead to stretching of the lingual nerve,

a)

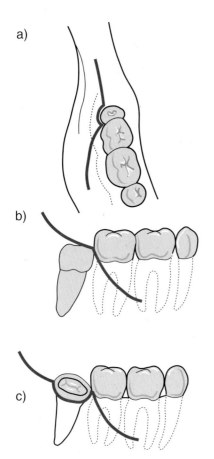

b)

c)

Fig. 27.4 Flap design for removing an impacted wisdom tooth: (a) occlusal view; (b) lateral view; unerupted; c) partially erupted.

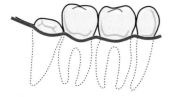

Fig. 27.5 Envelope flap (no vertical relief) for removing an impacted wisdom tooth.

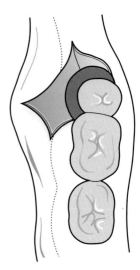

Fig. 27.6 Removal of pericoronal bone.

which is anatomically close to the lingual aspect of the lower wisdom tooth and, in many cases, can be avoided if sufficient visibility and access are gained without it.

Once the lower wisdom tooth is adequately exposed, consideration should be given to bone removal to facilitate delivery of the tooth. Bone removal is most commonly achieved using drills and burs and is carried out on the buccal aspect of the tooth and onto the distal aspect of the impaction. The intention is to create a deep, narrow gutter around the crown of the wisdom tooth (Fig. 27.6), and not a shallow, broad gutter. Bone should be removed to allow correct application of elevators on the mesial and buccal aspects of the tooth. The operator can then assess the possibility of removing the tooth in its entirety with the use of elevators or a combination of elevators and forceps. If it proves impossible to remove the tooth in this way and adequate bone has been removed, sectioning the tooth using burs is carried out (Fig. 27.7). Most commonly, the crown of the tooth is sectioned from the roots and the crowns and roots are then removed as individual items. Further separation of the roots with burs may also be necessary. Where the roots are separate, the tooth may be sectioned longitudinally, allowing removal of the distal portion of the crown and distal roots, followed by elevation of the mesial half of the tooth.

In younger patients under general anaesthesia, the lingual wall of the third molar socket may be removed using a hammer and chisel (the split bone technique). This often allows the tooth to be delivered in one piece by rotating it lingually. Clearly, this technique does require a lingual flap to be reflected but in skilled hands it can be a very successful and rapid technique.

When tooth removal is completed, any debris is cleaned out and any follicular tissue – especially that hidden behind the second molar – is curetted free. After smoothing any sharp bone, irrigation of the socket is carried out with saline. The flap is then sutured using either resorbable or non-resorbable materials.

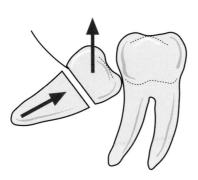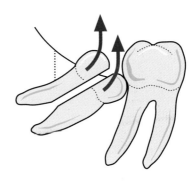

Fig. 27.7   Methods of sectioning an impacted wisdom tooth.

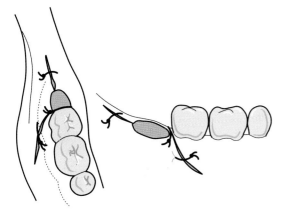

Fig. 27.8   'Anatomical' closure of a flap after surgical removal of an impacted wisdom tooth.

Although it is possible to suture the flap across the socket to the lingual side, many operators prefer to return the flap to its original position, leaving a socket that is more easily kept clean by the patient postoperatively, and may well also reduce swelling (Fig. 27.8).

Upper third molars

These teeth are generally easily removed by elevation from the mesiobuccal aspect using a curved Warwick James elevator or Coupland's chisel. If undue resistance to elevation is encountered then excessive force can cause fracture of the posterior aspect of the tuberosity, and forceps should be used if possible in this circumstance. If this is not possible due to only partial eruption of the tooth, a buccal flap can be raised with appropriate bone removal.

Upper third molar removal should not be underestimated and access to grossly carious, partially erupted examples with diverging roots in large patients can be more than a little challenging.

Postoperative care

The overuse of antibiotics is being recognised and, in particular, there is controversy about their use prophylactically in the removal of wisdom teeth. Some routinely prescribe antibiotics to the patient whereas others withhold antibiotics and use them only if infection occurs. No clear evidence is available to support either viewpoint. Some operators provide antimicrobials where there is a history of repeated episodes of pericoronitis or if there has been a recent acute episode. Others prescribe if extensive bone removal is necessary or there is extreme difficulty in removing the tooth.

The antibiotic may be administered preoperatively, perioperatively or immediately postoperatively. Regimes and choice of antibiotic vary but the most commonly used are amoxicillin or metronidazole, and they should be prescribed for as short a period as possible. The use of corticosteroids during the removal of wisdom teeth is more evidence-based and more clinicians are now using them to reduce postoperative swelling. The provision of postoperative analgesia is an integral part of treatment. Chlorhexidine mouthwashes twice daily and frequent hot saline rinsing is beneficial. Patients should be encouraged to keep moving the jaw, despite the swelling and discomfort, as this reduces stagnation and consequent infection.

Complications of surgery

These can be considered under perioperative and postoperative complications.

Perioperative complications are similar to those occurring with any other dentoalveolar surgery and include excessive bleeding (see Ch. 26). Certain complications are more specific to the third molar region and include fracture of the mandible, loss of a root in the lower jaw into the lingual space or in the upper jaw displacement of the tooth into the maxillary air sinus or into the pterygoid space (see Ch. 26). Direct trauma to the inferior dental neurovascular bundle may occur and can be difficult to avoid where anatomically the roots are intimately related to the canal tissues. The most obvious example of this is the rare situation where the inferior dental canal actually passes through the root. Even here, it may be possible to split the root around the neurovascular bundle leaving the bundle relatively undamaged.

Postoperatively, the majority of patients will have swelling at the angle region, trismus and discomfort. This generally peaks after 48 h and will resolve within a week to 10 days. Infection in the form of localised osteitis (dry socket) can occur and should be managed in the usual symptomatic way (see Ch. 26). Occasionally, the wound may become infected with pus production and this is more likely if there has been haematoma formation in the cheek or other adjacent soft tissue spaces.

Anaesthesia (complete loss of sensation), paraesthesia (partial loss) or dysaesthesia (an altered sensation often painful to the patient) are more worrying sequelae. Where lingual nerve damage has been sustained taste perception is also frequently altered and can be an additional distressing symptom. The prognosis for resolution is good but a small number of patients have to accommodate to permanent loss or alteration of sensation in the distribution of the particular nerve. Recovery of normal sensation may take from a few days to several months, but after a year little improvement will occur.

28 Cysts of the jaws

Introduction

A cyst, by definition, is a pathological cavity that is usually lined with epithelium and which contains fluid or semi-fluid.

The vast majority of cysts of the jaws form within bone and grow slowly. They may therefore attain a relatively large size because they are often initially symptom free. Diagnosis of a cyst is not uncommonly made when the cyst becomes acutely infected, or it is found by chance on routine radiography of the dentition. Table 28.1 shows a list of the cysts found in the jaws. Several are very rare. The most common will be considered in more detail here, discussing their clinical features, diagnosis and treatment.

Table 28.1	Features of cysts of the jaws			
Type	Site	Epithelial source	Frequency	Radiographic appearance
Radicular (apical or dental)	Any non-vital tooth	Debris of Mallassez	Most common of all	Round or oval radiolucency
Dentigerous	Unerupted teeth	Reduced enamel epithelium	Relatively common	Radiolucency around crown of unerupted tooth
Keratocyst	Angle of mandible but anywhere possible	Dental lamina	Relatively common	Multilocular when large
Periodontal	Periodontal pocket	Debris of Mallassez	Uncommon	Round or oval radiolucency
Nasopalatine	Midline anterior hard palate	Epithelium nests at nasopalatine fissure	Uncommon	Midline palatal radiolucency, lamina dura of centrals intact
Nasolabial	Nasolabial fold (not intrabony)	Possibly epithelium from the nasolacrimal duct	Very rare	May cause depression of nasal lateral wall
Solitary bone cyst	Mandibular body	Not epithelium lined	Rare	Radiolucency often scalloped around roots of lower molars
Staphne's idiopathic bone cyst	Mandibular body on lingual aspect	Not cystic but submandibular salivary gland inclusion	Very rare	Small round shadow below inferior dental canal
Aneurysmal bone cyst	Usually mandible	Not cystic	Rare	Multilocular, soap-bubble apearance

Radicular cysts

A radicular cyst is by far the most common cyst of the jaws. Its synonyms are dental cyst, periapical cyst or simply apical cyst. From time-to-time the teeth responsible for the formation of a radicular cyst may be extracted but the cyst remains and may well increase in size subsequent to the extraction. In this circumstance the name residual cyst is commonly used.

A radicular cyst develops when epithelial debris of Mallassez in a granuloma at the apex of a non-vital tooth is stimulated to proliferate. The epithelium forms a ball or mass of cells, which may break down centrally, perhaps due to lack of nutrients, to form a liquefied central area. Alternatively, the epithelium cells may form strands and sheets that encompass part of the granuloma, with a similar resulting breakdown of the enclosed granulomatous content to form the fluid centre of the cyst. Whichever method occurs, the effect is the formation of an epithelial semipermeable lining to the cyst content that allows fluids to enter the lumen by osmosis and leads to its gradual enlargement. This whole process is sometimes known as cystic degeneration.

Clinical features

Initially, the cyst will be contained within the alveolar bone around the apex of the non-vital tooth. At this stage the bone increases its density peripherally around the lesion in an attempt to wall it off. This is possible due to its slow rate of growth and explains why, radiographically, there is a sharp radio-opaque line surrounding the radiolucent shadow of the cyst.

With continued growth, the cyst eventually approaches the surface of the alveolar bone and as the apices of most teeth lie closer to the buccal than the palatal or lingual plates, it is the buccal plate which is usually first affected. Lying on the surface of the bone is the periosteum, and this layer of osteogenic tissue in turn reacts to the encroaching cyst by laying down new bone over its advancing front. The first real evidence of a cyst is therefore a bony swelling, known as bony expansion, in the buccal sulcus. Occasionally, especially with an upper lateral incisor, the expansion may be palatal, reflecting the palatal inclination of the apex. This expansion will feel hard to palpation and its presence may be convincing only on comparison with the contour of the bone on the other side of the jaw. With further growth, this enlargement will continue until the periosteum can no longer lay-down bone sufficiently rapidly and the cyst erodes through an ever-thinning bony buccal covering until it presents as a soft fluctuant (fluid-filled) swelling in the sulcus, which often appears slightly blue in colour. When the overlying expanded bone is very thin, palpation may elicit the characteristic eggshell crackling though this is rarely felt in practice.

Acute infection can supervene at any time during this process of evolution and this will convert the cyst, as far as its clinical features are concerned, into those of an acute apical abscess. If the acutely infected cyst bursts and discharges into the mouth, the continued discharge may lead to formation of a sinus.

Loosening or tilting of adjacent teeth is only encountered in very large cysts, and resorption of roots usually results from repeated infection of the cyst and is relatively uncommon.

Unless a radicular cyst becomes infected, it will remain painless and vital structures will be gently moved aside to accommodate it. This can be seen clearly in larger mandibular cysts, which push the inferior dental canal downwards to the lower border of the mandible. No anaesthesia will be noted of the lip or chin unless the pressure within the cavity rises rapidly as with an acute infection. With large cysts occasionally the tooth responsible for the lesion elicits a rather hollow note on percussion.

Diagnosis

As mentioned above, many radicular cysts are found either by chance radiographically or because of acute infection. However, other clinical features may present. Expansion of bone is usually buccal and hard to palpation. Later it is soft, fluctuant, and bluish in colour. The tooth will be non-vital. Radiographic features will show the classic appearance of a round or oval-shaped radiolucency (Fig. 28.1) surrounded by a sharply delineated thin white line of increased bone density. The affected tooth will show loss of its apical lamina dura. Very occasionally there may be evidence of resorption of adjacent teeth and this reflects repeated acute episodes of infection within the cyst. Similarly, such infection can cause a haziness in the sharp radio-opaque delineations of the margin of the cyst. In larger mandibular cysts there may be clear evidence of the inferior dental canal having been displaced downwards by the advancing lesion.

Aspiration of the cyst contents may be possible in larger cysts with little or no bony covering. Classically,

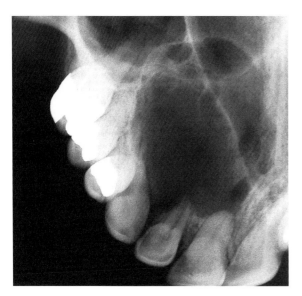

Fig. 28.1 A radicular cyst associated with a lateral incisor showing as a round radiolucency.

the fluid appears as straw-coloured in which a shimmer may be seen due to its cholesterol content. However, if the cyst has been infected, this characteristic appearance may be lost and the fluid may well consist of pus or blood-stained pus. Many authorities have alluded to the difference between the higher soluble protein content of the radicular cyst and the dentigerous cyst compared with the lesser amount contained in odontogenic keratocysts. Such analyses are in practice seldom, if ever, carried out because of their cost and due to the fact that the differences between aspirates are visible to the naked eye and the use of a simple cytological smearing of suspected keratocysts makes such expensive tests unnecessary.

With very large cysts, especially in the mandible, it may be prudent to obtain some lining for histopathological examination, as this may allow differentiation between a large radicular (or residual) cyst, a keratocyst or a cystic ameloblastoma, especially when considering the differential diagnosis of a radiolucency of the angle of the mandible.

Treatment

There are two main methods of treatment for cysts: enucleation (removal of the lining in total) and marsupialisation (creation of a permanent opening into the cyst cavity). The vast majority of cysts are treated by enucleation, with marsupialisation tending to be reserved for certain categories of patients, usually with larger cysts.

Enucleation

This is suitable for all small to moderate-sized cysts and the majority of large cysts.

Root-treating and conserving the tooth causing the cyst may be worthwhile and surgery may therefore be preceded by endodontic treatment.

A standard mucoperiosteal flap is raised buccally with the vertical relieving incision placed anteriorly (see Ch. 23). The thin bone is then removed with bone rongeurs (nibblers) or burs to allow surgical access to the fluid-filled sac. The cyst lining is then separated with periosteal elevators or curettes from its bony wall and 'shelled' out. The lining should be sent for histopathological investigation. After irrigating with sterile saline the flap is sutured back to its anatomical position. If the tooth has been root filled, an apicectomy should be performed at the same time with retrograde sealing of the canal if appropriate.

The operation is for all but very large cysts usually carried out under local anaesthesia with or without sedation according to the patient's preference. Postoperative complications are rare, although breakdown of the wound in large mandibular cysts can occur. The patient is normally recalled about 4–6 months postoperatively, when a radiograph should show evidence of bony infilling of the cyst cavity.

Marsupialisation

As the name implies, marsupialisation means creating a pouch. The rationale of this treatment is the permanent destruction of the integrity (wholeness) of the cyst. This, in effect, depressurises the cyst cavity, stops its continued expansion and encourages a shrinkage of the lining by new bone formation around its periphery. It is more suitable for large cysts where enucleation may endanger vital structures such as the inferior dental nerve or there is a risk of fracture during enucleation. The limited surgery involved is very suitable for outpatient care under local anaesthesia and it can therefore be particularly appropriate for elderly or medically compromised patients who would be at risk from a general anaesthetic. Any decision to marsupialise a cyst cavity should be preceded by histological evidence that confirms the lesion as a cyst

231

and this involves a small incisional biopsy or retrieving tissue from the cyst cavity at the time of the procedure.

Marsupialisation may be achieved most simply by extraction of the tooth responsible for the cyst, aspirating the contents through the socket, then irrigating the cyst lumen before packing the opening with a surgical pack. Sterile ribbon gauze soaked in Whitehead's varnish is excellent for this purpose, as the antiseptic content will protect the cyst cavity from infection. The pack is later substituted for a partial denture with a root-shaped acrylic bung extending into the cyst cavity from the socket. The patient is then given syringes with which to irrigate the cyst cavity with warm saline on a twice-daily basis. With the lining no longer complete, the bone heals inwards around the cyst, reducing it progressively in size. Some operators remove the cyst by enucleation when it has reduced to a more manageable size.

If no tooth is involved – as in a large residual dental cyst – then a small semilunar flap is raised over the most expanded part of the cyst to allow part of the lining to be excised, and the cyst contents to be aspirated and washed out. The flap is then turned into the cyst and sutured to its lining, and the opening maintained initially with a surgical pack and later by a denture or prosthesis with an acrylic bung.

Marsupialisation of a large cyst may take many months for healing to occur and the onus is therefore on the patient to maintain cleanliness by frequent irrigations of the cyst cavity, as described above.

Dentigerous cysts

These cysts are developmental odontogenic cysts, which arise when cystic degeneration occurs in the reduced enamel epithelium (dental follicle). They are seen around unerupted teeth and are therefore most frequently found in the third molar areas, both upper and lower, the upper canine region and, less frequently, around lower second premolars. They may also arise in relation to super-numerary or supplemental unerupted teeth.

Clinical features

These cysts grow slowly and have the same effect as radicular cysts on surrounding bone. A bony expansion occurs initially and at a later stage a soft fluctuant swelling over the area of the unerupted tooth will develop. As with radicular cysts, dentigerous cysts are usually asymptomatic until infected.

Diagnosis

Radiographic imaging and aspiration are often fairly conclusive (Fig. 28.2). A very large dentigerous cyst in the lower third molar area can displace the wisdom tooth and may require to be differentiated from other lesions such as a keratocyst or ameloblastoma. Although both these lesions are classically described as being multilocular radiolucencies on radiograph, it must be remembered that unilocular lesions do exist. Aspiration may not be sufficient to differentiate a dentigerous cyst from a keratocyst, particularly if there has been infection. Similarly, an ameloblastoma may have within it areas of cystic degeneration, even in the more solid tumours, and a variant of the ameloblastoma – known as the cystic ameloblastoma – can be very similar to the dentigerous cyst in its clinical appearance, radiographic image and aspirated fluid content. If any doubt exists, then biopsy of a small portion of the lining will be diagnostic in most cases, although in the cystic ameloblastoma the tumour may only be evident histologically in a small area of the cyst lining and the sample taken may therefore be misleading.

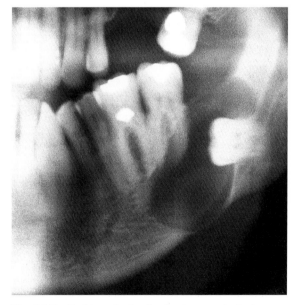

Fig. 28.2 Radiograph of a dentigerous cyst in the lower third molar area showing downward displacement of the inferior dental canal.

Treatment

Treatment will either be enucleation along with extraction of the unerupted tooth or marsupialisation. Marsupialisation is the method of choice if it is hoped to encourage eruption of the buried tooth, but it is remarkable how seldom the involved tooth is in a satisfactory position in terms of its angulation and depth to make this the preferred choice. The vast majority, therefore, are enucleated with the unerupted tooth.

Keratocysts (odontogenic keratocysts)

Keratocysts are believed to be derived from remnants of the dental lamina. They can be found anywhere in the jaws but the most common site is at the angle of the mandible. Unlike other cysts of the jaws, their epithelium is a keratinising stratified squamous epithelium and their contents are therefore filled with desquamated squames and keratin, which form a semisolid material that has been likened to cottage cheese. Their mode of growth is also different from the other cysts in that the lining appears to be more active, with passive fluid ingress of little significance. Keratocysts are also characterised by the formation of microcysts or satellite cysts which protrude into the surrounding fibrous tissue and tend to be left behind during enucleation. This increases the risk of recurrence and dictates a different management approach.

Clinical features

The active growth of keratocysts appears not to be evenly distributed, so the cyst does not expand uniformly as a sphere or oval-shaped lesion. Different rates of activity within areas of the lining probably account for the formation of locules, which, once the cyst has achieved a moderate size, will give rise radiographically to the typical multilocular appearance. They appear to grow selectively within the looser medulla of the jaw initially and although eventually the outer cortical plates do show expansion, the cyst may be by that time a considerable size. Lingual as well as buccal expansion is often noted.

Infection often only occurs when the cyst is quite large and where soft tissue trauma allows ingress of bacteria. It is not infrequent to find that with expansion the cyst communicates with the surface through the periodontal space of an adjacent tooth. It is important to realise that, unless infected, these sometimes very large lesions are painless and do not exert sufficient pressure on vital structures such as the inferior dental nerve to cause anaesthesia of the lip and chin. When infected, however, they can become very painful, cause anaesthesia and may discharge into the mouth, with consequent bad taste and bad breath as additional clinical features.

Diagnosis

As with other cysts, the diagnosis is based on clinical features, radiographic findings and the results of aspiration and biopsy. Two extraoral radiographic views at right angles to each other, such as an orthopantomogram and posteroanterior mandibular view, may be required with large keratocysts. Classically, the appearance is of a multilocular radiolucency with marked expansion of both buccal and lingual plates. Unerupted wisdom teeth may well be pushed into bizarre ectopic positions such as inverted high into the ramus of the mandible. The inferior dental canal may be difficult to see and may reflect the more active growth of these cysts around the canal with less evidence of significant repositioning as is seen with radicular cysts. Displacement or tilting of the teeth can be a feature, as can resorption of roots, although this is again probably a result of infection. Infection within a cyst also accounts for many becoming symptomatic.

As previously indicated, the soluble protein content of the aspirate obtained from a keratocyst is lower than that of other cysts and this is due to the fact that keratin is an insoluble protein. Aspiration will yield a 'dirty' cream-coloured semisolid material composed of keratinised squames. These can be confirmed histologically and provide good evidence that the lesion is a keratocyst.

As the differential diagnosis may well include odontogenic tumours such as ameloblastoma, many surgeons prefer to make a small flap incision and remove some lining of the cyst to confirm the diagnosis.

Treatment

Keratocysts have a higher recurrence rate than other cysts and especially when they are large and multilocular.

Enucleation is suitable for most keratocysts but may be difficult in large ones where, for example, they extend upwards into the vertical ramus of the mandible. Surgical access may be difficult and with the multilocular pattern of growth it may be impossible to ensure that the whole lining is removed. It is known that small clusters of epithelium known as microcysts, or satellite cysts can lie outside the epithelial lining and within the fibrous wall, and leaving even a small amount of this fibrous wall may well account for eventual recurrence. For this reason, some operators have in the past used chemicals such as mercuric salts or, more recently, cryotherapy techniques (particularly liquid nitrogen sprayed around the bony cavity) to try to ensure that no viable soft tissue remnants remain (see Ch. 38).

Marsupialisation can be used particularly with large keratocysts where it can be very effective (Figs 28.3 and 28.4). It has the same advantages as mentioned previously with radicular cysts and probably reduces the chance of recurrence. Again, it may be appropriate in some cases to use the technique to reduce the size of the lesion before enucleating it. Whatever method is used, follow-up is required for years to ensure that there is no recurrence, and this is mainly radiographic.

Gorlin–Goltz syndrome

Gorlin–Goltz syndrome, or multiple basal-cell naevi syndrome, is an inherited (autosomal dominant) condition in which multiple keratocysts of the jaws form part of the overall syndrome. Other aspects in these patients are the presence of many skin lesions in the form of basal-cell naevi or carcinomas, and skeletal abnormalities affecting the vertebral column and the ribs. Calcification of the falx cerebri is also a noteworthy feature.

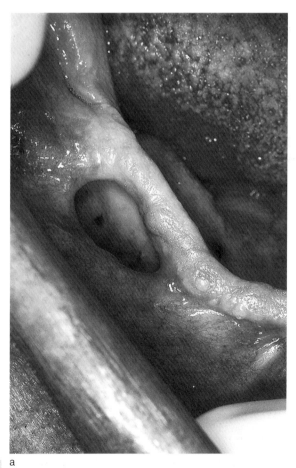
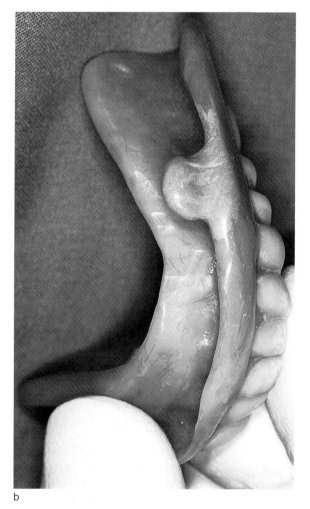

a
b

Fig. 28.3   Marsupialisation of a large keratocyst showing (a) cyst cavity; (b) denture with extension.

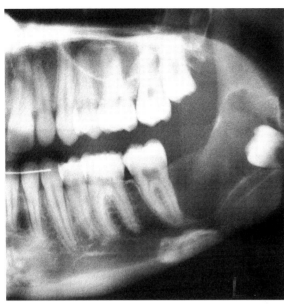

a

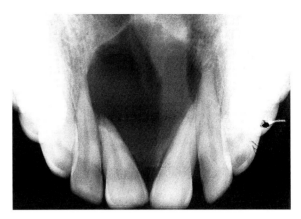

Fig. 28.5 A radiograph of a nasopalatine cyst causing displacement of incisor roots.

Clinical features

These cysts cause swelling of the anterior aspect of the midline of the hard palate. They may become infected and cause pain and overlying tenderness and can, on occasion, discharge forming a sinus. However, as with most cysts, they are painless unless infected and may grow to a considerable size.

Diagnosis

Presence of a midline anterior palatine swelling is the only usual clinical finding. However, many are again diagnosed through chance by radiographs of the teeth in this region. It can be difficult when such radiolucencies are found on routine radiographic assessment of the central incisors, to know if the image seen is within normal anatomical limits of the nasopalatine foramen. A radiolucency of approximately greater than 8 mm in diameter is more likely to represent cystic degeneration but, where doubt exists, a further radiograph 6 months to 1 year later may be more conclusive. The normal radiographic image is a round or inverted pear-shaped radiolucency with sharp radio-opaque margins (Fig. 28.5). When they are large, they can cause separation of the central incisor roots, but the laminae dura of the teeth remain intact. If there is doubt whether the cyst is a radicular cyst related to one or other incisor, pulp testing can be carried out and close examination of the apices radiographically should show an intact lamina dura.

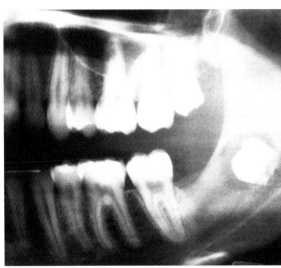

b

Fig. 28.4 Radiograph of keratocyst at left angle of mandible: (a) at presentation; (b) 6 months after marsupialisation.

Nasopalatine cysts

These cysts arise from epithelial remnants within or near to the nasopalatine foramen. They are not odontogenic but are classified as fissural cysts, and they represent by far the most common example of fissural cysts of the jaws.

Treatment

These cysts should be enucleated – never marsupialised because marsupialisation in this area can lead to a

235

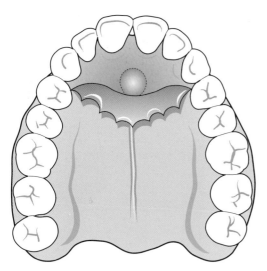

Fig. 28.6 Palatal flap raised to expose a nasopalatine cyst.

permanent cavity that will show no evidence of restoration of the normal contour. Normally, enucleation is carried out with a palatal flap taken around the gingival margins of the premolars on one side to the premolars of the other (Fig. 28.6). After enucleation, interdental interrupted sutures are used to replace the flap and in larger cysts. It is sometimes useful to have constructed a palatal plate from preoperative impressions to support the flap and prevent the formation of a painful haematoma.

Other cysts

The other cysts of the jaws are very uncommon and, as they are so rare, it is only necessary to know a few facts about them.

Nasolabial cyst

This is a fissural cyst that is thought to form by cystic degeneration of epithelium from the lower part of the nasolacrimal duct during embryological development. Clinically, they may present as painless swellings in the nasolabial fold, where they may be palpated either externally on the skin surface or intraorally high in the buccal sulcus anteriorly. Radiographically, although they are not intrabony cysts they may, if they attain a reasonable size, cause a depression of the radio-opaque margin of the floor and lateral wall of the nose, which is best viewed by an oblique anterior occlusal radiograph.

This bony surface is normally very gently convex in appearance but may show concavity where the cyst has caused saucerisation of the bone in this region. Confirmation may be obtained by aspiration and the normal treatment would be surgical enucleation.

Solitary bone cyst

This used to be known as a traumatic bone cyst or a haemorrhagic bone cyst. It is usually found in the mandibular body and appears radiographically as a radiolucency that not infrequently shows scalloping around the roots of the lower molar and premolar teeth. It causes no expansion of the bone and even on radiographic examination the outline of the radiolucency is less well defined than would be obtained from other cysts. This cyst is not a true cyst in so far as it has no epithelial lining and, in fact, the majority have apparently no content whatsoever. When surgically explored, they tend to heal spontaneously after the surgery.

Staphne's idiopathic bone cyst

Although usually discussed with cysts of the jaws, this is not in fact cystic at all. It consists of submandibular salivary gland tissue that occupies a recess on the lingual aspect of the mandibular body. These cavities are usually found by chance on routine radiography of the lower jaw where they appear as round or oval-shaped radiolucencies

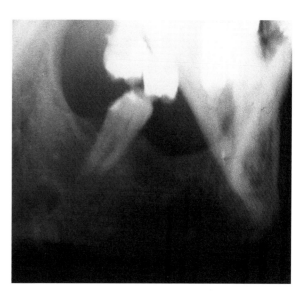

Fig. 28.7 Staphne's idiopathic bone cyst.

lying below the image of the inferior dental canal (Fig. 28.7). Surgical exploration is not advised and most clinicians would take a further radiograph 6 months to 1 year later to confirm that the shadow of this cavity remains unchanged.

Aneurysmal bone cyst

This is discussed in Chapter 36.

Globulomaxillary cyst

This cyst was originally thought to be a separate clinical entity. It was believed to be a fissural cyst formed between the upper lateral and canine teeth, but many now consider it to be a radicular cyst derived from the lateral incisor.

29   Periradicular surgery

Introduction

The term 'periradicular surgery' has superseded the older term of 'apicectomy' and reflects the fact that the surgery might not always be related to an apical problem but can affect the side of the root, as when a post has perforated into the periodontal space. Virtually any tooth can be treated in this way although anterior teeth, being strategically and aesthetically more important, are more common. The indications for periradicular surgery will be discussed, followed by a consideration of surgical techniques and post perforations.

Indications for surgery

In general, too many teeth are treated by periradicular surgery and this is a direct result of inadequate endodontic techniques. There are, however, several indications for periradicular surgery, including endodontic failure, which may be unavoidable. These will be discussed in turn (Table 29.1).

Endodontic failure

Obstructions to instrumentation, such as calcified root canals, dilacerated (hooked or curved) roots, broken endodontic instruments or root fractures may occur; root-filling problems may also arise. Underfilling of the canal often reflects preparation of the root canal short of the true apex with necrotic tissue perpetuating the infection (Fig. 29.1). Overfilling of the canal may occur and the material used and the quantity of material through the apex will determine the likelihood of the need for surgery. A small amount of relatively non-irritant material, provided the patient is symptom-free, can often be left (Fig. 29.2). An open apex may require both endodontic and surgical sealing if the apex is funnel-shaped.

Miscellaneous examples of endodontic failure include significant lateral canals, often near the apex, poor natural drainage and difficult canal morphology. This can lead to difficulty in controlling infection and may need apical surgery in addition to endodontics.

Table 29.1   Indications for periradicular surgery
Endodontic failure:
canal obstruction
problems with root filling
other, e.g. canal number and shape
Pathology
Post-crowned teeth

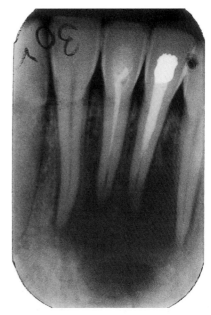

Fig. 29.1 Radiograph of an underfilled root canal.

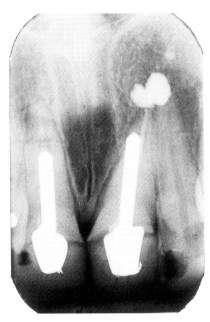

Fig. 29.2 Radiograph of an overfilled root canal (and lateral perforation).

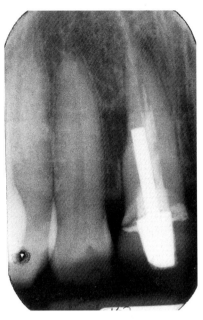

Fig. 29.3 Lateral perforation of a root with a post.

Pathology

The presence of a radicular cyst requires enucleation after endodontic sealing of the canal. Also there may be associated pathology such as infection from an upper lateral incisor spreading to the follicle of an unerupted canine.

Post-crowned teeth

Post-crowned teeth can fail due to any of the above reasons and there may be additional considerations in the decision to carry out periradicular surgery. Often, the correct treatment would be to root treat the tooth again, but this would involve destroying the existing crown and removing the post. This may be unattractive to the patient, especially if the crown is good functionally and aesthetically. The pragmatic solution may therefore be to leave the crown and post undisturbed and carry out the surgery, unless the endodontic filling is very poor.

Minimising the risk of post perforations and their management will be discussed later (Fig. 29.3). It is, however, likely that the infection is initiated by the acidity of the cement used to retain the post causing tissue necrosis in the periodontal space and this subsequently becoming infected.

Surgical technique

Periradicular surgery is a simple minor procedure and is outlined in Table 29.2.

Anaesthesia

Infiltration with an adrenaline (epinephrine)-containing solution is preferable and significantly improves visibility by its haemostatic effect. Even where a block anaesthetic is given, additional infiltration is wise. Palatal or lingual infiltration is needed for full gingival margin flaps to allow suturing but may be necessary for larger lesions in any case, e.g. upper lateral incisor where the infection has eroded palatal bone.

Table 29.2   Periradicular surgical technique
Anaesthesia
Flap design
Bone removal
Apex removal
Curettage
Retrograde root filling
Wound closure
Follow-up

Flap design

An 'L' or inverted 'L'-shaped flap from the gingival margin is the flap of choice (see Ch. 23). Only one vertical incision is normally required and the access afforded is excellent (Fig. 29.4). The only perceived disadvantage may be gingival recession postoperatively, but this can be minimised by careful suturing.

The older semilunar flap avoids the risk of recession but has several disadvantages (Fig. 29.4). It gives less surgical access, is more difficult to suture accurately and, by cutting across the gingivae, can lead to dysaesthesia (painful altered touch sensation) of the gingivae, which may be long lasting.

Bone removal

It may be necessary to remove bone over the apex of the tooth to gain surgical access. This is relatively easy when the pathology has destroyed bone, but accurate assessment of the location of the apex is required when the area of infection is smaller, and good radiographs may be very helpful. The apical third of the root should be found by using a fast-rotating round bur with good suction and light, and bone then removed over the apex and sufficiently above it to allow access.

Removal of apex

Normally, 3 mm of apex is removed using a narrow-tapered fissure bur. Ideally, the cut across the root should be at right angles to the long axis of the root and this stage should be carried out early in the procedure to clear the field for curettage of the existing infection.

Curettage

Large to medium-sized caries excavators are ideal for curettage. The cavity should be clean but it is probably unnecessary to spend too much time removing every fragment of soft tissue. Ideally, curettings should be sent for histopathology.

Retrograde root filling

The vast majority of teeth treated require retrograde sealing of the root canal. This need may be obvious from the outset with good radiographs but visual inspection

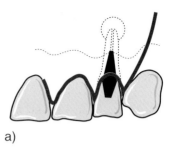

a)

Fig. 29.4 Flap design for apicectomy: older L-shaped flap.

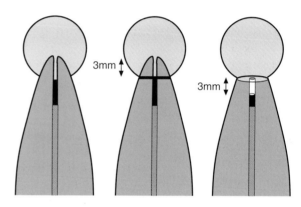

Fig. 29.5 Retrograde sealing of a root canal.

and probing will almost inevitably indicate the requirement.

The root canal needs to be prepared and cleansed to a depth of 3 mm (Fig. 29.5). In practice, this can be accomplished with a small rose head bur (a small contra-angle hand-piece may be helpful) or by ultrasonic preparation using specially designed tips.

After drying the canal, various sealants can be used, including zinc oxide and Eugenol® preparations, ethoxy benzoic acid cement (EBA) and, more recently, mineral trioxide aggregate (MTA). No material will produce a hermetic seal, although this must be regarded as the ultimate objective of the procedure. Excess filler should be removed carefully to reduce foreign body reactions.

Wound closure

After thorough irrigation with sterile saline the wound should be closed. In the anterior region, especially, a finer gauge of suture and smaller needle may facilitate a neater result. Great care should be exercised to ensure that the interdental papillae are repositioned accurately.

In many cases, the knot can be tied over the contact point, allowing the suture to act as a pulley in this context (Fig. 29.6). Where there is no contact point, a vertically arranged mattress suture can be very helpful in holding the papilla firmly on either side of the tooth. Time spent in the closure of these wounds is well spent as the aesthetics of the end result can depend largely on accurate suturing.

Follow-up

Sutures are usually removed 5–7 days postoperatively and patients are normally seen 3–6 months after this to assess the longer-term results. Absence of pain, tenderness of the sulcus sinus formation and undue mobility are indicative of success. Radiographs should show the retrograde seal in good position and a reduction in the radiolucency compared with the preoperative film.

Reasons for failure

The reasons for failure of periradicular surgery are listed in Table 29.3.

The procedure will fail if the apical seal is inadequate and release of toxins and bacteria continues. The seal may be poorly placed at surgery or it can be displaced when, for example, a new post is being prepared for the tooth. The possibility of extra root canals or bifid root apices may be missed and hence not sealed.

Inadequate support may cause undue movement of the tooth and may cause reinfection. This may result

Table 29.3 Reasons for failure of periradicular surgery
Inadequate apical seal
Inadequate tooth support
Vertical tooth fracture

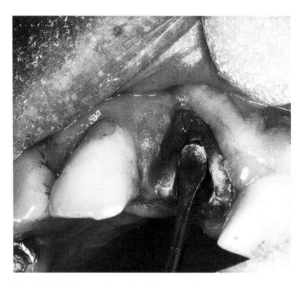

Fig. 29.7 The root of a tooth supporting a post crown showing a vertical split.

from an existing periodontal lesion, undue forces acting on the tooth or overzealous removal of the root apex.

A vertical split in the tooth may be the result of excessive forces acting on a large post (Fig. 29.7). A vertical fracture may be suggested if the post has had to be recemented on several occasions and the radiolucency evident on the radiograph may correspond with the post rather than the apex of the tooth. If a vertical fracture is diagnosed, the tooth must be extracted.

Post perforations

The risk of post perforation during preparation of the root canal for the posts can be minimised by ensuring the preparation is carried out without local anaesthetic. If an inadvertent perforation occurs, the patient will feel pain and bleeding may be evident from the canal. In addition, root-filling material should be removed carefully using hand-driven non-dentine cutting instruments. Finally, good quality radiographs should always be available.

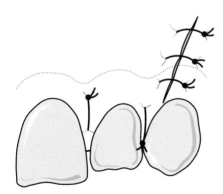

Fig. 29.6 Suturing of an L-shaped apicectomy flap. Suture between 23 is interrupted and tied over the contact point. The suture between 12, having no contact point interdentally, is a vertically arranged mattress suture.

Perforations which do occur should be gently irrigated, dried and the correct alignment re-established. The false channel should normally be sealed on filling the canal.

Diagnosis

This may be obvious if the post has perforated mesially or distally, when the rarefaction can readily be seen on periapical radiograph (Fig. 29.3). If the perforation has been labial or palatal (or lingual) then the use of a 'profile' (i.e. lateral) periapical radiographic view may be useful. The site of the radiolucency can be a valuable clue, as it will generally appear on the lateral side of the root at the level of the top of the post. This appearance can also be seen where there is a vertical split.

Management

To curette the abscess and seal the perforation from the surgical aspect will normally be unsuccessful in the long term. Better results demand removal of the post and thorough cleansing of the false channel. Root filler should then obliterate this channel and, as excess filler may be extruded into the abscess cavity, curettage should be arranged very soon afterwards. Sealing the defect can lead to complete healing and resolution of the defect. If the original post is otherwise satisfactory, it may be reduced in length before recementing, or a new post could be fitted along the correct line of the root canal. Surgical access is achieved in the usual way, the cavity curetted of infected tissue together with any excess root filler. If the perforation is directly palatal or lingual, access may be virtually impossible and the prognosis will hence be poorer.

Some clinicians have extracted inaccessible perforated roots, sealed the perforation outside the mouth and reimplanted it with appropriate splinting. This is clearly 'last chance' treatment but can be remarkably successful, at least in the short term.

30 Preprosthetic surgery

Introduction

In the normal course of events, the extraction of teeth will be the final surgical procedure undertaken before the provision of a prosthesis, whether this is a full or partial removable appliance or a fixed system. The presence of 'hidden' pathology in the form of unerupted teeth or roots, or residual infections or cysts, should also be ascertained and dealt with appropriately before prosthodontic work is undertaken, as this may well avoid embarrassing complications at a later date, which might compromise the prosthesis. However, certain situations – often anatomical rather than pathological – will benefit from minor surgical modifications, which can greatly improve the provision of a more stable and comfortable prosthesis. Additionally, dental implants have opened up new horizons for increased stability and hence patient acceptability of both fixed and removable crowns, bridges and dentures, and this topic will be discussed in more depth in Chapter 38.

Preprosthetic surgery can conveniently be divided into three subtopics: extraction of teeth; soft tissue surgery and bone surgery (Table 30.1), and these will be discussed in turn.

Extraction of teeth

Standing teeth

Standing teeth should be extracted with an awareness that preservation of the bony socket and attached gingiva will materially promote healing by preserving the maximum amount of tissue on or within which future replacement of the lost unit(s) will be based. Good technique ensures that soft-tissue damage by forceps is minimal, as does firm digital support of the alveolus during extraction. Compression of expanded buccal plate

Table 30.1   Preprosthetic surgical procedures
Extraction of teeth
standing teeth
unerupted teeth
Soft tissue surgery
fraenal attachments
vestibular denture-induced hyperplasia
palatal hyperplasia
leaf fibroma
fibrous tuberosities
flabby ridges
Bone surgery
alveolectomy or alveolotomy
bony exostoses and bone undercuts
sharp bony ridges
torus palatinus
torus mandibularis
sharp mylohyoid ridge
genial tubercles
ridge augmentation and vestibuloplasty

and judicious use of sutures over the socket margins, or where minor soft tissue tears have occurred, can also benefit the healing process.

It is clearly beneficial that teeth are extracted without root fracture, but this may be unavoidable. Surgical removal of any such roots requires awareness by the operator that the ridge form can be influenced by the technique employed to remove the fragment. It is unwise to persist in attempting to elevate a root through the socket if this causes damage to the soft tissue margins or destroys bone in an uncontrolled fashion. A mucoperiosteal flap can often not only preserve soft tissue health but also reveal the underlying root in such a way as to minimise bone loss. In some cases, bone may be preserved around the coronal aspect of the socket by gaining application points for elevators further apically, in a manner similar to bone removal for apicectomy. This will help to

243

preserve the ridge height. Careful wound debridement is essential and the flap should be sutured back anatomically to maximise ridge form. Drawing a buccal flap over the socket on completion will effectively reduce both ridge height and also the stronger attached gingiva, which is better able to cope with future prostheses. In some situations, periodontal bone loss and gingival recession may combine to leave spurs of interradicular bone lying proud to the socket margin, and careful trimming with bone rongeurs will allow the blood clots to cover all the underlying bone.

Unerupted teeth

Before provision of any prosthesis, it must be ascertained that no buried teeth that could compromise longer-term success are present. The most commonly found are wisdom teeth, upper canines and lower premolars, and an orthopantomogram is an ideal radiograph to reveal such potential problems. A judgement is needed as to whether it is likely that an unerupted tooth could, within the lifetime of either the patient or the proposed prosthesis, cause a problem that would prejudice the appliance. This assessment may be relatively easily made where there is related pathology such as dentigerous cyst formation around the crown or evidence of communication, however minimal, with the surface. In many cases, however, it may well be in the patient's best interests to leave such a tooth, especially where its depth makes it improbable – even with resorption over many years – that it will ever interfere with a prosthesis. Further, its surgical removal might risk damage to nerves or involve a considerable amount of bone removal resulting in a poorer ridge form. If removal is deemed necessary, planned removal of bone in which sectioning of the tooth may well reduce this need can better preserve the ridge contour and height. So-called osteoplastic flaps can, in a limited number of situations, help to preserve bone. This technique usually involves hinging the buccal plate (with its periosteum intact) from the underlying tooth to gain surgical access, and then suturing the intact plate of bone, still with its blood supply through the periosteum, back to its anatomical site.

Soft-tissue surgery

Several soft-tissue impediments to provision of a good, stable prosthesis can be rectified surgically and are relatively minor surgical procedures.

Fraenal attachments

These anatomical fraenal bands are composed not of muscle but of fibrous tissue. They may form an attachment on the ridge, which is near the crest, and cause instability to removable appliances when adjacent muscles are in function and they become tense.

Surgically, they may be excised (see Ch. 31) or their attachment to the ridge may be incised close to the alveolar ridge and a surgical pack sutured over to prevent reattachment. Alternatively, if the patient has an existing prosthesis, this may be lined with gutta percha or a zinc oxide-based periodontal pack to hold the incised fraenum away from the ridge during the healing phase.

Vestibular denture-induced hyperplasia

Several forms of denture-related hyperplastic soft-tissue lesions are recognised but they all arise as a result of loss of denture fit and are therefore more often seen in the 'old denture' wearer, who is often the satisfied denture wearer.

Aetiology and clinical appearance

The most common form is the result of alveolar resorption over a considerable number of years. This causes the periphery of the flange of the denture to impinge on the sulcus depth or adjacent lip or cheek tissue. As this is a very gradual process, the tissues have time to react to the irritation by a protective hyperplastic reaction. This results in a characteristic sausage-shaped roll of excess tissue, which can lie in function either on the outer aspect of the flange or between the flange and the alveolar ridge where there is a space (Fig. 30.1). This can result, on occasion, in two parallel rolls of tissue lying across the sulcus region, and sometimes – when progressive loss of fit causes trauma further into the lip or cheek – in several flaps of redundant tissue. Hyperplasia of this kind can occur anywhere along the periphery of a denture, and even along the line of the post-dam, but it is most common in the lower labial anterior sulcus, reflecting the more extensive resorption of alveolar bone in this region.

A less common but distinctive group of patients with this problem are the immediate denture wearers, whose dentures have not been adjusted appropriately for the more rapid loss of fit that is caused by initial resorption. These patients often complain of pain – in marked contrast to the 'old denture' wearer – because the tissues,

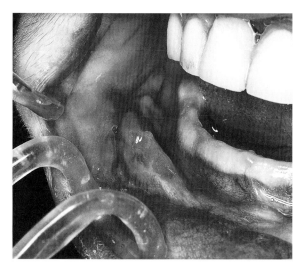

Fig. 30.1 Denture-induced hyperplasia of the lower labial sulcus in a patient with a loose-fitting denture.

having had less time to react to the loss of fit, ulcerate in addition to forming a hyperplastic protective overgrowth.

Management

In the established denture wearer, the roll of tissue is usually composed of very mature connective tissue, which, even if the flange is trimmed back, will not shrink appreciably and resolve. However, trimming of the flange should always be carried out at the time of presentation, with or without the use of a tissue-conditioning lining to maximise the retention of the prosthesis. Surgical trimming of the excess tissue is almost always needed and this is usually done under local anaesthesia. The surgeon can manipulate the roll of tissue better by passing a suture through the lesion, allowing accurate incision along its margins. When the incision on the outer and inner aspects of the role of tissue is completed, its base can often be simply lifted and separated using a scalpel. It is undesirable to cut down to deeper tissues, as this can cause excessive scarring on healing thus reducing sulcus depth. When the base of the wound extends into lip or cheek, superficial 'tack' sutures can be used after careful undermining of the margins, but in some cases the base is left open and covered by a surgical pack, or the previously trimmed old denture lined over the wound with gutta percha or a zinc oxide-based periodontal pack.

In the more 'acute' immediate denture hyperplasia, denture adjustments with appropriate soft lining can often obviate the need for surgery, because the hyperplasia is often oedematous and elimination of further trauma produces a dramatic resolution.

In both cases, provision of new dentures is the ultimate aim.

Palatal hyperplasia

Aetiology and clinical appearance

This reactive condition results from movement and loss of even contact of the upper denture base on the palatal epithelium and underlying connective tissues. The clinical appearance can vary between a multitude of small papillary projections, to an appearance of cobblestones, to areas of surface hyperplasia with slit-like clefts between the 'blocks' of hyperplastic mucosa. This latter form is more commonly seen under partial dentures. This clinical appearance represents a hyperplastic type of denture stomatitis (Newton's classification Type III) and is infected with *Candida*. The tissues may be significantly red and inflamed.

Management

Treatment of the candidal infection involves:

- leaving the denture out during sleep
- thorough scrubbing of the fitting surface of the denture
- leaving the denture in Milton's solution (sodium hypochloride) or, in the case of metal-based dentures, in chlorhexidine solution overnight
- brushing the palatal soft tissue with a toothbrush night and morning
- the use of systemic antifungals, such as fluconazole.

The dentures should be lined with tissue conditioner for daytime use.

Total resolution by such means is unusual and removal of the hyperplastic tissue either with diathermy loop or laser may be needed. The resultant raw surface created by surgery is best covered with the denture lined with a zinc oxide-based periodontal pack.

Leaf fibroma

Aetiology and clinical appearance

This lesion is not, as its name implies, a true neoplasm but is again the result of chronic frictional irritation of the palatal soft tissues by movement or irregularity of the

245

palatal coverage of an upper denture. Were it not covered by the denture, it would grow evenly as a rounded exophytic non-ulcerated swelling but, because of its position, it is flattened into a leaf shape by the denture. It is a perdunculated lesion, which means that it has a stalk-like attachment, and on occasion can be of considerable size, having lain unseen in the vault of the hard palate (Fig. 30.2). Gentle probing can often cause it to lose its adhesion to the true vault and it then hangs from its narrow attachment and is very obvious.

Management

Excision biopsy under local anaesthesia is very simple. Bleeding can be a problem from its feeder arteriole, which may need to be cauterised.

Fibrous tuberosities

Aetiology and clinical appearance

These excess masses of fibrous gingival enlargement of the upper molar regions are usually bilateral, although often asymmetrical. They may be so bulky that they contact the lower alveolar process in edentulous patients and hence prevent provision of adequate dentures. Grossly enlarged tuberosities may be due to bony overgrowth rather than fibrous tissue and it is important to ensure by clinical examination and radiographs which tissue is present in excessive quantity. Fibrous over-growth may often be moveable on palpation, unlike bony overgrowth, but if doubt exists as to the extent of the soft tissue component, a sharp probe can be used for assess-ment after appropriate local anaesthesia has been given.

Management

Surgical reduction can be undertaken in which a wedge of soft tissue is excised through an elliptical surface incision (Fig. 30.3).

After removal of this wedge of tissue, the margins require to be undermined by further cuts and 'filleting' on either side of the original excision to allow the edges to be approximated and sutured without undue tension.

'Flabby' ridges

Aetiology and clinical appearance

Flabby ridges are the result of fibrous replacement of the bony ridge. This is most commonly seen in the upper

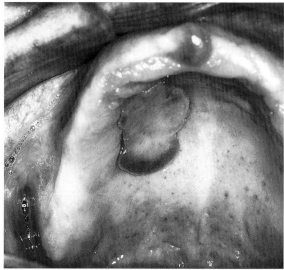

a

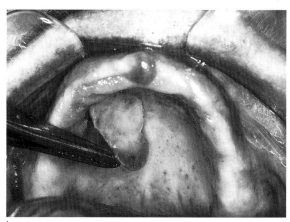

b

Fig. 30.2 Leaf fibroma: (a) lying against hard palate; (b) demonstrating pedunculated attachment.

anterior segment where a full upper denture is opposed by natural lower teeth but with free end saddles not compensated with a partial lower denture. The resultant tipping action induced by the protrusive chewing action results in bony resorption and fibrous replacement of the ridge. The ridge becomes excessively mobile reflecting the lack of underlying hard tissue.

Management

Surgery is seldom indicated, as most prosthodontists would prefer more rather than less of this tissue given that the bone is by then lost. In the grossest situation it

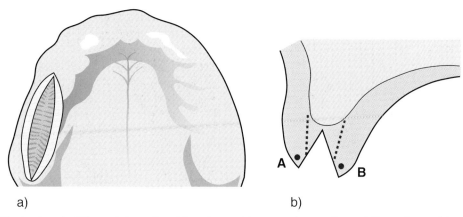

a)   b)

Fig. 30.3   The treatment of fibrous tuberosities: (a) wedge excision removing an ellipse of fibrous tissue; (b) cross-section showing undermining of the wedge to allow suturing without tension from 'A' to 'B'.

can be 'tightened' by a wedge excision similar to the fibrous tuberosity reduction.

Bone surgery

Alveolectomy or alveolotomy

Aetiology and clinical appearance

The indications for these procedures are rare but may be of value where excessive anterior projection of the ridge in the upper premaxillary area might pose problems for future denture aesthetics or stability. Class II, division I malocclusions are therefore most likely to benefit from such surgery.

Management

Alveolectomy involves reduction in both the height and width of the ridge and is mainly accomplished by reduction of the labial plate. The mucoperiosteum is best raised with a 'U'-shaped incision to allow access. Bone rongeurs or larger 'acrylic' burs can be used to reduce the labial plate prominence and, on occasion, also the interdental septae. The bony margin is then smoothed with a file and the wound closed with sutures.

Transeptal or interseptal alveolotomy reduces the labial prominence but maintains the height of the ridge. Following extraction of the incisors and canines, the interdental septum is removed between each socket and the labial plate is then fractured inwards with firm digital pressure. A vertical cut may be needed over the canine

prominence labially to facilitate this fracture. The labial plate will still be attached to its overlying periosteum and should therefore remain viable.

These operations may be facilitated by cooperation with the prosthodontist, who can provide the surgeon with a template of acrylic that is made on the cast trimmed to the desired contour. Unless the patient desires an aesthetic change, these procedures are becoming less frequent.

Bony exostoses and bone undercuts

Aetiology and clinical appearance

Surgery is indicated where the bony morphology, either through localised excessive growth or as a result of unusual resorption of the ridge, gives rise to impediments to denture construction.

Management

A simple mucoperiostial flap is taken, the bone impediment is reduced with rongeurs or burs, and the flap is closed with sutures.

Sharp bony ridges

Aetiology and clinical appearance

These are usually found in the lower anterior region where resorption of bone has produced a pointed, often razor-sharp, bony ridge, described as a knife-edge or feather-edge ridge.

Management

The incision to gain surgical access is often best made on the buccal aspect of the crest of what is often a very thin line of attached gingiva forming the soft tissue crest of ridge. This allows the underlying bone to be smoothed but prevents undue disruption to the stability of the overlying soft tissues when the wound is closed.

Torus palatinus

Aetiology and clinical appearance

This presents with a midline bony swelling (Fig. 30.4) which is normally symmetrical and, unless traumatised, symptom free. The overgrowth is composed of normal bone but its presence may make palatal coverage with a denture impossible or, if a denture is made over, it can cause fracture of the denture. In some dentate patients, repeated trauma caused by the swallowing action on its posterior aspect may result in ulceration of the overlying soft tissues and this would merit surgical reduction.

Management

A preoperative impression allows construction of a palatal splint in dentate patients or the existing denture, if available, can be used as a postoperative covering. An incision is made anteroposteriorly along the midline of the torus and relieving 'Y'-shaped incisions are made at the anterior and posterior extensions (Fig. 30.5). The overlying mucoperiosteum should be reflected with care as it is often very thin. The bony mass is then divided

with one anteroposterior fissure bur cut and crossed by several lateral cuts. This conveniently divides the mass into smaller blocks, which can be chiselled free. A final smoothing with a round 'acrylic' bur precedes wound closure. Some soft tissue reduction of the margins may be needed, as there will be excess soft tissue. Suturing may be difficult and the prior construction of a plate to cover and hold the flap is very helpful, as this will reduce the chance of a painful palatal haematoma and will help the patient to eat in the first few days after the operation. Large palatal tori are better removed under general anaesthesia or at least under local anaesthesia with sedation.

Torus mandibularis

Aetiology and clinical appearance

Mandibular tori present on the lingual aspect of the alveolar process in the premolar region (Fig. 30.6). Often bilateral, they may or may not be symmetrical and the excess bone may be a single dome-shaped mass or several

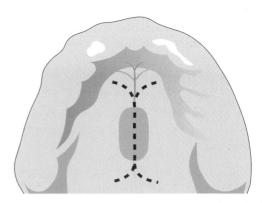

Fig. 30.5 Incision to allow surgical trimming of a palatal torus.

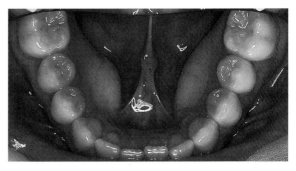

Fig. 30.6 Bilateral torus mandibularis.

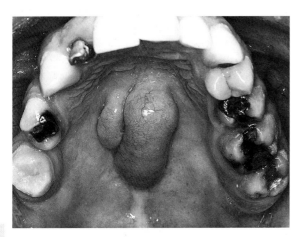

Fig. 30.4 A torus palatinus.

protuberances. Surgical reduction is only indicated if they impede denture design.

Management

In the edentulous patient, a straight incision over the crest of the ridge with no relieving incision is needed. This allows the raising of the mucoperiosteum from the torus. The excess bone can then be trimmed using a combination of a narrow fissure bur with a chisel or simply with a flame-shaped acrylic smoothing bur. Flap retraction should be combined with protection of floor of mouth and underlying soft tissue. The flap is then sutured back with no need for trimming.

In dentate patients, the procedure is essentially the same but surgical access caused by the presence of teeth in the area can make for difficult surgical access.

Sharp mylohyoid ridge

Aetiology and clinical appearance

With continued alveolar resorption in the lower molar region, most of the alveolar process may eventually be lost, with the denture base then being constructed over more basal bone. On the lingual aspect of the molar region, the mylohyoid ridge of bone can be covered by the lingual flange of a denture, which may cause discomfort and even overlying soft tissue ulceration due to its sharp upper surface.

Management

If the denture cannot be relieved adequately to reduce pressure on the ridge it may be surgically reduced.

A straight-line incision over the crest of the ridge, extending back into the retromolar pad from the premolar region, allows a lingual flap to be raised to expose the sharp upper aspect of the ridge. Often, minimal smoothing using a bur, or even a hand file, without stripping the muscle off the affected area is successful and can be judged by running a finger over the ridge. If muscle stripping is thought necessary, this will undoubtedly

increase postoperative swelling and haematoma formation is more likely. Patients require to be warned preoperatively of this possibility.

Genial tubercles

Aetiology and clinical appearance

Gross alveolar resorption following extractions can cause the upper tubercles to be traumatised by the lingual flange of a lower denture in the midline. Recurrent ulceration, hyperplastic tissue formation or simply discomfort may be the stimulus to surgery.

Management

An incision along the midline of the crest of the alveolar ridge allows a lingual flap to be raised to expose the bony tubercle. Simple smoothing with a bur is normally sufficient, and stripping of the genioglossus should be unnecessary because it is important to maintain the function of this muscle.

Ridge augmentation and vestibuloplasty

These minor surgical procedures can be of great benefit to the patient. It will be apparent that many problems arise as a result of alveolar resorption and surgeons have in the past devised many surgical procedures to make good this loss of ridge, either by augmenting the ridge or by deepening the sulcus (vestibuloplasty). Augmentation using bone, hydroxyapatite or allelograft material often failed due to infection or the inability of the soft tissues to accommodate the increased ridge bulk. Vestibuloplasties were probably more successful in that they increased sulcus depth rather than trying to increase the resorbed bony ridge. In recent years, however, such operations have largely been superseded by the use of dental implants. The success rate with implants is high and involves relatively minor surgical operative procedures. This rapidly growing field will be discussed in Chapter 37.

31 Orthodontics and oral surgery

Introduction

When jaw relationships such as severe skeletal base abnormalities result in a malocclusion that is beyond the scope of orthodontic treatment, orthognathic surgery or distraction osteogenesis should be considered to effect correction. These are described in Chapter 13.

Dentoalveolar surgery may be required, often in conjunction with orthodontic treatment, to deal with specific localised problems of eruption or crowding. Where several options exist, the risks of surgery, and perhaps general anaesthesia, must be weighed against the benefits of a successful outcome. It is for the surgeon and orthodontist together to explain the options and advise when a surgical approach is in the best interest of the patient.

The most common orthodontic problems with surgical treatment options are crowding, failed eruption, spacing and ankylosis. The orthodontist may have several treatment options so it is important for the surgeon to have a good appreciation of the orthodontic problem. A good history is essential. Clinical and radiographic examination reveal the nature of the malocclusion or orthodontic problem and the state of oral and dental health. Discussion of the surgical aspects with the patient and parents reveals their attitude to treatment, and helps to finalise the treatment plan.

Some causes of the orthodontic problems alluded to above are listed in Table 31.1.

Treatment options

A number of surgical treatments exist for orthodontic problems and these should be considered as part of the treatment-planning exercise. These include extractions, surgical removal of teeth, surgical exposure of teeth, fraenectomy and tooth transplantation.

Table 31.1   Causes of orthodontic problems
Crowding and impaction
teeth relatively large for arch size
early loss of deciduous teeth allowing mesial drift
supernumerary and supplemental teeth
odontomes
Failed eruption
crowding or early loss of deciduous teeth
retained deciduous teeth
congenital absence
supernumerary teeth/odontomes
fibrous tissue (scar) due to previous trauma, surgery or infection
ectopic development or dilaceration due to trauma
cysts and other pathology
cleft palate
cleidocranial dysostosis
Down syndrome or hypothyroidism
gingival hyperplasia or fibromatosis
Spacing
tooth size/arch size disproportion
small teeth
prominent fleshy frenum
proclined incisors
partial anodontia
Ankylosis
trauma
infection

Non-surgical extractions

Extractions are the most common requirement for relief of crowding. There may be an indication for general anaesthesia in very young or nervous children, and those with learning difficulties. Local anaesthesia, with or without sedation, should be used wherever possible, bearing in mind that in most cases orthodontic treatment is elective. In some cases, it is better to delay treatment until the patient is more cooperative. On the other hand, correct timing of extractions can be a significant advantage, often removing the need for later orthodontic appliance treatment. For example, timely removal of carious or heavily restored or hypoplastic first permanent molars may not only relieve crowding but also removes teeth of doubtful long-term prognosis.

Surgical removal of teeth

Surgical removal may be indicated when a tooth is unerupted. There is no need to remove a buried tooth unless there is a positive indication such as interference with the orthodontic movement of other teeth, or associated pathology such as cyst formation, or resorption of an adjacent tooth.

Surgical exposure of teeth

Surgical exposure is used to encourage eruption or to allow access for orthodontic traction. It involves removal of overlying soft tissue, bone and scar tissue. It is important to use a technique that will result in good gingival contour and minimise postoperative scarring. Adequate exposure is important otherwise the tissues will cover the tooth again. Orthodontic traction using a gold chain bonded to the exposed tooth can also be used.

Fraenectomy

Fraenectomy may be requested when there is a diastema or a localised periodontal problem. Upper labial fraenectomy or lingual fraenectomy are the most common of these procedures. A prominent fraenal attachment can cause a diastema, which is most common where there is a thick, fibrous, upper labial fraenum. When this is present, blanching of the palatal gingiva when the lip is pulled up to create tension confirms the need for fraenectomy, as does the presence of 'V' notching interincisally on a maxillary anterior occlusal radiograph. A radiograph should always be taken to exclude a midline supernumerary tooth or any other pathology. A tight lingual fraenum can pull on the gingival margin and cause a pocket or contour defect together with tongue restriction.

Tooth transplantation

Tooth transplantation can be considered when orthodontic movement cannot achieve the desired result, or sometimes to expedite the outcome in impacted canine cases. There are, however, inherent problems in the transplantation of teeth.

A transplanted tooth must not be left in traumatic occlusion or it will quickly fail. Unfortunately, transplants have a high failure rate. After a promising start many develop internal and external resorption after about 4 years. This often progresses to abscess formation despite root canal therapy. Root treatment soon after transplantation is advocated by some but the failure rate is still high. Alveolar bone is removed when the socket is created and abscess formation can cause further damage. The resulting depression in the alveolus causes a cosmetic problem with a subsequent denture or bridge, and leaves insufficient bone for an osseointegrated implant. For the above reasons, transplantation is now rarely the best option. It is often better to temporise and consider an adhesive bridge or implant later. Autotransplanation, where a tooth is extracted from one site, such as a lower premolar, and inserted into the upper central region after traumatic loss, has a good success rate, however, and should be considered.

Surgical management of specific orthodontic problems

The aforementioned treatment options can be applied to several teeth with orthodontic problems related to crowding and impaction. The problems of spacing and ankylosis will also be discussed followed by a consideration of the individual surgical procedures.

Incisors

Maxillary central incisors may be impacted. There may be lack of space but trauma is the most common factor. Young children often fall onto their deciduous incisors, causing displacement or damage to the permanent tooth germs. The tooth may subsequently develop in an ectopic position and the crown or root may be deformed. Also, trauma to the alveolar mucosa or bone may result in scar tissue, which later prevents eruption. Supernumerary teeth and odontomes are another common obstacle to eruption. Scar tissue formed following their surgical removal may also result in eruption problems. Further space can be lost by drifting of adjacent teeth if eruption is delayed.

Occasionally there are systemic factors such as cleidocranial dysostosis, Down syndrome or chemotherapy to cause a delay in eruption. Also, gingival overgrowth due to hereditary fibromatosis, or secondary to drugs such as phenytoin or cyclosporin may inhibit eruption.

Scar tissue or a supernumerary tooth frequently holds the incisor in a fairly normal pre-eruptive position, but following intrusion trauma it is more often displaced upwards and forwards and lies horizontally under the anterior nasal spine. Very occasionally there is a palatal inclination. It is important to realise that a tooth will only erupt through attached mucosa. If gingival mucosa has been lost through previous trauma or the tooth is attempting to erupt under the unattached sulcus mucosa, surgical exposure will be required.

The choice of treatment depends on the position of the tooth, the space available and patient cooperation. If the patient is unlikely to accept appliance therapy, or if oral hygiene is poor, it may be better to accept the space and construct a partial denture. Alternatively, the space could be allowed to close as far as possible and the defect disguised by building up, by restorative means, adjacent teeth. The tooth can be left in situ unless there is any associated pathology, but surgical removal is often indicated.

Ideally, the incisor should be aligned unless radiographs suggest that the tooth is hypoplastic, markedly dilacerated or in an unfavourable position. Surgical exposure is performed to encourage eruption and create orthodontic access. This would normally be by a labial flap, either apically repositioned, or replaced after attachment of a gold chain.

Removal of supernumerary teeth normally requires a palatal flap as they are almost always palatally situated relative to the permanent incisors.

Canines

Impacted maxillary canines have a prevalence of about 1.7% in Caucasians. Ideally, they should be detected before the teenage years, as timely interception can reduce the severity of the problem. Canines can be palpated in the labial sulcus at around 10 years of age. Eruption is expected at about 12 years of age in girls and 13 years of age in boys. Any deviation from this normal pattern warrants investigation. Extraction of the deciduous canine can encourage the successor to resume a normal path of eruption in more than 60% of cases depending on several factors such as canine height, inclination, mesiodistal position and crowding.

Unfortunately, resorption of the roots of adjacent permanent incisors can occur and it is claimed that the incidence may be as high as 12% for incisors adjacent to ectopic canines. It would not be practical or defendable to remove every buried canine for this reason and the best advice is to be vigilant. Root resorption, if it is going to happen, generally occurs at 10 or 11 years of age and it is rare for this complication to occur after 14 years of age, unless there is a general delay in dental development.

The management of the unerupted upper canine can be in one of four ways.

No surgery

The most common option is to leave the buried canine alone. The first premolar can be disguised by reducing the palatal cusp or by its orthodontic alignment provided this is not obstructed by the unerupted canine. The deciduous canine may be kept and often lasts for many years where alignment of the permanent tooth is not feasible. Later, an adhesive bridge or implant can be considered, although overeruption of an opposing tooth can cause difficulty.

Surgical exposure

Surgical exposure may be requested where space is readily available or where it is decided this will provide the optimum aesthetic result. The position of the tooth must be ascertained by clinical examination and radiography. The tooth may be palpable on the buccal or palatal aspect and the position and inclination of adjacent teeth often gives guidance. For example, the lateral incisor may show undue prominence of its root outline on the labial aspect and be almost retroclined due to the palatal presence of the canine crown exerting pressure on it. A panoramic film is most useful but other radiographs such as periapical or occlusal views may be required for localisation. It can be difficult to know whether the canine is inclined buccally, palatally or lies in the line of the arch. Parallax methods may help localisation but clinical assessment is often more reliable. Approximately three-quarters of impacted canines lie with crowns palatal to the arch line.

The principle of parallax is that the image of two parallel objects will alter with differing angulations of radiographic views. If, on comparing the image of the unerupted canine relative to the lateral incisor on a panoral film with its position on an oblique occlusal film, the canine appears to move upwards, then it is palatal to the lateral incisor. Put more simply, if the buried tooth moves with the position of the tube (i.e. the source of the X-rays), then it is palatal. The depth and inclination are relevant not only to the difficulty of surgery but also to the prospect of successful orthodontic alignment in reasonable time. Availability of space and overeruption of opposing teeth must also be considered.

Surgical removal

Surgical removal is required when the buried canine is not suitable for alignment and there is an indication, such as interference with proposed orthodontic treatment, or associated pathology, such as dentigerous cyst formation or resorption of the roots of the incisors. Often, a first or second premolar would need to be extracted to make space for alignment of the canine and the patient may prefer to avoid more prolonged appliance therapy by accepting space closure. As with exposure, the position of the tooth must be assessed by clinical and radiographic examination. Difficulties such as dilaceration of the root and proximity of adjacent teeth must be assessed.

Reimplantation

Reimplantation of canines is another option. If space is available or can be created and the impacted canine can be removed intact and with minimal trauma, it may be reimplanted into a surgically prepared socket. The transplanted tooth may need to be stabilised with a cemented splint or an orthodontic bracket. This technique is usually successful in the short term, although it is often difficult to place the canine in the optimum position unless additional space to that previously occupied by the deciduous canine is obtained preoperatively by orthodontic means. Commonly, the lower canine has over-erupted and this can also lead to difficulty in positioning free of occlusal contact. As described previously, the failure rate is high and transplantation is seldom the preferred option.

Premolars

In the maxilla the second premolar is occasionally excluded from the arch due to crowding. It is usually found in the palate, where it may remain harmlessly or eventually erupt. The tooth can be left unless it interferes with orthodontic treatment or if it erupts and becomes a threat to periodontal health by encouraging food trapping.

In the mandible, premolars may be impacted due to crowding and can be buccal, lingual or in the line of the arch. The second premolar is usually lingually inclined, in which case it can be left in situ or removed if there is a good indication. Surgery on the lingual aspect of the mandible can be awkward because of difficulty of access and of reflection of the delicate lingual mucosa. Generally, therefore, a lingually inclined premolar is removed via a buccal approach.

If lower first permanent molars have been lost early, the adjacent premolars have a tendency to drift backwards and may even become horizontally impacted against the root of the second molar. Surgical exposure and ortho-dontic alignment may be appropriate in a well-motivated patient.

First and second permanent molars

If one or more carious first permanent molars require extraction it is often beneficial to carry out balancing extractions. Ideally this should be done in children around the age of nine years.

Removal of second permanent molars at an appropriate time during development is still accepted as a method of encouraging wisdom teeth to erupt into a functional position but this is not always successful especially where there is severe crowding. Removal of second molars in late adolescence to allow eruption of wisdom teeth is not wise, as the eruption of third molars is unreliable and these teeth may be of poor quality.

Third molars

Imbrication of lower incisors often occurs around 20 years of age but prophylactic removal of third molars is no longer regarded as effective in preventing lower anterior crowding. There are only rare occasions when wisdom teeth should be removed for orthodontic reasons. Possible indications are proposed distal movement of second molars or orthognathic surgery involving the mandibular ramus.

Guidelines advise that the risks of damage to inferior alveolar or lingual nerve, as well as the trauma of surgery, should be undertaken only when there are valid indications. In our present state of knowledge it is not possible to predict the behaviour of lower third molars. If it were possible to predict which ones would need removal, this could be done much more easily during the teenage years, before their roots are fully formed and difficult impactions have developed.

Removal of lower third molar tooth germs at around 12 years of age, before calcification of enamel and dentine, used to be fairly common practice. This procedure, known as lateral trepanation, was fairly simple but a general anaesthetic was required. There is no evidence that this operation was worthwhile. Extraction of third molars is considered further in Chapter 27.

Spacing

Spacing is normal in the deciduous dentition and as the jaws increase in size to accommodate the permanent teeth. Spacing of permanent teeth may be due to small teeth or partial anodontia. There are usually restorative treatment options but implants may also be indicated.

Ankylosis and submerged deciduous teeth

Although most commonly seen in the upper incisors, ankylosis of other teeth also occurs. The causes are trauma and infection.

Upper incisors are frequently traumatised and ankylosis is especially common after reimplantation. An ankylosed tooth does not move as jaw growth progresses, so that, if reimplantation occurred at an early age, the reimplanted tooth is significantly palatally and apically displaced by adulthood. The tooth can function normally for many years, but frequently internal and external resorption results in abscess formation or complete loss of the root. An implant should be considered if no simple restorative option is available.

Submerged deciduous molars are also a result of ankylosis. Some children have submerged teeth in several areas, the cause of which is often unknown. It has been suggested that there is a lack of growth potential in these areas. The ankylosed tooth remains static while alveolar bone growth continues, so that it may become completely buried. The adjacent permanent teeth erupt and often the submerged tooth becomes impacted between them. The submerging tooth is prone to caries and eruption of the permanent successor is prevented. Removal becomes more difficult as they become more deeply embedded so it is better to extract them early.

Failure of a permanent molar to erupt may be due to ankylosis. The cause is again unknown but trauma to the

Table 31.2   Orthodontic surgical procedures
Upper labial fraenectomy
Removal of supernumerary teeth
Exposure of incisors
Exposure of palatal canines
Exposure of buccal canines
Removal of impacted premolars

area by a mouth gag during dental extraction or other surgical procedures under general anaesthesia is a possibility, as is primary failure of eruption. Surgical exposure is sometimes successful if there is soft tissue obstruction or a small odontome preventing eruption, but results are poor if there is true ankylosis or long delay after normal eruption time. These teeth are often partially erupted and develop caries and surgical removal is then indicated. Cyst formation can also occur.

Several of the surgical procedures discussed above are described in other chapters. Some, however, are specifically used only as an adjunct to orthodontic treatment (Table 31.2) and these are described below.

Surgical procedures

Upper labial fraenectomy

When the lip is pulled upwards, a fibrous band between the inner surface of the upper lip and the crest of the maxillary alveolar ridge can be palpated just underneath the mucosa. An incision is made around the fibrous band and the fraenal attachment on the ridge. The incision is superficial on the lip and fraenum but extends down to bone between the central incisors. The fraenum is grasped with forceps and detached by sharp dissection from the lip. The fibres entering the bone are detached with a small excavator or curette. Some operators mill the crestal bone surface with a bur.

When the fraenum has been removed, further dissection is required to recontour the sulcus. A Z-plasty can be performed but this can cause excessive swelling. It is simpler and kinder to hitch the midline of the incision to the periosteum overlying the anterior nasal spine with a resorbable suture. The fatty tissue on the anterior aspect of the alveolus is mobilised by inserting scissors superficial to the periosteum and opening the blades. This allows the bulky tissue to be displaced laterally so that a good sulcus depth can be achieved when the suture is placed. The incision is then closed with interrupted sutures. A Whitehead's varnish pack may be placed between the incisors and this will also cover the adjacent small defect in the alveolar mucosa, but this is often unnecessary.

Removal of supernumerary teeth

Supernumerary teeth may occur anywhere in the maxillary or mandibular alveolus but it is most common to find one or two in the midline of the anterior maxilla. They are almost always on the palatal aspect. A parallax view should confirm the position, but occasionally a lateral radiograph of the anterior maxilla is helpful.

It is better to wait until there is some root formation in the permanent centrals before surgery than to risk damage to the tooth germ. Bear in mind that many supernumeraries erupt and a surgical approach is then avoided. There is no need to remove those that have no associated pathology and are not in the way of orthodontic tooth movement.

The normal surgical approach is by a palatal flap using a gingival margin incision. The incisive vessels and nerve can usually be preserved. Larger supernumeraries are usually easy to find due to altered bone contour. Small ones can be very difficult to find, especially if the follicle is small or the enamel is hypoplastic. It is a mistake to look too high because the root of an inverted supernumerary is often found between the roots of the centrals, near the amelocemental junction. Bone overlying the buried tooth is removed with a chisel or bur, creating a window large enough for its elevation.

If there is an associated buried incisor, a decision should be made on whether surgical exposure is indicated. It may well be opportune to avoid a further anaesthetic but many orthodontists prefer to wait for eruption, as the gingival contour may be uneven following surgical exposure. Healing after removal of a large supernumerary often produces a barrier of scar tissue, however, and patients may require surgery if the incisor fails to erupt.

Exposure of incisors

Upper permanent centrals are usually on the labial aspect of the alveolus. The object of surgery is to leave a portion of the crown exposed to allow natural eruption or orthodontic traction. Alternatively, if the tooth is high and simple exposure is not possible, an attachment such as a gold chain can be cemented via a surgical approach.

A labial flap with parallel sides is taken. The horizontal arm of the incision must include attached mucosa, as this will be used to form the gingival margin when the flap is repositioned. The flap is carefully dissected away from any bulky follicle or scar tissue. Soft tissue and bone are removed from around the crown. It is sometimes necessary to excise a wedge of palatal mucosa and follicle to ensure that the incisal edge remains exposed. The flap is then repositioned apically and sutured in position. It is important to place the flap high enough to ensure that the tissues do not heal over the tooth. In this situation, the flap can be inverted so that the attached mucosal edge of the flap is brought close to the amelocemental junction of the incisor. A resorbable mattress suture placed high in the vertical incision will usually stabilise the flap. The flap will have less tendency to slide back over the crown if this suture enters and exits on the mucosal surface, as this helps to invert the margin.

When the above technique is not feasible a gold chain may be attached. There are alternatives, such as brackets or wire loops, but these are less effective. Gold chain is used only because stainless steel chain is not readily available. A small circle of stainless steel mesh is welded to one end of the chain to facilitate bonding to the enamel. Corrosion between gold and stainless steel can result in detachment of the chain and so it is better to add a ligature of fine wire around the weld.

Attachment of the chain is easy if the enamel surface is isolated. A section of a surgical rubber glove makes a convenient sterile 'rubber dam'. The enamel is etched in the normal way and the surface is irrigated with sterile water and dried using the surgical suction. The mesh is attached to the tooth using a light-cured orthodontic bonding agent. After testing the bond with a gentle tug, the flap is replaced with the chain emerging in the proposed path of eruption (usually at the crest of the ridge).

With normal healing, orthodontic traction can begin after a couple of weeks. If there is a long delay, scar tissue forms around the chain and makes alignment more difficult. Patients should be warned that traction might take many months.

Exposure of palatal canines

The hard palate is covered by keratinised mucoperiosteum so that it is not necessary to preserve and reposition a flap to achieve a gingival margin.

If the surgeon is confident that the crown of the unerupted tooth lies palatally, an ellipse of overlying mucoperiosteum can be excised. The amount of further tissue to be excised becomes clear as the operation proceeds. Alternatively, a palatal gingival margin flap is raised and an ellipse of tissue is excised after the tooth has been uncovered. Overlying bone is removed with a bur or hand chisel, taking care not to uncover root dentine or damage adjacent teeth. The amount of soft tissue and bone removal should be sufficient to prevent mucosa reforming over the canine. The crown of the tooth should be visible within a saucerised cavity.

There may be brisk haemorrhage from the palatal aspect. Digital pressure or artery forceps will control this during the procedure. A suture should be placed around any identified vessel if bleeding persists at the end. A Whitehead's varnish pack is held in place using non-resorbable sutures. The pack is left in situ for 1–2 weeks, depending on the extent of the surgery. The orthodontist often waits for some eruption before commencing appliance therapy.

An alternative method is to attach a gold chain once the tooth is uncovered and replace the palatal flap without excising the overlying mucoperiosteum. This is technically more challenging due to difficult access and haemorrhage, which makes creating a dry field for attachment of the chain more problematic.

Exposure of buccal canines

It is sometimes difficult to get a good result, particularly if the tooth is high in the buccal sulcus. Ideally, an apically repositioned flap should be carried out, as for buried incisors. Unfortunately, the only attached mucosa may be the gingival margin of the lateral incisor, but this cannot be used as it would leave an unsightly defect. If there is a gap, however, sufficient mucosa may be available on the ridge.

Overlying mucosa in the sulcus may be excised and a pack inserted, but often the tissues close over or the tooth is tethered by unsightly scar tissue. A better option is to take a normal flap and attach a gold chain as described above or simply to close the flap over the surgically exposed crown.

Removal of impacted second premolars

The impacted maxillary premolar is normally palatally placed and may be removed by raising a palatal mucoperiosteal gingival margin flap. Elevation is then often sufficient to remove the tooth but occasionally bone may need to be removed to gain adequate elevation.

Impacted lower premolars are usually lingually inclined and, if sufficiently erupted, can be removed by gentle elevation and forceps. Fine beaked upper forceps are often ideal for this purpose. If a surgical approach is needed, a buccal flap is raised and bone removed to expose the crown buccally and several millimetres of the root. The crown can then be sectioned and delivered lingually and the root subsequently elevated into the space vacated by the crown.

32 Tissue sampling and soft tissue lesions

Introduction

A biopsy is defined as a procedure whereby tissues are sampled from a patient for the purpose of histopathological, microbiological, or other laboratory analysis. Results from such investigations may confirm a provisional diagnosis or establish one. They may also help in the determination of a prognosis, which in turn is defined as a likely outcome of the disease encountered and is based on previous knowledge.

The word biopsy may have unwanted connotations for many patients, who regard this procedure as a test for malignant disease, and it may be better avoided or explained more fully. Any abnormal tissue removed from the mouth should undergo routine analysis, with the possible exception of caries or periodontally infected teeth, where selection of particular cases may at times also be worthwhile. If a surgeon considers that removal of soft tissue is indicated even though the nature of the pathological process is certain, this is best confirmed with appropriate histological examination. Various methods may be used to sample tissue and some representative examples will be discussed (Table 32.1). This will be followed by consideration of individual soft tissue lesions.

Table 32.1 Tissue sampling techniques
Aspiration techniques
blood
pus
cysts
radiolucencies
fine-needle aspiration
Surgical biopsy
excision
incision
punch
frozen sections

Tissue sampling

Aspiration techniques

Aspiration of blood, cavity fluids and solid tissue can all provide diagnostic information, as discussed below.

Blood

A venous blood sample can yield a vast amount of information on disease processes relevant to oral surgical practice. Most common is the full blood count, which indicates total numbers of red cells, white cells and platelets. The differential count of white cells will indicate the numbers of neutrophils, lymphocytes and eosinophils within the white-cell population. The haemoglobin level is also included in this analysis.

Blood serum can also be examined to determine biochemical parameters such as electrolytes, proteins and enzyme levels, which may alter significantly in disease. Within the globulin fraction of the serum, antibody levels may be determined, which may reflect a patient's previous exposure to viral or bacterial infection. Glucose levels, if raised, may raise suspicion of diabetes mellitus and indicate further investigation.

Aspiration from pathological lesions

The most common example of this is the aspiration of an abscess presenting either in the soft tissues of the submandibular or submental regions, or intraorally in the buccal sulcus or palate. The advantage of aspirating a pus sample is that the technique avoids gross contamination of the aspirate by other organisms, especially in the mouth where there is a commensal population. Additionally, by drawing the pus into the partial vacuum of a sterile syringe, the viability of the anaerobic bacteria is protected and they are therefore more likely to grow in the laboratory. Anaerobes are extremely common in dentoalveolar infections and their survival from any sampling procedure is important, allowing a more accurate assessment of the antibiotic sensitivity of the infection.

Cystic lesions are also often easily aspirated to determine both their fluid nature and contents. Keratocysts, which contain keratin and shed epithelial squames, can be differentiated from inflammatory or other odontogenic cysts, which contain a proteinaceous fluid. More sophisticated assessment of the contents of keratocysts and of other cysts involves assessment of soluble protein content (the keratocyst has less than the dental cyst) although, in practice, this is seldom needed (see Ch. 28).

Aspiration of radiolucent areas of the jaw may also indicate that a presumed pathological cyst cavity is not, in fact, cystic. If no fluid is present then the aspiration will yield nothing, which may indicate a need for an incision biopsy of the tissues within the cavity because the implication is that the lesion is solid. Occasionally, in the maxilla, air may be aspirated from a radiolucent image. This might indicate that the maxillary air sinus has been penetrated and incorrectly diagnosed as a pathological cavity. Very occasionally blood may be aspirated from a lesion, which may indicate the presence of an intrabony haemangioma or arteriovenous shunt.

Fine needle aspiration biopsy

This technique, which aspirates cells from solid lesions, can be useful in less accessible swellings or lumps such as in salivary glands or the neck. Cytology is more difficult to interpret than an incisional biopsy but it can be a valuable guide as to the nature of a swelling.

Surgical biopsy

Two types of biopsy can be taken from abnormalities of the soft tissues of the mouth: the excision biopsy and the incision biopsy, using either a scalpel or a punch biopsy.

Excision biopsy

This procedure removes all the clinically abnormal tissue that is evident. It is therefore normally carried out on relatively small swellings or lumps for which the clinician would have normally made a confident provisional diagnosis. Lesions such as papillomas, fibrous hyperplastic overgrowths and mucocoeles are common examples of lesions normally removed in total by this means.

Incision biopsy

A representative piece of tissue is removed from a lesion whose total removal would not be practicable as an outpatient procedure, either because of its size or because its nature is not known and requires to be identified histologically to allow a correct treatment plan to be formulated. Such lesions as widespread erythroplakia or leukoplakia, larger swellings either arising as soft-tissue lumps or within bone are examples of the appropriateness of this technique.

Punch biopsy

This may be a useful way of sampling a lump before deciding on its definitive treatment. The punch is a hollow trephine of 3–4 mm in diameter, which can remove a small 'core' of soft tissue with minimal damage and does not normally require suturing.

Sample disposition

Accurate orientation of the sample may be important when sending the specimen to the histopathology laboratory, especially if the lesion is thought to be neoplastic. Correct disposition into 10% formalin is also needed to preserve the tissues in the best possible condition and undue trauma during the surgery should be avoided for the same reason. All relevant clinical information should be included on the specimen form for the information of the pathologist.

In widespread lesions it may be prudent to take more than one biopsy sample, especially where there is a clinical variation in the appearance in different areas of the abnormal tissue. An example of this would be a white patch but within which there are areas of redness denoting atrophic epithelium or superficial ulceration.

At one time, it was considered necessary to provide an incision biopsy that contained the transitional area between clinically normal and abnormal soft tissue. This is now considered of less importance than providing an untraumatised, representative sample of the lesion itself.

Where there are extensive areas of soft tissue abnormality and there is therefore a choice of site for incision biopsy, certain areas should be avoided. The orifices of the parotid and submandibular ducts may cause fibrosis and contraction if surgically traumatised, and this in turn may lead to obstruction of salivary flow and resultant swelling with or without ascending infection. The tip of the tongue is very sensitive and should, where possible, be avoided, as should areas close to larger blood vessels or nerves such as in the region of the mental foramen or the deep lingual veins on the ventral surface of the tongue.

Almost instant histopathological assessment can be achieved by freezing the specimen rapidly rather than fixing it in formalin. This is known as a frozen section and can provide information to the clinician within minutes. It can be a very appropriate way of ensuring that margins of tumour excision are clear during the operation and can therefore be acted on while the patient is still anaesthetised. However, the clarity of the prepared specimen may not be as good as the paraffin prepared sections. For this reason, frozen sections are not indicated for routine diagnostic biopsies. Immuno-fluorescence cannot be performed on formalin-fixed tissue and so fresh tissue for frozen sections is required for immunopathology using fluorescent techniques.

Soft tissue lesions

Soft tissue lesions that may present on the buccal mucosa or gingivae are listed in Table 32.2. Oral carcinoma is discussed further in Chapter 17 and denture-induced hyperplasia is considered in Chapter 30. Minor salivary gland swellings are considered in Chapters 14 and 34.

Fibrous epulis

An epulis may be defined as a swelling or lump arising from the gingivae, and the fibrous epulis is the most common type. The lesion is basically a hyperplastic response to irritation to the attached gingivae. In some cases, the stimulus or irritant is very obvious, such as an overhanging restoration or subgingival calculus. In others, however, it may be more difficult to detect and only careful examination may reveal a small develop-mental defect in the enamel or dentine of the tooth at the gingival margin. Clinically, they present as smooth-surfaced, rounded swellings, normally pink in colour and often pedunculated in attachment (Fig. 32.1). In older, more mature lesions, the surface may show stippling reflecting the attached gingival origin of the overgrowth. Treatment is by surgical excision, with removal of any irritant focus found. The base of the wound is often dressed with a periodontal pack or if larger with a ribbon gauze impregnated with Whitehead's varnish. This may be sutured over the raw surface.

Table 32.2   Oral soft tissue lesions
Carcinoma
Denture-induced hyperplasia
Fibrous epulis
Fibrous overgrowth
Giant-cell epulis
Haemangioma and lymphangioma
Lipoma
Pregnancy epulis
Pyogenic granuloma
Squamous cell papilloma
Salivary gland lesions

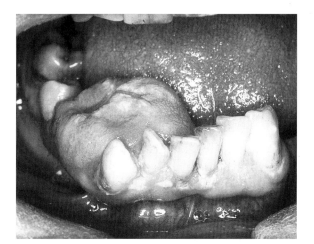

Fig. 32.1   A fibrous epulis.

Fibrous overgrowth

Fibrous overgrowths or fibroepithelial polyps are relatively common in the mouth and are usually the result of trauma or frictional irritation. By contrast, fibromas, which are benign neoplasms, are extremely rare. They are most often seen in the cheeks or lips where such irritation from the dentition can be encountered. Some-times known as polyps, they may be semi-pedunculated or sessile in their attachment and are similar in colour to the surrounding normal tissue unless they have been traumatised frictionally, when they may show a whitened keratinised surface. They do not, however, have the cauli-flower hyperkeratotic surface of the papilloma, being smooth-surfaced and hence easily distinguished from the papilloma (Fig. 32.2). Treatment is simple surgical excision. As, histologically, they are simple hyperplasias, there is no requirement to remove a margin of normal tissue nor to extend the excision deeply into the under-

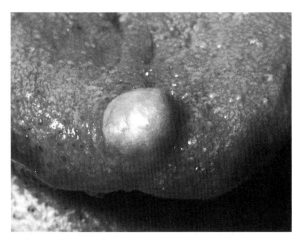

Fig. 32.2 A fibroepithelial polyp of dorsum of tongue.

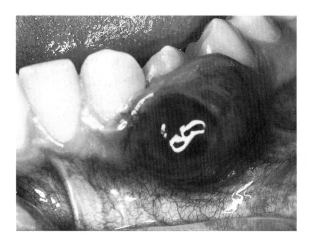

Fig. 32.3 A giant cell epulis.

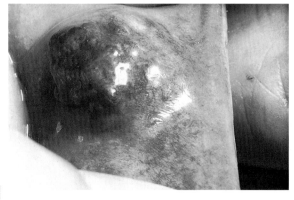

Fig. 32.4 A haemangioma of cheek.

lying tissues. A suture may be needed to ensure adequate haemostasis in the larger lesions.

Giant cell epulis

This epulis is sometimes known as a peripheral giant-cell granuloma and, as its name implies, the tissue consists of a mass of multinucleated giant cells in a vascular stroma. Many are seen in teenagers or adolescents and are usually found in the anterior regions of the mouth. They may represent an overgrowth of osteoclasts derived from the resorptive process encountered during the loss of the deciduous dentition. They can, however, arise in the older patient. These lesions are typically deep red or even purplish in colour and are often quite broadly based, unlike the paler coloured, often pedunculated fibrous epulis (Fig. 32.3). If suspected of being a giant-cell lesion, radiographs should be taken to ensure that it is a peripheral and not a centrally, i.e. bony, originating lesion, which would appear as a radiolucent area (see Ch. 36). If it is a peripheral epulis then surgical excision with curettage or cautery to its base is normally curative. The base of the lesion can be covered by a periodontal pack if small, or a Whitehead's varnish packing may be used for larger lesions. If a central giant-cell lesion is evident on the radiograph, it must be distinguished from the brown tumour of hyperparathyroidism by appropriate assessment of blood calcium, phosphate and para-thormone levels (see Ch. 36).

Haemangioma and lymphangioma

These lesions, which may appear in any of the soft tissues of the mouth, are regarded as hamartomata. They are developmental overgrowths of either blood vessels or lymphatic vessels. In some patients they may achieve a considerable size, particularly in the tongue. Typically, however, the haemangioma will appear as an exophytic multilobular swelling, deep blue in colour, and often likened to a small bunch of grapes (Fig. 32.4). Gentle finger pressure on the surface of the haemangioma empties the blood-filled vessels leaving the swelling flat and pale in colour. If the malformation is likely to be, or has been, traumatised repeatedly, it may either be removed surgically or treated by cryotherapy. This latter method may be very successful but, as no pathological confirmation of the diagnosis is possible, the clinician must be quite sure of the diagnosis before treatment is carried out in this way (see Ch. 38). Provided they are symptom free and not subject to direct trauma, some are simply kept under observation.

Lipoma

This is a benign neoplasm of fat; true intraoral lipomas are quite rare. They may present with a soft swelling, which is often pale or yellow in colour, and they are normally sessile. These lesions may, on occasion, grow into muscle layers and be quite difficult to dissect out surgically. The treatment, however, is normally that of excision.

Pregnancy epulis

This lesion is histologically indistinguishable from the pyogenic granuloma, being essentially a vascular over-growth of granulation tissue. It may be related to an obvious focus such as calculus but it may equally arise from an extraction socket. Hormonal changes during pregnancy are believed to enhance the reactive tissue response to irritation and although many lesions remain small and do not require surgical intervention, some can grow alarmingly fast and attain considerable size even to the point of being traumatised by the opposing teeth. These lesions are therefore surgically excised with appropriate curettage or diathermy to their bases. If small they tend to resolve following the pregnancy.

Pyogenic granuloma

The pyogenic granuloma is a lesion that arises from a failure of normal healing causing an exuberant over-growth of what is essentially granulation tissue. They may grow in relation to extraction sockets or from traumatic injuries to soft tissues, most often tongue or palate. They can be regarded as reactive lesions and obvious irritational factors may be evident clinically or from the patient's history. Foreign bodies related to extraction sockets, such as fragments of filling material or indeed of small bony sequestra, may form the stimulus, whereas in soft tissues there is occasionally a history of self-medication with a variety of remedies that could be attributed as causal. Clinically they appear as red or speckled-red overgrowths of tissue that closely resemble granulation tissue on visual examination (Fig. 32.5). Treatment is surgical excision with curettage or diathermy to the base of the lesions where appropriate.

Squamous cell papilloma

This is not an uncommon lesion of the oral mucosa and may arise at virtually any site, but more commonly on palate, buccal mucosa or lips. It is a benign neoplasm of epithelial tissue and most squamous cell papillomata present as pedunculated (stalked attachment) lesions with characteristic white, hyperkeratinised, crenated surfaces, which can be likened to a cauliflower (Fig. 32.6). They are normally small, usually less than 0.5 cm in diameter. Treatment is simply excision at the base of the stalk

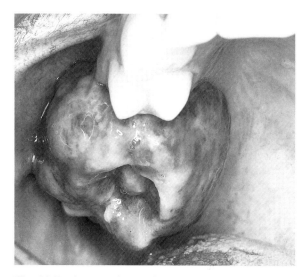

Fig. 32.5 A pyogenic granuloma.

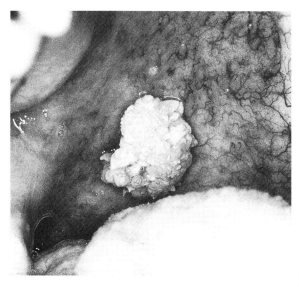

Fig. 32.6 A squamous cell papilloma of the soft palate.

attachment. A very similar lesion may be attributed to a viral origin and is sometimes known as a viral wart. In these cases it is sometimes possible to see finger warts that have clearly been responsible for transmitting the virus to the oral cavity. These can also be treated effectively with cryotherapy (see Ch. 38).

33 Pyogenic dental infection and its spread

Introduction

Dental disease, both caries and periodontal disease, is an infective process occurring in a bacterial oral environment. It is therefore not surprising that pyogenic dental infections are common. The most common causes of pus-producing infection in the mouth are listed in Table 33.1.

A dental abscess, otherwise known as an apical abscess or periapical abscess, arises from an infected pulp, which is most commonly the result of caries but may also be due to trauma, either physical or chemical. A periodontal abscess arises from a periodontal pocket and may involve the bifurcation or trifurcation of molar teeth. Pericoronitis results from infection involving the follicle and overlying gingivae (operculum) of a partially erupted and usually impacted tooth. This infection was discussed in Chapter 27. Salivary gland infection is usually the result of obstruction to a major salivary gland, most commonly the submandibular gland. The infection is said to be 'ascending' from the oral cavity along the duct. Management was discussed in Chapter 14.

Dental abscess

The dental abscess accounts for the majority of pyogenic infections in the mouth. Acute infection may arise directly from spread of acute pulpal infection or it may represent re-ignition of an existing chronic abscess or granuloma

by more virulent bacterial contamination or through a lowering of the patient's natural resistance as, for example, after influenza. Dental abscesses are normally polymicrobial. This means that there are several organisms present and anaerobic bacteria predominate.

Clinical features

Pain

The dominant symptom is pain, which can be described variously as throbbing, unremitting or unresponsive to simple over-the-counter analgesics. Unlike pulpal-derived pain, thermal irritation tends not to be a feature. Severity is usually sufficient to cause sleep loss. In function, the pain is made worse as the abscess will be under considerable pressure because of the acute inflammatory reaction. Interestingly, the pain may be slightly reduced by gentle occlusal pressure from the opposing tooth and this may be due to pressure increasing to the point that nerve endings become non-functional. When the abscess has achieved sufficient size, it breaks out of the bone into the soft tissues and at this point the pain reduces dramatically as the pressure eases.

As the soft tissue reacts to the infection, acute inflammation within these tissues will eventually again cause pain as swelling in the soft tissues increases and pressure even in the more lax soft tissue spaces rises. This may take up to 2–3 days to occur.

Swelling

Early abscesses are confined within the unyielding alveolar bone and at this stage no swelling is evident. It is only when the abscess bursts through alveolar bone that swelling may become apparent, together with redness and surface tenderness. The site of the swelling varies and may be intraoral and/or extraoral. The sulcus

Table 33.1   Common pus-producing oral infections
Dental abscess
Periodontal abscess
Pericoronitis
Salivary gland infection

263

on the labial or buccal aspect of the tooth is the most common intraoral site of swelling because the apices of most teeth are closer to the buccal plate surface. The minority of upper lateral incisors have apices closer to the palatal bone surface and can therefore present as palatal swellings. In later presentations, the sulcus swelling may become soft and fluctuant, or even have discharging pus through a sinus, and this heralds reduction in both swelling and pain.

Spread of infection

When dental abscesses escape the confines of alveolar bone, the infection passes into soft tissues and in turn provokes in these tissues an acute inflammatory reaction and eventually pus formation. Where this happens depends largely on the anatomy of the region in which the apex or apices lie. The length of the root is therefore relevant, and how it relates in certain cases to muscle attachments. In acute abscesses of deciduous teeth, therefore, the short roots often dictate that the infection passes not into the facial structures but intraorally, forming a so-called 'gumboil'. Where spread of infection causes facial or cervical swelling it is often characteristic of the quadrant of the mouth involved, and these will be considered in turn.

Maxilla

Anteriorly from incisor to canine, the patient may show upper lip swelling, obliteration of the nasolabial fold and puffiness of the lower eyelid. In extreme cases, the eye may be almost totally closed with oedematous swelling (Fig. 33.1).

Posteriorly, the swelling will be evident in the upper part of the cheek, with swelling around the eye occasionally but will not distend the nasolabial fold or cause significant lip swelling (Fig. 33.1). Spread upward from molar or premolar infection seldom passes into the maxillary air sinus. The buccinator muscle attachments in the molar region may determine whether the infection passes above it into the cheek or below into the sulcus, although both are frequently present, as this muscle will form only a partial barrier.

Mandible

Spread from incisors or canine teeth may cause mental or submental swelling (Fig. 33.2). Lower canine infections

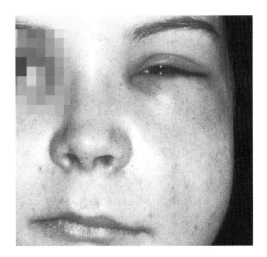

Fig. 33.1 Facial swelling and closure of the eye due to infection spreading from an upper incisor.

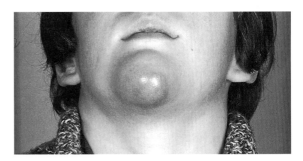

Fig. 33.2 Mental abscess arising from infection associated with a lower incisor.

do sometimes pass into the floor of mouth, resulting in swelling here in addition to the swelling of the chin.

Posterior teeth infections may pass either buccally or lingually through the bone, and the attachments of buccinator laterally and mylohyoid lingually will have a bearing on the direction of spread. If buccal spread occurs above buccinator, the swelling will largely be seen in the sulcus but, if below, it will cause swelling on the lateral aspect of the jaw externally, which may gravitate downwards into the upper part of the neck. Occasionally, infection may spread deep to the masseter muscle. This usually arises from a pericoronal infection around a wisdom tooth, as described in Chapter 27. If the infection passes lingually, the swelling will be in the submandibular space if below the mylohyoid or in the floor of mouth if above this muscle. Although the muscles direct the route of spread into the various tissue compartments, it is important to be aware that both intraoral and extraoral spread can occur from any tooth. It is therefore not unusual to see swelling in both the sublingual and sub-mandibular space from a lower molar tooth or, for that matter, both sulcus swelling and facial swelling from an upper tooth.

When infection spreads into whichever of the soft tissue spaces, the initial reaction of these tissues will be an acute inflammatory reaction. The fluid exudate of this reaction causes the early swelling, which is therefore mainly oedematous, and this phase can be known as a cellulitis complicating the original bony abscess. As the soft tissues continue to react to the infection, pus will be formed, which may collect within the compartment, giving rise to, for example, a submandibular or a sub-mental abscess (Fig. 33.3). A well-recognised compli-cation of lower jaw dental infection is the rapid spread of submandibular and sublingual infection across the midline of the neck. This is a life-threatening situation known as Ludwig's angina and requires immediate hospital admission for appropriate drainage and intensive antimicrobial therapy.

Pus within the soft tissues of the upper part of the face seldom presents as a facial external abscess but usually collects within the upper buccal sulcus.

Management

Management of the acute dental abscess is shown in Table 33.2.

Drainage

Provision of drainage remains the most important measure where pus has formed.

Extraction

Extraction of the tooth is usually carried out if it is unconservable or if the acuteness of the condition warrants it. This provides excellent drainage, especially in upper teeth. If the abscess is still confined to the alveolar bone, or even where spread to soft tissues is in its early oedematous phase, extraction is often sufficient to allow resolution. There is no justification whatsoever in delaying the extraction on account of swelling because this is one of the best ways of achieving good drainage, and thereby speeding resolution.

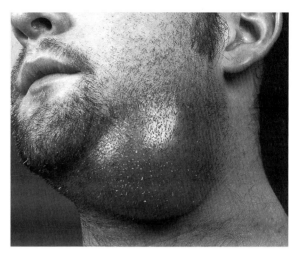

Fig. 33.3 A submandibular abscess.

Table 33.2   Management of an acute dental abscess
Drainage
tooth
extraction
root canal drainage
incision
intraoral
extraoral
Removal of source of infection
endodontic treatment
extraction
periradicular surgery
Supportive antibiotic therapy
severe spreading infection
systemic toxicity
medically compromised

Root canal drainage

Opening of the root canal can, in the early intrabony abscess, be sufficient in itself. When opened and pus is obtained, it is prudent not to close the canal immediately but allow sufficient time for adequate drainage to occur. This may take only 12–24 h but gross contamination and even caries within the root canal can occur if the tooth is left open for too long.

Incision of intraoral abscesses

The presence of pus is usually detected by a palpable 'bounce' in the swelling within the buccal sulcus. Local

265

anaesthesia within the outer wall only of the abscess is normally sufficient to allow incision with a pointed scalpel blade (number 11), which should be used with a stab action and a cut of suitable size made on withdrawal. If the pus is deeper, fine artery forceps may be introduced to explore the abscess and gently open it to encourage free flow of pus. This may require more extensive local anaesthesia. Palatal abscesses may require excision of a small ellipse of soft tissue or insertion of a small drain after incision as this mucoperiosteum tends to rebound and seal following the release of pus, thus preventing further free drainage.

Incision of extraoral abscesses

This is usually carried out by a specialist surgeon and, unless the abscess is very superficial, under general anaesthetic. Provision of a general anaesthetic for some of these patients is a skilled procedure when trismus is a marked feature and laryngeal oedema masks the normal anatomy (see Ch. 10).

The presence of pus is confirmed clinically by eliciting fluctuation on careful palpation of the swelling. Finger pressure of one hand on one side of the swelling causes fluid movement to be detected by the pulps of the fingers of the other hand. This can be difficult to determine, especially in deeper lying pus collections. Generally, the abscesses requiring such treatment will be submental or submandibular.

The key points of treatment are that the skin overlying the abscess should be prepared with surface antiseptic and isolated with sterile drapes. A wide-lumen needle should be introduced into the abscess cavity to obtain an uncontaminated sample, and it may also help to 'find' the pus. An incision is made below the maximum convexity of the swelling, parallel to the lower border of the mandible, if possible using a skin crease line to minimise later scar visibility (see Ch. 15). The incision should be through skin only and normally an incision of about 2 cm is sufficient. Blunt dissection is then carried out with blunt scissors or Hilton-type forceps into the cavity, which should be explored thoroughly with the blunt instrument or a finger. A drain is then inserted into the abscess and sutured to the skin surface. A dry sterile dressing is finally taped over the drain. This allows frequent assessment of the continuing discharge. The drain is removed after the dressings are seen to contain no further pus.

Removal of source of infection

This will be accomplished immediately if the tooth is extracted in the process of gaining drainage but may be a later procedure in the form of either endodontic treatment or periradicular surgery.

Supportive antibiotic therapy

The decision to prescribe antibiotics for acute abscesses will depend upon a number of factors and is not invariable. Extraction of a maxillary tooth or incision of a well-localised sulcus abscess may well be sufficient to allow resolution of the acute infection without antibiotic supplemental treatment. Clinical experience is invaluable but some features may well influence the decision to prescribe an antibiotic (Table 33.3).

The swelling may encroach on the airway as, for example, in a submandibular or sublingual infection. Difficulty in swallowing normally implies that the tongue, floor of mouth or parapharyngeal spaces are affected. If incision and drainage have yielded poor quantities of pus, this suggests that management may be inadequate without antibiotics. Regional nodes are often late to react to acute dental infection or are masked by the swelling. If present, this is good evidence of spreading infection, which would require supplemental antibiotic treatment. If the patient is medically compromised, and particularly if the immune system is compromised, patients may not have the capability to respond adequately to this type of infection. Patients with conditions such as diabetes mellitus, HIV infection, or who are receiving treatment with corticosteroids or cytotoxic drugs, can be included in this group. Where infection is evident in the floor of the mouth, there appears to be an increased likelihood of rapid spread. The patient may feel unwell, with an elevated temperature and a tachycardia, signifying systemic toxicity. Most severe infections will cause a

---

Table 33.3   Factors influencing antibiotic therapy in the management of acute dental abscess

Airway
Dysphagia
Lack of drainage
Medically compromised
Site of spread
Systemic toxicity
Trismus

degree of trismus by simply stretching the soft tissues, but profound trismus often implies infection affecting muscles either directly or indirectly involved in jaw movement.

The choice of antibiotic is initially empirical, as the results of antibiotic sensitivity testing will not be available. The penicillin group is often chosen in non-allergic patients, with the wider-spectrum amoxicillin being a common choice. Metronidazole is becoming more popular as a first choice antimicrobial because anaerobes are the predominant pathogens. Cephalosporins, erythromycin and, where antibiotic sensitivity indicates, clindamycin are all possible useful agents. In severe acute infections, it is sometimes considered necessary to prescribe two or more antibiotics. Metronidazole and amoxicllin have proved to be a popular choice where two antibiotics are deemed necessary.

Finally, management of the acute abscess requires meticulous follow-up to ensure that the treatment is having the desired effect. In the early stages, this may be as an outpatient and require daily assessment until it is evident that resolution is being achieved. If the dentist, from the initial presentation, feels that the infection is very severe, early referral to a specialist is appropriate, because a number of patients will require admission to hospital for appropriate drainage and perhaps intravenous antibiotic therapy.

Complications

A number of complications may arise from a dental abscess as listed in Table 33.4.

Cavernous sinus thrombosis

Spread of infection through emissary veins from the periorbital region and upper face can, in theory, cause thrombus formation within the cavernous sinus. With modern antibiotics, this complication is seldom seen nowadays.

Table 33.4	Complications of dental abscess
Cavernous sinus thrombosis	
Ludwig's angina	
Necrotising fasciitis	
Orofacial sinus	
Osteomyelitis	
Septicaemia	

Ludwig's angina

This severe complication has been described above and requires immediate admission to hospital for drainage and appropriate intravenous antibiotic therapy.

Necrotising fasciitis

This combination of virulent pathogens can cause massive soft tissue necrosis with formation of multiple sinuses. It can arise from a dental infection.

Orofacial sinus

This complication arises when the pus has discharged onto the face or neck, either through lack of treatment or inadequate treatment (Fig. 33.4). If the condition remains untreated it can cause disfiguring soft tissue fibrosis around the intermittently discharging sinus. Epithelium from the skin can grow into the sinus, complicating the treatment in that surgical revision of the opening may be necessary. The dental source must be removed as soon as possible.

Osteomyelitis

This is very rare and may be an indication of an immuno-compromised state or previous irradiation of the jaw, which has reduced the blood supply to the bone (see Ch. 36).

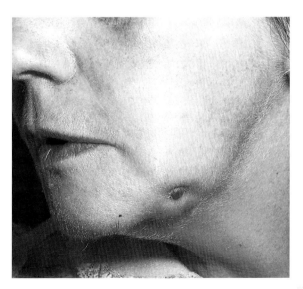

Fig. 33.4 An orofacial sinus arising from a lower premolar abscess.

Septicaemia

This is discussed in Chapter 8.

Periodontal abscess

This arises from a periodontal lesion and the clinical features are therefore different from the apical lesion.

Clinical features

Pain and swelling

The swelling in this type of abscess being further coronal than the apical abscess normally discharges eventually through a periodontal pocket or through a sinus in the alveolar process. Spread to soft tissues is therefore relatively rare but can involve particularly the floor of mouth.

Mobility of the affected tooth

This feature may not be particularly helpful in diagnosis if other teeth also have mobility reflecting a generalised periodontal loss of bone. The tooth in question, however, will be uncomfortable on testing its firmness.

Vitality

The tooth in question will normally be vital to pulp testing.

Management

Extraction is often the logical treatment. This provides good drainage and also removes the source of infection. Occasionally, if the abscess involves a strategically important tooth and the patient's general periodontal condition is considered capable of control, then curettage and root planing may be appropriate.

Less common pyogenic oral infections

Less common infections that produce pus are cervico-facial actinomycosis and submandibular staphylococcal lymphadenitis of childhood. Although these infections are rare, they are important to recognise and manage successfully. Both are somewhat unusual in that they are due to one organism rather than the polymicrobial nature of most pyogenic oral infections.

Cervicofacial actinomycosis

Different species of actinomyces microorganisms can be found in mixed dental abscesses related to infected teeth, and do not require particular management other than appropriate drainage with additional antibiotic therapy if considered necessary. Cervicofacial actinomycosis is a distinct clinical entity and arises subsequent to either mandibular extractions or jaw fracture.

Aetiology

The infecting organism is the strictly anaerobic *Actinomyces israelii*. This microorganism is found in dental plaque and appears to gain access to the soft tissues through an extraction socket or fracture through the tooth-bearing area of the mandible.

Clinical features

Most commonly, a swelling forms either at the lower border of the mandible or in the neck. It classically presents a week or so (and up to 6 weeks) after the wound in the mouth, which will normally appear to have healed well. Severe pain is not a feature and, if not treated, the infection may develop with several swellings and skin sinus formation. The related skin is said to have a dusky, bluish tinge. Tissue planes are not followed and the tissues respond by forming a granulomatous reaction around the infected area. If a sinus is active, closer examination of the pus may reveal small, yellow, seed-like granules in the discharge. These are known as sulphur granules.

Diagnosis

Microscopic analysis of a granule by crushing it between glass slides and Gram staining shows typical Gram-positive branching mycelia with related pus cells. Anaerobic culture will later reveal the typical 'molar tooth' colonies of *Actinomyces israelii* on blood agar. Occasionally, another small Gram-negative bacillus may be found: *Actinobacillus actinomycetemcomitans*.

Management

Where pus is formed, incision and drainage should be carried out. Antibiotics should be prescribed for 6 weeks because they take a considerable time to penetrate the granulomatous fibrous tissue reaction in the soft tissues. Shorter courses may result in a recurrence of the infection and it is therefore important to stress to the patient the importance of continuing the antibiotic for the full prescribed period. *Actinomyces israelii* is sensitive to most commonly used antibiotics and, being a narrow-spectrum antibiotic, penicillin is a sensible choice. If cervicofacial actinomycosis presents late or is treated inadequately, it can gravitate from the neck into the mediastinum, and this is clearly a serious complication. Less serious but disfiguring is the scarring that results from the fibrotic reaction in the neck.

Acute submandibular staphylococcal lymphadenitis

This acute infection occurs in children between the ages of 2 and 12.

Aetiology

The cause of the infection is *Staphylococcus aureus*, which probably arises from the nasal passages or from infection of the skin hair follicles and which passes down the lymphatics to settle in submandibular lymph node. The child may not have been previously exposed to a staphylococcal infection and, the immune reaction being insufficient to deal with this challenge, the node is overwhelmed and becomes an abscess itself.

Clinical features

This is similar to any acute inflammatory swelling at the lower border of the mandible. There may be surface reddening and it will be tender to palpation; the temperature may be elevated. Dental examination shows no carious focus and this generally will raise suspicions of a staphylococcal infection. There may be evidence of infection of a hair follicle on the face on that side or a history of recent nasal congestion such as a head cold.

Management

If there is evidence of accumulation of pus, such as fluctuation, then incision and drainage is necessary. Aspiration prior to the incision, will allow an accurate microbiological analysis. If no pus is formed, then a beta-lactamase-resistant form of penicillin, such as flucloxacillin or erythromycin, may be effective in allowing resolution.

34 Salivary gland diseases

Introduction

Surgery of the major salivary glands has already been discussed in Ch. 14, but there are some conditions that are treated by minor surgery within the oral cavity. These procedures are mainly related to pathology of the minor glands but, where the major gland ducts are involved, it is often possible to treat the condition by less radical surgery intraorally.

When the major gland ducts are involved, it is often possible to treat obstructive sialadenitis intraorally. Obstruction of the minor salivary gland ducts can also be managed by minor surgery and these conditions are considered here, after a review of their applied anatomy.

Applied anatomy

An awareness of the location of the minor glands and the anatomical course of the ducts of the major glands is needed and these will be considered in turn. The gross anatomy of the major glands has been discussed in Chapter 14.

Parotid duct – (Stenson's duct)

This duct is approximately 6 cm in length and is formed within the anterior part of the gland by the joining of two main branches. After emerging from the gland it runs horizontally forwards over the surface of the masseter muscle to the anterior border of that muscle and then turns inwards, passing through the buccinator and buccal pad of fat, before ending in a slightly raised papilla adjacent to the upper first or second molar tooth on the buccal mucosa. The accessory parotid gland lies closely related to its initial third and the buccal branches of the facial nerve may be in close relationship to it.

Submandibular duct (Wharton's duct)

This duct is between 5 and 6 cm in length. It originates from the deep surface of the gland just behind the posterior limit of the mylohyoid muscle. It runs upwards and forwards between mylohyoid and hyoglossus, and then between the sublingual gland and the genioglossus muscle, before ending on the sublingual papilla beside the fraenulum of the tongue and just behind the lower incisor teeth. Its important relation is the lingual nerve, which crosses its lateral surface on its earlier course before running upward on its medial side where the nerve is already beginning to divide into its smaller terminal branches. As the duct runs forwards, it becomes progressively more superficial.

Sublingual ducts

The sublingual gland lies fairly superficially beneath the mucosa of the floor of the mouth, which it raises to form the sublingual fold. It has many ducts (around 12), some of which run directly up to open onto the floor of mouth, whereas others may join the submandibular duct.

Minor salivary glands

Around the mouth are aggregates of minor salivary glands, which are mucus secretors. They lie superficially in the submucosal regions and are most easily felt by passing the tongue along the inner aspect of the lower lip, where they are felt as a multitude of small lobules. They are most numerous in the lower lip but are plentiful in the upper lip, buccal mucosa and floor of mouth. In lesser numbers, however, they may also be found in the palate, the posterior aspect of both the hard palate and soft palate, and also on the ventral surface of the tongue. They open onto the surface of the mucous membrane by tiny ducts and their secretion is an important contribution to the lubrication of the soft tissues.

Obstructive sialadenitis

Obstructive sialadenitis in a major gland is due either to a stone or, less commonly, stenosis of the duct. Minor gland obstruction gives rise to a mucocoele.

Major gland obstruction

Aetiology

Obstruction to the free passage of saliva from a major gland can clearly cause problems to a patient. The most common cause of this is blockage of the duct by a stone that is sometimes known as a sialolith. This is relatively uncommon in the parotid gland and is more frequently seen close to the orifice of the duct. In the submandibular gland, the stone may form either within the duct or the gland itself, but duct stones are more common. A certain number of obstructions within the duct are poorly calcified, if at all, and are referred to as mucous plugs.

Other less common causes of obstruction are stenosis (probably a developmental occurrence) and pressure effects from space-occupying lesions, such as malignant disease, arising either from the epithelium of the floor of mouth or within the gland itself. In the parotid gland, there may be another cause related to the trapping of the duct as it pierces the buccinator muscle, and this has been described as more often occurring in children or adolescents.

Submandibular duct stones are relatively common and their presentation may vary from patient to patient.

Clinical features

Characteristically, the stone may become apparent by swelling and discomfort in the submandibular gland region. The swelling is palpable at the lower border of mandible in the submandibular triangle. It is often made worse at meal-times and, typically, pain may last for a couple of hours. Although this can occur at each meal-time for several days, it often settles and the patient may report being quite symptom free for weeks or months. It is not unknown for large stones occupying most of the floor of mouth to present with no history whatsoever of discomfort or swelling in the gland.

More dramatically, however, infection may supervene because the duct is not being 'washed out' with saliva. Bacteria from the mouth may pass along the duct and gain access to the gland around the obstruction. This is known as ascending infection and it can give rise to acute sialadenitis of the submandibular gland. When this occurs, the patient experiences severe pain and swelling of the gland, which becomes extremely tender with dysphagia and, often, high temperature. Pain is made worse on attempting to eat or drink and the patient may complain of a bad taste in the mouth. Intraorally, the floor of mouth may be severely swollen with a raised, red, wheal-like line along the length of the duct. Small amounts of pus may be expressed from the orifice of the duct on occasion.

Diagnosis

This is made fairly straightforward with a clear history but clinical examination by visual inspection of the floor of the mouth may show a yellowish coloured, rounded or fusiform-shaped lump of varying size along the line of the duct. This is more often seen when the stone is close to the orifice of the duct or is fairly large. If it cannot be seen, bimanual palpation of the floor of the mouth with the 'outside' hand pushing the floor of the mouth upwards while the line of the duct is palpated with the index finger of the 'inside hand' may reveal a hard lump. Saliva from the orifice of the duct may be absent, sparse, or slightly turbid in appearance.

Radiographs are usually confirmatory with a lateral view (lateral oblique jaw or orthopantomograph) and occlusal view, the latter being most useful (see Fig. 14.4). If no stone is noted on the radiograph, it may indicate that the obstruction is not calcified. In these circumstances, a sialogram – where a radio-opaque dye is passed along the duct prior to the radiograph being exposed – may reveal this type of obstruction and also strictures within the duct (see Fig. 14.5).

In the acute presentations, the clinical features are fairly conclusive but radiographs should be taken to allow accurate location of the stone.

Management

Acute sialadenitis should be treated vigorously with aspiration, incision and intraoral drainage if possible, and antibiotics. Amoxicillin is commonly prescribed with a high initial dosage, and this can usually be administered orally. Clindamycin may be appropriate in cases unresponsive to more commonly described antibiotics, as it is secreted through the salivary glands and perhaps has a more direct effect.

Removal of the stone may often be done on an outpatient basis with local anaesthesia. However some patients have great difficulty in relaxing their tongue sufficiently to allow the surgery, particularly if the stone is further back in the mouth. Large stones are normally easy to treat but some small stones can be very difficult technically. The nearer to the duct orifice the stone lies, the less difficult it will prove to remove. Anaesthesia is best carried out with a lingual nerve block, as infiltration can often distort the surgical site and with small stones may obscure them from easy vision and palpation.

The technique involves passing a suture behind the obstruction underneath the duct and tightening this sufficiently to prevent the stone being pushed inadvertently backwards during the procedure. There is often dilatation of the duct up to the point of the obstruction and this displacement therefore is a real possibility, with the added complication that it may pass from the duct into the gland itself.

An incision is then made over the stone parallel to the duct and slightly lateral to it. A blunt dissection is then carried out to expose the duct. An incision is made in the duct over the stone, which is removed. There is often a release of pus and saliva at this point. The wound should not be sutured. It is accepted that the saliva may not 'use' the duct but may form a false opening through the wound. Suturing may additionally cause excessive fibrosis on healing, which may itself cause obstruction. Patients should be encouraged to rinse copiously postoperatively and a free flow of saliva should be encouraged with citrus drinks.

Mucocoeles

Mucocoeles are the most common cause of minor salivary gland problems. Neoplasms arising from minor salivary glands are relatively uncommon but both benign and malignant varieties can be found. They can occur at any site where minor glands are found but the most common intraoral location is at the junction of the hard and soft palates. Swellings in the upper lip are usually neoplastic rather than mucocoeles, which are rare in the upper lip.

Aetiology

Mucocoeles are caused either by damage to the minor duct leading to leakage of saliva into the submucosal layer (mucous extravasation cyst) or by blockage of the duct, normally by a mucus plug (mucus retention cyst). By far the more common is the extravasation cyst.

On occasion, small stones can cause obstruction to minor salivary glands. This is more commonly seen on the upper lip or buccal mucosa and secondary infection of the gland can occur, causing a localised raised tender swelling. On the top of this dome-shaped swelling it may be possible to see or feel the small stone. Treatment is simply surgical excision of the lesion.

Clinical appearance

Clinically, mucocoeles present as soft, bluish, fluid-filled swellings that often burst or leak, only to reform, and patients normally are little inconvenienced by them. The most common site is the lower lip (Fig. 34.1), probably reflecting its greater tendency to trauma and ductal damage, but the floor of mouth is also quite a common site.

In the floor of mouth, they may be related to the sublingual gland and can rapidly assume quite a large size. The ballooning lesion in the floor of the mouth may be described as a ranula (frog's belly) and may be a nuisance to the patient, although they frequently rupture.

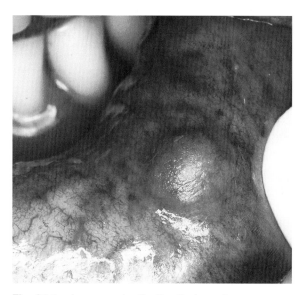

Fig. 34.1 A mucocoele affecting the lower lip.

More precisely, however, a ranula merely implies a sublingual swelling regardless of aetiology.

Diagnosis

The diagnosis is very straightforward, as the history is usually typical. Occasionally, mucocoeles resemble minor salivary gland tumours, especially if they have become fibrosed and more walled off. Their bluish colour can make them similar to a superficial haemangioma but they tend not to deflate on sustained digital pressure, as would most haemangiomas.

Management

The majority of mucocoeles are surgically excised but some in the floor of mouth may be marsupialised.

Excision is carried out under local anaesthesia. An incision over the swelling must be executed with care or the lesion will burst and the subsequent removal may be more complicated. Extravasation cysts do not have epithelial lining and, if the cyst is ruptured, it may be difficult to visualise. A blunt dissection around the cyst frees it very simply if it remains intact and minor glands at its base are usually also removed. One or two sutures may be needed to close the wound.

Marsupialisation of a larger floor of mouth mucocoele is preferable to dissecting the lesion out and removing it. This may be done by passing a suture through the lesion to lift it. A small incision can then be made over the maximum convexity and the contents aspirated. Sterile ribbon gauze is then packed into the now empty cavity through the small incision to 'reconstitute' the swelling, and the mucosal roof can then be removed with scalpel or scissors. The opening into the cavity must be kept patent by suturing its margins to the oral mucosa, or the pack may be soaked in Whitehead's varnish and sutured to the side walls. The aim, whichever technique is used, is to prevent the opening sealing up and closing. Despite this, some do recur as the floor of mouth wound does close over rapidly. If floor of mouth mucocoeles do repeatedly recur, it may be necessary to remove the sublingual gland. (see Ch. 14).

Minor salivary gland biopsy

In Sjögren's syndrome, it has become established that the lymphocytic aggregates around minor glands are a direct reflection of the pathology in the major glands that causes the reduction in saliva production. Histological examination of minor salivary glands therefore avoids the more invasive major gland biopsy. An incision is made in the mucosa of the lower lip – along the lines of the mental nerve branches rather than across them, to minimise nerve damage. The minor mucous glands will extrude through the open wound and can be excised before wound closure (Fig. 34.2).

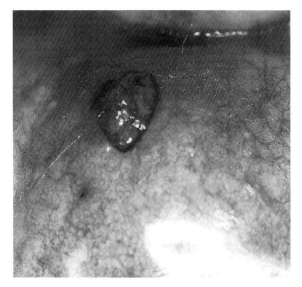

Fig. 34.2 An incision in the lower labial mucosa showing the minor salivary glands protruding through the wound.

35

Oral surgery in the medically compromised patient

Introduction

Patients who require an oral surgical procedure will have their medical status questioned as a matter of routine during the history taking. Certain conditions have a direct bearing on the management and treatment of these patients, which may have to be altered or modified as a result. Thus the treatment plan may have to be modified for the patient's safety.

Most medical conditions do not interfere with minor oral surgical procedures carried out under local anaesthetic. The major problems are with patients who have bleeding tendencies, allergies, are on corticosteroids or have cardiac disease.

Those requiring general anaesthetic will be treated in the secondary care system under the supervision of a consultant anaesthetist.

Not only can systemic disease influence the oral management of a patient, but systemic disease may arise from the mouth, usually as a result of infection. An example of this is infective endocarditis arising in a patient with valvular or other cardiac disease; immunocompromised patients, such as those taking cytotoxic chemotherapy, are also at special risk of infection. Moreover, a number of acute medical emergencies may arise while oral surgical procedures are being carried out and the surgeon must have the necessary agents available for the appropriate management of the patient. The main systemic diseases that impact on the practice of oral surgery are listed in Table 35.1, and these will be discussed in turn.

Blood disorders

Haematological disease, particularly anaemia, is not uncommon. Except in severe cases and those requiring general anaesthesia, anaemia is not a significant problem

Table 35.1 Systemic disease and oral surgery
Blood disorders: haemorrhagic disease
Cardiovascular disease
Endocrine disease
Liver disease
Neurological disease
Pregnancy
Radiotherapy
Renal disease
Respiratory disease

because blood loss during minor oral surgical procedures should be controlled and not excessive.

A number of bleeding disorders can occur (see the discussion in Ch. 6) and the specific management of postextraction haemorrhage is considered in detail in Chapter 26. In addition, it should be noted that aspirin is being taken by an increasing number of patients for prophylaxis against thrombotic disease such as coronary artery disease or cerebrovascular thrombotic incidence. Normally, a dose of 75 mg daily is prescribed, which has the desired effect of reducing platelet adhesiveness. In theory, this should also cause more bleeding after oral surgery, but in practice it seldom seems to have a significant effect. Occasionally, continued oozing may prompt haemostatic measures such as suturing or use of regenerated oxidised cellulose but in most cases firm pressure is all that is necessary.

When patients are taking higher doses of aspirin for chronic pain (e.g. patients with osteoarthritis or rheumatoid arthritis), then more major oral surgery may require the use of alternative analgesics for about 2 weeks before surgery, as the effects on platelets might prove more troublesome in these circumstances.

Patients taking anticoagulants, such as warfarin, for cardiac arrythmias or those with prosthetic heart valves, should have their INR (International Normalised Ratio) estimated on the day of surgery. A higher INR can be accepted before minor oral surgical than before general surgery (Ch. 6). Some suggest that an INR of <4 can be accepted, but most oral surgeons would wish the INR to be between 2–3 for elective procedures other than single tooth extractions. Haemostasis should be secured with local measures including Surgicel®, suturing and pressure packs.

Surgeons must also be aware of the effect of prescribed drugs on anticoagulated patients. Most antibiotics and some antifungals will enhance the anticoagulant effect of warfarin, and non-steroidal anti-inflammatory drugs such as aspirin not only enhance the activity of warfarin but risk more severe bleeding from the stomach by their action on the gastric mucosa.

Cardiovascular disease

From an oral surgical viewpoint, patients with cardio-vascular disease can be considered in two groups.

Those with vascular disease

Hypertension is probably the most common consequence of peripheral vascular disease. Patients may be taking a variety of medications, ranging from diuretics to beta-blockers, calcium-channel-blockers or angiotensin-converting-enzyme (ACE) inhibitors. In general terms, treatment of the hypertensive patient will be largely unaltered other than under a general anaesthetic. Most dentoalveolar surgery can be carried out with no problems under local anaesthesia, although adrenaline (epinephrine)-containing local anaesthetics are known to cause a reduction in the blood potassium level and, in patients taking potassium-losing diuretics, an adrenaline (epinephrine)-free local anaesthetic may be preferred. This is a theoretical risk.

Those with cardiac disease

Those with cardiac disease can be conveniently considered under two headings.

Valvular disease

Although rheumatic fever is now extremely rare, valvular disease of the heart is still seen in the older population as a consequence of its effects on the valves. Although damage is not invariable, these patients are regarded as 'at risk' unless there is proof to the contrary. This should include those with developmental septal defects and those with prosthetic heart valves following cardiac surgery. Patients with cardiac pacemakers are not at risk and anti-biotic therapy is not required. The remainder are at risk of endocarditis as a result of bacteraemia, which will be resultant upon oral surgery. Antibiotic cover is, therefore, a preoperative requirement and the regime is dependent on whether the patient is being treated under local or general anaesthesia, whether the patient is allergic to penicillin and whether penicillin has been prescribed on more than one occasion in the previous month. Patients at a particular high risk are those who have had a previous episode of endocarditis. The appropriate regime for managing these patients is listed in Table 35.2.

Ischaemic heart disease

Patients at particular risk are those with severe hyper-tension, those with angina or those who have had a previous myocardial infarction. Anxiety or pain can cause an outpouring of adrenaline, which can increase the strain on the heart and also precipitate dangerous arrhythmias. The patient should, therefore, be exposed to minimum stress and prescribed sedation if required (see Ch. 11).

The most effective agent for local anaesthesia is lidocaine (lignocaine) 2% with adrenaline (epinephrine) (see Ch. 24). Doses of local anaesthetics should be kept to a minimum and treatment sessions should not be prolonged.

If it is unavoidable, general anaesthesia should be given by an expert anaesthetist in a hospital setting, because cardiovascular disease is the chief risk of death under anaesthesia.

A number of measures should be considered when treating patients in an outpatient environment under local anaesthesia. Patients should be advised to continue their normal medication before and after procedures. Patients should bring their glyceryl trinitrate (GTN) spray to the surgery, if they use one, because they may wish to use it prophylactically. Oxygen should be available on a continuous flow delivery system and staff should be trained in the appropriate care for the collapsed patient.

Where possible, surgical treatment is best deferred for 3–6 months after myocardial infarction, depending on

Table 35.2   Prevention of endocarditis[1] in patients with heart-valve lesion, septal defect, patent ductus, or prosthetic valve

Dental procedures[2] under local or no anaesthesia, patients who have not received more than a single dose of a penicillin in the previous month, including those with a prosthetic valve (but not those who have had endocarditis), oral amoxicillin 3 g 1 h before procedure; CHILD under 5 years quarter adult dose; 5–10 years half adult dose

patients who are penicillin-allergic or have received more than a single dose of penicillin in the previous month, oral clindamycin[3] 600 mg 1 h before procedure; child under 5 years quarter adult dose; 5–10 years half adult dose

patients who have had endocarditis, amoxicillin + gentamicin, as under general anaesthesia

Dental procedures[2] under general anaesthesia, no special risk (including patients who have not received more than a single dose of a penicillin in the previous month), either i.m. or i.v. amoxicillin 1 g at induction, then oral amoxicillin 500 mg 6 h later; CHILD under 5 years quarter adult dose; 5–10 years half adult dose

or oral amoxicillin 3 g 4 h before induction then oral amoxicillin 3 g as soon as possible after procedure; CHILD under 5 years quarter adult dose; 5–10 years half adult dose

or oral amoxicillin 3 g + oral probenecid 1 g 4 h before procedure

Special risk (patients with prosthetic valve or who have had endocarditis), i.m. or i.v. amoxicillin 1 g + i.m. or i.v. gentamicin 120 mg at induction, then oral amoxicillin 500 mg 6 h later; CHILD under 5 years amoxicillin quarter adult dose, gentamicin 2 mg/kg; 5–10 years amoxicillin half adult dose, gentamicin 2 mg/kg

patients who are penicillin-allergic or who have received more than a single dose of a penicillin in the previous month,

either i.v. vancomycin 1 g over at least 100 min then i.v. gentamicin 120 mg at induction or 15 min before procedure; CHILD under 10 years vancomycin 20 mg/kg, gentamicin 2 mg/kg

or i.v. teicoplanin 400 mg + gentamicin 120 mg at induction or 15 min before procedure; CHILD under 14 years teicoplanin 6 mg/kg, gentamicin 2 mg/kg

or i.v. clindamycin[3] 300 mg over at least 10 min at induction or 15 min before procedure then oral or i.v. clindamycin 150 mg 6 h later; CHILD under 5 years quarter adult dose; 5–10 years half adult dose

---

[1] Reproduced from the *British National Formulary* (March 1997), with the permission of the British Medical Association and the Royal Pharmaceutical Society of Great Britain.
[2] Dental procedures that require antibiotic prophylaxis are: extractions, scaling and surgery involving gingival tissues. Antibiotic prophylaxis for dental procedures may be supplemented with chlorhexidine gluconate gel 1% or chlorhexidine gluconate mouthwash 0.2%, used 5 min before procedure.
[3] If clindamycin is used, periodontal or other multistage procedures should not be repeated at intervals of less than 2 weeks.

---

the severity of the attack and the patient's rate and degree of recovery.

Endocrine disorders

A number of endocrine disorders can complicate the management of the patient undergoing minor oral surgery. The most prevalent of these conditions is diabetes mellitus, which can occur in the insulin-dependent form or in the non-insulin-dependent, maturity-onset form. In addition, an increasing number of patients take corticosteroid drugs for the management of autoimmune conditions. The management of these groups of patients will now be discussed.

Diabetes mellitus

If oral surgery requires a general anaesthetic, the requirements of preanaesthetic starving and the difficulties with postoperative food intake will need appropriate management. This needs to be carried out on an inpatient basis in cooperation with the patient's physician and using a balance of dextrose infusions and soluble insulin.

Under local anaesthetic, patients should be encouraged to maintain their normal regime with regard to eating and insulin injections. Effort should be made not to delay treatment such that the normal dietary intake is disrupted.

Diabetic patients have a compromised response to infections. Certain procedures may, therefore, warrant an antibiotic prescription to cover them over the initial healing period. For the straightforward extraction in a well-controlled patient, however, this is not necessary, particularly where good oral hygiene can be relied upon.

Certain non-steroidal anti-inflammatory drugs have an effect on blood sugar levels and paracetamol, with or without codeine, may be a wiser analgesic choice.

Corticosteroid treatment

Corticosteroids have important effects when given in sufficiently large doses, and these include depression of adrenocortical function, which will lead to collapse under stress. Depression of the inflammatory and immune responses may lead to an increase in opportunistic infections and impaired wound healing.

The need to give additional steroids for those patients taking systemic corticosteroids, or having used them in the previous 2 years, is controversial. Where clinical concerns exist regarding the risk of hypotensive shock, patients should be treated by increasing oral steroid therapy or by intravenous or intramuscular hydrocortisone.

Liver disease

Normal liver function is essential for production of several blood-clotting factors and for the metabolism and detoxification of many drugs. Viral disease also has implications in terms of cross-infection (see Ch. 7). It is important to assess coagulation defects preoperatively to ensure that adequate haemostasis will occur (see Ch. 6), and to be aware of the possibility of reduced drug break-down when administering or prescribing agents. The *British National Formulary* contains valuable information on prescribing for such patients and should be consulted appropriately.

Neurological disease

The most significant neurological problem presenting routinely in minor oral surgical practice is that of grand mal epilepsy.

Most patients with epilepsy will be taking antiepileptic drugs such as carbamazepine or phenytoin for the control of the seizures. Oral surgery can be carried out under local anaesthesia without any problems if control is satisfactory and patients should be advised to continue their normal antiepileptic drug unchanged. If general

Table 35.3   Oral surgical considerations in pregnancy
Risk to mother
increased gingivitis and epulis formation
risk of hypotension if supine
risk of hypertension
vomiting especially with general anaesthesia
aspirin may cause neonatal haemorrhage
Risk to fetus
radiography hazardous
respiratory depression with sedatives
tooth staining with tetracyclines
prilocaine rarely causes methaemoglobinaemia
some drugs are teratogenic

anaesthesia is required, the anaesthetist should be made aware of the history to allow for the use of appropriate volatile agents for anaesthetic maintenance.

Pregnancy

Minor oral surgical procedures can be carried out during pregnancy, which, it should be remembered, is a physio-logical state. The potential risks to the mother and fetus are outlined in Table 35.3.

In the later stages of pregnancy, patients should normally receive treatment in a more upright position rather than supine because the weight of the fetus and uterus can interfere with blood return via the inferior vena cava.

Although radiographs in the region of the jaws do not cause direct irradiation of the abdominal area, these should be restricted to clinical necessity, as should all radiographs. Patients who have non-acute problems should defer radiographic imaging until after pregnancy. Protective shielding where radiographs are needed should be used as much for reassurance as for their actual benefit. In acute conditions, radiographs will often be necessary and patients should be reassured that the risk is minimal.

Prescription of drugs should be carefully considered and reference to the *British National Formulary* is necessary to allow a choice of drugs that have been proven safe during this period. Lidocaine (lignocaine) plus adrenaline (epinephrine) is an appropriate anaesthetic and some clinicians prefer to avoid prilocaine with felypressin, which may (in theory) have a mild oxytocic effect. During the first trimester of pregnancy, particular care should be taken with any prescription as this is the time when drugs administered to the mother can have the most serious consequences on the child's development.

Necessary dental treatment should continue during pregnancy, especially such measures as extraction of unrestorable, grossly carious teeth where delay could lead to acute pain and spread of infection. Prompt treatment under local anaesthesia may well avoid the need for later use of antibiotics and painkillers, and even the need for general anaesthesia where gross infection precludes the use of a local anaesthetic. For less urgent surgery, such as removal of wisdom teeth or periradicular surgery, it is better that the surgical treatment is carried out during the middle trimester of pregnancy or deferred until after the pregnancy.

Most pregnancies are trouble free, but if there are related problems surgeons should communicate with the consulting obstetrician if there is any doubt as to the appropriateness of dental treatment.

Radiotherapy

Radiotherapy in the head and neck region may not only cause mucosites and xerostomia but also reduces the vitality of bone, which increases susceptibility to osteoradionecrosis. This is discussed in Chapter 36.

Renal disease

Renal disease is becoming more important to the dental surgeon as more patients are now receiving renal dialysis or renal transplantation. Patients receiving regular haemodialysis are heparinised before dialysis and haemostasis is impaired for 6–12 h thereafter. These patients are also at greater risk of carrying hepatitis viruses. Furthermore, the permanent fistula formation that is required for haemodialysis is susceptible to infection and antibiotic cover should be provided for these individuals.

In addition, the kidney is a major organ of excretion and many drugs may have reduced elimination leading to possible toxic effects if renal function is impaired. The *British National Formulary* should be consulted before prescribing drugs for any patient with a history of renal disease.

Respiratory disease

Long-standing or severe obstructive pulmonary disease poses general anaesthetic problems not only because of the compromised gaseous exchange but also because of the possible related right-sided heart failure problems. The conditions most likely to cause chronic obstructive pulmonary disease are bronchitis, bronchiectasis and asthma.

Treatment that is to be carried out under local anaesthetic should be staged to reduce stress and fatigue. Asthmatic patients should be counselled to bring their salbutamol or corticosteroid inhalers to the surgery and to use them if the need arises. Salbutamol and oxygen should be kept in the surgery, with a suitable method of delivery as an emergency measure.

Worsening of asthma can be related to non-steroidal anti-inflammatories and caution should be exercised in their prescription.

36 Diseases of bone

Introduction

The health of the bone of the jaws is important to the integrity of the oral cavity and the teeth. Among them, a number of conditions, primarily of bone, exist which may be genetic, metabolic or due to some other aetiology. Often, however, bone disorders have a mixed aetiology which makes their classification problematic: cherubism is a genetic condition but is also a fibro-osseous metabolic bone disease. A list of bone disorders, categorised according to their known aetiology is shown in Fig. 36.1. These will be discussed in turn.

Achondroplasia

Achondroplasia is the most common genetic skeletal disorder and is characterised by failure of epiphyseal cartilage growth. This leads to short limbs and a retrusive middle third of the face due to defective growth at the base of the skull. The facial deformity leads to malocclusion.

Aneurysmal bone cyst

This very rare condition affects the mandible rather than the maxilla. It is characterised by expansion of the mandibular inner and outer cortical plates with a very vascular fibrous tissue that contains osteoclasts and areas of immature bone. The lesion may appear radiographically as multilocular radiolucencies with a soap-bubble type of appearance and with evidence of marked expansion in larger lesions. Treatment is by curettage locally and some operators prefer to freeze the periphery of the bony cavity with liquid nitrogen. Occasionally, very aggressive aneurysmal bone cysts may require more radical treatment in the form of local resection of the affected part of the jaw.

Central giant-cell granuloma

The clinical appearance in the jaws of this lesion may be exactly the same as the brown tumour described later in hyperparathyroidism. However, it is not a parathyroid-related problem but appears to be an endosteally originating resorptive process causing a cyst-like lesion filled with a very vascular fibrous tissue rich in multinucleated giant cells.

Clinical presentation

There is normally a bony expansion of mandible rather than maxilla and there may be mobility of related teeth and resorption of roots.

Diagnosis

Radiographically and histologically, the giant-cell granuloma is indistinguishable from the brown tumour, and bone biochemical tests must be carried out to exclude hyperparathyroidism. The diagnosis is therefore made on histological grounds supplemented by negative serological findings of parathyroid disease.

Management

These lesions are treated conservatively by local curettage. They do have a tendency to recur and many operators now freeze the bony walls of the cavity with liquid nitrogen after curettage in an attempt to prevent this recurrence. In children, where there may be quite gross deformity, the lesions may respond to calcitonin injections, which are given over a prolonged period such as a year. When successful, such treatment may avoid the need for extensive surgery and the consequent aesthetic problems that can, in turn, require later surgical reconstruction in the form of bone grafting.

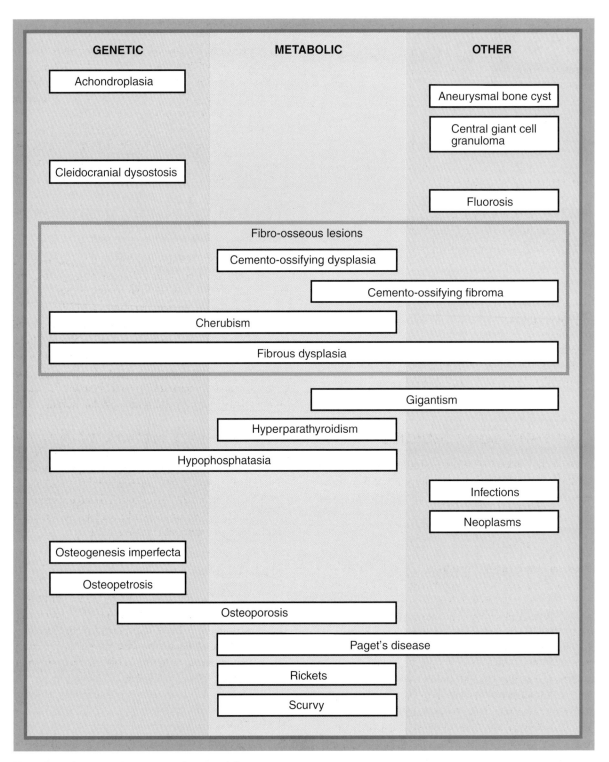

Fig. 36.1 Diseases of bone according to aetiology.

Cleidocranial dysostosis

This is also a very rare inherited disorder. It is characterised by partial or complete agenesis of clavicles, by frontal bossing, ocular hypertelorism (excessive spacing between the orbital cavities) and late closure of skull fontanelles. Dentally, there may be multiple supernumerary teeth, lack of eruption of teeth generally and thin dilacerated roots. It would appear that normal resorptive activity during eruption is compromised leading to the unerupted teeth lying in crypts covered with overlying bone which does not resorb. Dental treatment involves exposure of teeth and removal of obstructing supernumeraries where these are impeding normal eruption. However, even after exposure, the teeth may not erupt satisfactorily.

Fluorosis

Excessive intake of fluoride can lead to mottling of the teeth. Skeletal sclerosis can also occur and this is histologically similar to Paget's disease.

Fibro-osseous lesions

These form a group of lesions with diverse aetiologies with a range of clinical presentations. Fibrous dysplasia is the most important.

Fibrous dysplasia

This condition affects children and is, as the name implies, a replacement of normal bone by an immature bone not unlike woven bone with extensive vascular fibrous tissue elements. The abnormality may affect many bones (polyostotic) or one bone (monostotic), and the maxilla is far more commonly affected than the mandible. Two rare variants are also identified, one being cherubism and the other Albright's syndrome, which is a form of polyostotic fibrous dysplasia with additional features of skin pigmentation and precocious puberty in females. Fibrous dysplasia is usually self-limiting and tends to 'burn out' on completion of skeletal growth. It can, however, cause quite marked disfigurement in severe cases and in the polyostotic form can encroach on bony foramina leading to compression of nerves.

Clinical appearance

In the monostotic form, the usual presentation is of a painless enlargement of the maxilla on the affected side. Buccal and palatal aspects of the alveolar bone may be enlarged and expanded and this may cause spacing between the teeth compared to the unaffected side. The occlusion, however, is seldom significantly affected other than the spacing and the teeth erupt normally and are not unduly mobile. The overgrowth can usually be seen as a facial asymmetry with fullness of the cheekbone and nasolabial fold.

Diagnosis

The diagnosis is normally made on three grounds: the age of the patient and clinical features described; the radiographic appearance and the histopathology. Radiographs of the affected bone or bones typically show a granular appearance that has been likened to ground glass. There is an obvious excess of this abnormal bone and it merges with the normal appearance of bone without a clearly defined separation. A bone biopsy will generally show the typical histological picture of islands of irregularly shaped bone with vascular fibrous tissue interspersing.

Bone biochemistry is normally unhelpful, with calcium, phosphate and alkaline phosphatase levels within normal limits. The alkaline phosphatase level, which is a measure of osteoblastic bone formative activity, may be raised if the sample is taken during an active growth phase of the child, and its relevance is therefore almost impossible to determine.

Management

Unless there is unacceptable disfigurement, most surgeons prefer to defer treatment until growth is complete. The surgery is normally in the form of recontouring of the excess bulk of bone. In more gross cases, surgery may be needed at an earlier stage but may require to be repeated when maturity is reached.

Cherubism

This is regarded as a form of fibrous dysplasia that is familial and carried by a dominant gene. It is characterised by an increased width and fullness of the angles of mandible bilaterally. The bone itself is immature in these regions with areas of vascular fibrous tissue. Radiographically, it appears as bilateral multilocular cyst-like radiolucencies. Although normally seen in the mandible, the maxilla can be affected also. The condition is first seen in childhood and becomes less active on maturity.

Cemento-ossifying fibroma

These rare lesions can grow to a considerable size. They are essentially fibrous overgrowths that become filled with either a bony or cement-like calcification. They are generally painless and are found as swellings usually in the buccal sulcus. They may be encapsulated but these capsules are not invariably present. Surgical removal of the lesion may be difficult as the boundaries of the lesion may be almost impossible to ascertain. They are more common in the mandible and generally present in young adults.

Cemento-ossifying dysplasia

This process is similar to fibrous dysplasia but lesions resemble cemento-ossifying fibromas and probably arise in the periodontium. The condition may be multifocal or generalised. Single lesions are called cementomas and florid lesions are termed gigantiform cementomas. They are more common in women and black patients and undergo progressive periapical calification. This leads to difficulties with extractions and the subsequent risk of osteomyelitis.

Gigantism

Excess growth hormones arising from a pituitary adenoma will cause increased growth in height before the epiphyses are closed. Subsequent growth causes acromegaly with prognathism and increased soft tissue growth leading to coarse facial features and macroglossia. The bone quality is normal.

Hyperparathyroidism

This may be primary and due to overproduction of parathormone often by an adenoma in the parathyroid glands or secondary to conditions that reduce calcium levels in the blood, such as chronic renal disease. Where increased levels of parathormone are present, calcium is mobilised from the bony skeleton to raise blood levels of

calcium. In the primary form of the disease, this leads to hypercalcaemia, and renal calculi may develop if the problem is not identified. In the bone, however, where the jaws can be affected, cyst-like spaces known as 'brown tumours' may develop. The bone in these tumours is resorbed by vascular fibrous tissue with multinucleated giant cells in profusion. This has given rise to the other name of this condition, osteitis fibrosa cystica. In the jaws, the mandible is more commonly affected by such lesions than the maxilla.

Clinical features

In the mandible, the presence of a brown tumour may give rise to expansion of the outer and/or the inner cortical plates of bone. Occasionally, the soft tissue of the brown tumour may grow through the upper border of the alveolar process and appear as a dark red or purple-coloured mass under the oral mucosa. The lesion is usually non-painful but may be tender to palpation.

Diagnosis

Radiographs will show a well circumscribed area of radiolucency with a less defined lamina dura surrounding it than is normally found in a true cystic lesion. The outline may have a scalloped margin and some authorities also describe a lack of definition of the lamina dura around all the standing teeth. This, in fact, is difficult to discern and tends to be a rather subjective finding.

An incision biopsy of the lesion reveals the typical histological appearance of fibrous vascular tissue with large numbers of multinucleated giant cells.

Serum biochemistry will reveal elevated parathormone levels and, in the primary form of the disease, this will be accompanied by a raised serum calcium and lowered phosphate level.

Management

Primary hyperparathyroidism is normally treated surgically by removal of usually an adenoma of the parathyroid gland. The bone lesions usually resolve spontaneously following this surgery.

Hypophosphatasia

This rare recessive genetic disorder can be of early or late onset. It is characterised by bony fragility and a rickets-like condition. Defective cementogenesis can lead to shedding of the teeth.

Infective bone conditions

Infection in bone is relatively uncommon in the jaws given the large number of dental abscesses that occur and also the amount of bone exposed by extractions that heal without apparent problems. It is probably a reflection of the good blood supply in the mouth generally, and particularly in the upper jaw, which seldom becomes infected. The use of antibiotics also limits the occurrence of bone infection compared with preantibiotic days. Osteomyelitis is so rare nowadays that most clinicians look for underlying reasons for its occurrence. Conditions that have rendered the patient immunocompromised, such as diabetes mellitus, HIV infection, immuno-suppressive drug therapy and blood dyscrasias should be excluded. Local factors, such as previous radiotherapy to that region of the jaw or lack of a normal blood supply (as encountered in osteopetrosis), are also relevant as predisposing factors. A number of distinct bony infections can occur (Table 36.1) and these will be considered here.

Localised osteitis (dry socket)

This is discussed in Chapter 26.

Acute osteomyelitis

By definition, this is an acute inflammatory reaction to infection within the medulla of the affected bone. It rarely affects the maxilla, which has a more profuse blood supply, being primarily a mandibular infection. It is comparatively rare and may well be an indication of other disease that reduces the normal defence mechanisms. The source of most mandibular osteomyelitis is dento-alveolar infection and the microbial profile is similar to

Table 36.1   Infective bony conditions
Localised osteitis
Acute osteomyelitis
Chronic osteomyelitis
Chronic sclerosing osteomyelitis
Subperiosteal osteomyelitis
Osteoradionecrosis

that found in dental abscesses with anaerobes predominating. It differs in this from osteomyelitis in a long bone, which is often of staphylococcal origin and is said to be haematogenous, meaning that the bacteria have circulated in the bloodstream from other sources such as skin infections.

Clinical features

These reflect the results of a sudden increase in pressure within the medulla of the bone in which the intact cortical plates do not allow any release in the early stages. This rapid increase in pressure is brought about by the inflammatory reaction in response to the presence of infection. Patients therefore complain of severe throbbing pain, trismus, swelling over the mandible and paraesthesia or anaesthesia in the distribution of the mental nerve. More variably, a bad taste or discharge through sinus formation may be seen. In severe cases there may be pyrexia with consequent malaise and anorexia. Lymphadenitis may be relatively late but may be palpable and tender in the submandibular and upper cervical chain of nodes. Later features may include sinus formation on the skin and shedding intraorally of necrotic bone.

Radiographic features

Initially, there may be little evidence of changes within the bone, other than possible dental foci of infection. In the later stages, areas of patchy radiolucency are present, within which there may be irregular areas of increased density that signify bony sequestra (Fig. 36.2). Sequestra are areas of dead bone formed by thrombus formation in the nutrient blood vessels to these areas of bone brought about by the increased pressure on these vessels. The areas of necrotic bone further enhance the inflammatory reaction, as the body attempts to shed them in the same way as any foreign body.

Management

Initially, the management of osteomyelitis follows the principles of any acute pyogenic infection: incision and drainage of any collection of pus together with appropriate vigorous antibiotic therapy. If possible, pus should be sampled by aspiration for culture and antibiotic sensitivity testing but antimicrobial prescriptions should not be delayed for this laboratory analysis. Commonly, metronidazole and amoxicillin are used together but

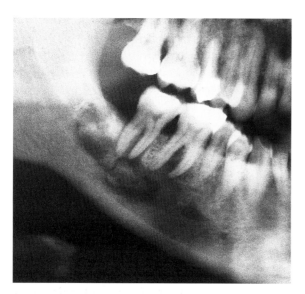

Fig. 36.2 Radiograph showing acute osteomyelitis 3 months after removal of an infected lower third molar.

these can be changed to reflect the bacteriological findings if required. Clindamycin has good bone-penetrating qualities and is effective in many anaerobic infections, it is therefore a useful drug if there is a poor clinical response. Once the acute phase has been brought under control, surgical sequestrectomy, which removes any areas of dead bone and curettage, is carried out. If significant loss of bone has occurred, bone grafting may be considered at a later stage but only after total resolution of the infection.

Chronic osteomyelitis

Features of chronic infection are less florid that in the acute form, and hence pain is less marked, disturbance of nerve transmission is much less likely and generally the presentation is more subtle. Management is normally by surgical means with sequestrectomy and curettage.

Chronic sclerosing osteomyelitis

This is a rare and ill-understood condition in which areas of bone in the mandible show radiographic evidence of rarefaction often giving patchy round or oval radiolucencies in the affected region. It does not appear to be due to bacterial infection although there is some dispute over this, and surgical curettage reveals chronic inflammatory changes but no histological evidence of microbial presence. The condition may cause swelling

and pain that responds to non-steroidal anti-inflammatory drugs, which are often used together with antibiotics, although the latter are usually prescribed before any accurate diagnosis is made. Systemic corticosteroids can also be helpful in controlling the acute symptoms. Some investigators have suggested that the condition, which is chronic and intermittent in character, may be related to excessive tooth clenching or grinding, and will therefore respond to interocclusal splinting of the teeth. Surgery often involves decortication of the outer lamellar bone and this is normally followed by an osteosclerotic reaction. The condition frequently remits spontaneously with the affected region or regions showing increased radiodensity on radiographic examination.

Subperiosteal osteomyelitis

This is more commonly seen in children or young adults where infection usually through an infected tooth causes pus to form under the periosteum of the bone. The periosteum is hence lifted off the bone and reacts by forming a layer of new bone known as an involucrum. Patients have a fairly hard bony swelling formed of this new bone beneath which pus may be trapped. Radiographically, this is often best illustrated by occlusal or posteroanterior mandibular views, which show the outer cortical plate with a thin overlying wafer of new bone where the periosteum has been raised from the surface and formed new bone in an attempt to wall-off the infection. Treatment consists of removal of the source of infection, normally a tooth, and curettage of the area with appropriate removal of the overlying involucrum bone.

Osteoradionecrosis

Irradiation to the jaws may occur as a result of radiotherapy for malignant disease of the mouth, pharynx or salivary gland regions. Damage to the cells within the bone, the osteocytes, and to the nutrient blood vessels within bone, renders the bone less vital and hence more open to infection. In the blood vessels there is an endarteritis and periarteritis that significantly reduces the blood supply to the bone and this particularly affects mandibular bone, which has a less profuse vascular network than the maxilla. Where irradiation has been extensive, which is now less commonly seen due to better zoning of the beam and protection of adjacent tissues, a form of avascular necrosis can occur with exposed bone failing to sequestrate normally and heal with granulation tissue. Creation of a wound such as an extraction wound can, therefore, result in infection very easily, and this may be difficult to control. Added to this problem is a dry mouth and high caries rate if the salivary glands have been affected by the radiation.

Management

Prevention is preferable to treating exposed or infected bone and careful preradiation assessment of restorative needs is essential. Unrestorable teeth should be extracted, if possible 3 weeks before the start of radiotherapy. Strict oral hygiene measures should be stressed to reduce the chance of subsequent caries and tooth loss and this should be in conjunction with regular dental treatment including preventive measures.

When extraction is unavoidable after radiation, most clinicians use antibiotics for a week to 10 days after the extraction. Care should be taken to cover any exposed bone such as interradicular septa and, if necessary, such uncovered areas need to be protected with a Whitehead's varnish ribbon gauze pack or covered with a surgical flap. More recently, hyperbaric oxygen therapy has been used with some success in the management of these problems. The treatment involves the patient entering a pressure chamber where the atmospheric pressure is increased to about 2.5 atmospheres for a period of 90 min. This has to be done daily for several weeks but does appear to help the healing process significantly. It has also been shown that surgery to remove necrotic bone following hyperbaric oxygen treatment increases the chance of successful healing. The success of hyperbaric oxygen therapy underlines the ischaemic cause of the problem consequent to radiotherapy.

Neoplasms

Neoplastic disease

Neoplasms derived from bone itself are relatively infrequent in the jaws. The benign osteoma and the malignant osteosarcoma are very uncommon. However, the jaws may be affected by neoplasms of dental origin, such as odontogenic tumours, secondary metastatic deposits in bone from primary tumours such as breast, thyroid or lung, or more commonly from direct invasion of the oral squamous cell carcinoma arising from the overlying mucosal epithelium. Neoplasms in bone give rise to radiographic changes in the form of radiolucencies

Table 36.2 Neoplasm in bone
Osteoma
Osteosarcoma
Cemento-ossifying fibroma
Odontogenic neoplasms

and therefore bone loss unexplained from the more common infective causes should always arouse suspicion. In these situations, a biopsy of the area is the only satisfactory method of eliminating the possibility of neoplastic disease. The neoplasms to be discussed are listed in Table 36.2.

Osteoma

This is a benign tumour of bone and, unlike bony exostoses, is very uncommon. It can arise from compact or cancellous bone in the form of a painless hard swelling. Radiographically, a round or oval-shaped radiodense image is seen and although a capsule is classically found in benign tumours it is seldom seen clearly on such radiographs. If the swelling is interfering with function it can be surgically removed.

A more rare condition, Gardner's syndrome, is characterised by multiple osteomata of the jaws. The condition is important because the syndrome exhibits multiple intestinal polyposis and these polyps have the potential for malignant transformation. Urgent referral to a gastroenterologist is therefore needed.

Osteosarcoma

This is – fortunately – a rare malignant tumour of the jaws. It is more common in young people under the age of 30 but can occur in older patients and a small number of people with Paget's disease develop osteosarcoma as a rare complication. The age of presentation of the disease appears to be significantly older in the jaws than in other bones, and it may affect maxilla or mandible. Jaw lesions also appear to differ from those in other bones in that metastases usually to lung or brain are less prevalent. The poor prognosis of the disease appears to be more related to local aggressive recurrence.

Clinical appearance

This varies according to the site of origin but normally consists of a fairly rapidly enlarging swelling, which can be painful and cause loosening of related teeth. Anaesthesia may also occur if the tumour grows in relation to the inferior dental canal or infra orbital canal causing altered sensation peripheral to the point of tumour pressure or infiltration.

Radiographs may show clear evidence of bone destruction although areas of radio-opacity, which may be quite dense, can be seen within the radiolucent region. The periphery is indistinct reflecting the rapid growth and both widening of the periodontal membranes and resorption of the roots of teeth may be evident.

Diagnosis

This is confirmed by incision biopsy of the lesion.

Management

The lesion is treated by radical excision of the affected bone and wide margins of soft tissue are also removed. More recently, better responses have been claimed by presurgical chemotherapy and, if necessary, postsurgical chemotherapy or radiotherapy.

Cemento-ossifying fibroma

This neoplasm has been discussed in the section on fibro-osseous lesions.

Odontogenic neoplasms

This is a collection of neoplasms derived from tooth-forming tissue and may arise from epithelial or mesenchymal tissue. They are rare, although the most aggressive of them – the ameloblastoma – is the most common. At the other end of the spectrum of these neoplasms are the odontomes, which are best considered hamartomas (which means that they are abnormal tooth-like structures that generally do not continue to grow once their development is complete). There are many histological types of odontogenic tumour, the more common of these are listed in Table 36.3.

Ameloblastoma

The ameloblastoma is the most common of the odonto-genic tumours and can present at any time from child-hood to older age groups but is more often seen in the middle-aged adult population. It occurs in both mandible and maxilla but is far more common in the lower jaw,

Table 36.3 Odontogenic tumours and odontomes
Epithelial in origin
Ameloblastoma
Calcifying epithelial odontogenic tumour (Pindborg tumour)
Adenomatoid odontogenic tumour
Mesenchymal in origin
Odontogenic myxoma
Cementoma
Odontomes
Invaginated odontome (dilated composite odontome and 'dens in dente')
Compound composite odontome
Complex composite odontome
Germinated odontome

with an approximate ratio of 3:1. In the lower jaw, the angle and ramus is the most frequent site, with over two-thirds of occurrences.

The tumour is variable in its aggressiveness and spreads by local destruction of bone. If untreated, it will eventually spread into soft tissues and this may make it very difficult to eradicate surgically. It does not tend to metastasise other than the extremely rare malignant ameloblastoma variant. There are several histological variants of this tumour, the two most common being the plexiform and the follicular forms, but these different appearances do not appear to produce differences in behaviour or prognosis.

Clinical features

Gradual swelling of the jaw is the usual initial symptom of this tumour, although it may be diagnosed through a radiograph before this becomes apparent. Loosening and displacement of teeth can occur, although pain or altered sensation is not usually reported. In the earlier stages, the swelling will be in the form of expansion of buccal and/or lingual cortical plates and is hence hard to palpation. With further growth, however, the swelling may be softer but firm denoting that the lesion has eroded through the bone into the adjacent soft tissues.

Radiographs classically show a multilocular 'soap bubble' round or oval-shaped radiolucency with well-demarcated radio-opaque margins (Fig. 36.3). The sharp delineation of the radiolucent areas reflects the slow rate of growth of these neoplasms. It may displace the outline of the inferior dental canal and may also cause displace-ment and/or resorption of the roots of the teeth.

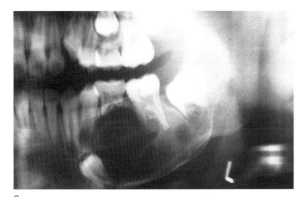

a

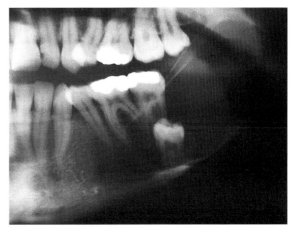

Fig. 36.4 Radiograph of a cystic ameloblastoma.

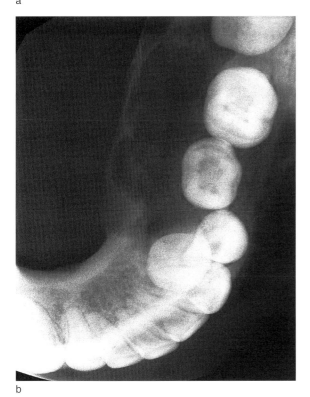

b

Fig. 36.3 Radiograph of an ameloblastoma showing (a) soap-bubble appearance; (b) expansion.

One recognised variant of the ameloblastoma is the cystic ameloblastoma, which most frequently occurs at the angle of mandible. Radiographically, this is indistinguishable from a dentigerous cyst related to an unerupted wisdom tooth and is a fluid-filled cystic cavity with nodules of ameloblastoma within certain areas of the lining of the cyst (Fig. 36.4). Even if an incision biopsy of the cyst lining is taken following aspiration of

the fluid content, it may not be taken in an area that is showing neoplastic change and it is therefore important that, when any presumed cyst is enucleated, the whole pathological specimen is examined by a pathologist who is aware of such variations of the ameloblastoma (see Ch. 28).

Treatment

Irrespective of histological differences in this neoplasm, most authorities advise total resection with around 1 cm clearance of the affected bone. In smaller lesions this may still allow preservation of the lower border of the mandible and this clearly has significant advantages with regard to aesthetics. The resultant defect may be filled with a bone graft and, where necessary, supported by a reconstruction plate.

Calcifying epithelial odontogenic tumour (Pindborg tumour)

This rare neoplasm can occur at any site in the upper or lower jaw but is most commonly found in the mandible. It causes painless expansion of the affected area and is frequently related to an unerupted tooth. Radiographs show a radiolucency, which may be multiloculated, and there may be areas of radiodensity within the central area of the radiolucency. Demarcation of the tumour from normal bone is not always clear. The lesion is locally invasive into the surrounding bone and is treated by a localised resection with a small margin of normal bone around it to reduce the chance of recurrence.

Adenomatoid odontogenic tumour

This benign neoplasm is commonly found in the maxilla and is often related to an unerupted canine tooth. Radiographically, it can be indistinguishable from a dentigerous cyst around the crown of the unerupted tooth. Conservative curettage is its method of treatment.

Odontogenic myxoma

These slow-growing tumours are benign and are most frequent in the second and third decades. They occur in either jaw but are more common in the mandible. They erode bone and enlarge to form multilocular, radiolucent regions that can be very difficult to differentiate from other multilocular lesions such as ameloblastoma or odontogenic keratocysts. Treatment is conservative by thorough bony curettage. Recurrences can occur and, therefore, although the treatment is generally conservative, follow-up is required. These tumours do not appear to metastasise.

Cementoma

These lesions are composed of cementum and may occur singly or may affect many teeth in the dentition. They are a form of cemento-ossifying dysplasia. They are asymptomatic and are usually diagnosed by radiographic appearance. In the early stages they cause radiolucency, which later mineralises into cement-like tissue. The teeth affected are vital throughout this process.

Odontomes

Odontomes are relatively infrequent occurrences in the dentition but, when they do occur, they often impede the normal eruption of adjacent teeth or, in the case of the invaginated form, directly affect the vitality of the tooth. They are best regarded as malformations of development of the tooth from its dental lamina or as hamartomas, which cease their growth at completion of their formation and do not alter thereafter.

Invaginated odontome

This malformation is most often seen related to the upper lateral incisor tooth. It is formed by an ingrowth of enamel epithelium forming a blind-ending, enamel-lined pouch that is in direct communication with the surface of

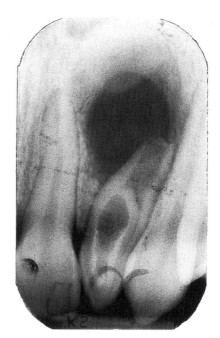

Fig. 36.5 Radiograph of an invaginated odontome with related radicular cyst.

the tooth, most commonly at the cingulum. The labial surface of the tooth may look entirely normal and the entrance to the invagination may be a minute pit, but the ingress of saliva and bacteria usually results in pulpal death and the development of an apical lesion. Such invaginations may be so small as to be difficult to image even with good radiographs but in some cases the malformation may be so great that the whole clinical crown is taken up by the dilated nature of the ingrowth and the appearance on radiograph can then be likened to a tooth within a tooth or 'dens in dente' (Fig. 36.5).

When the invagination is small the tooth may well be amenable to conventional root canal treatment and, where an apical cyst has developed, periradicular surgery. However, the malformation may be so gross that extraction is the only practical solution.

Complex odontome

This developmental aberration results in a random laying-down of all the dental elements in a totally haphazard fashion. Radiographically, it gives rise to an irregular radiodense image. Enamel, dentine, cement and pulpal tissues are all represented and the radiographic image obtained may well reflect these different tissues

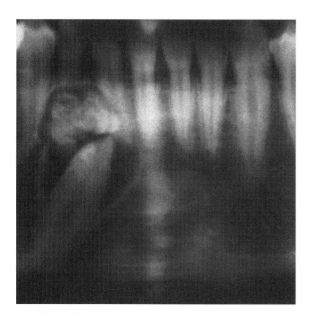

Fig. 36.6 Radiograph of a complex odontome.

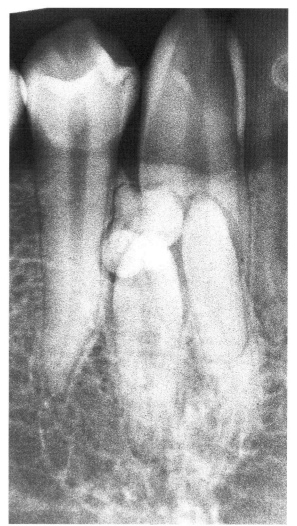

Fig. 36.7 Radiograph of a compound odontome.

with varying degrees of opacity and radiolucency (Fig. 36.6). Complex odontomes may obstruct adjacent teeth from normal eruption and they are better removed as early as possible to reduce this chance.

Compound odontome

In this abnormal manifestation of development, there is more organisation of the dental tissues and the lesion consists of numerous small denticles massed together within an outer capsule (Fig. 36.7). The odontome may be small, with only a few tiny teeth, or it may be of considerable size and contain many denticles. As with the complex odontome, the compound form should be removed where it is affecting normal eruption of the dentition.

Germinated odontome

This defect of development arises from either a complete or partial fusion of adjacent tooth germs or by a splitting or dichotomy of one germ. The result is a fusion of the resultant tooth that may affect only the crown or the crown and root together. They can pose both aesthetic and orthodontic problems and, where extraction is necessary, they may cause difficulties due to the complex nature of

the root form. Management of this problem will largely be dependent upon aesthetic and orthodontic criteria.

Although not a developmental problem, fusion of teeth by excessive production of root cementum can lead to what is referred to as pathological germination or concrescence. The most common teeth to be joined in this fashion are upper second and third molars, especially where the upper wisdom tooth has developed with a disto-oblique angulation. Concrescence of teeth is fortunately very rare as they pose considerable problems in removal since they are usually only detected at extraction.

Osteogenesis imperfecta

This is a group of rare, usually autosomal dominant conditions of varying severity affecting the formation of all bony tissue. The condition is sometimes referred to as brittle-bone disease because the inherent weakness of the structure of the tissue can lead to fracture of the bone with even minimum trauma. The condition arises due to defective biosynthesis of type I collagen, leading to inadequate amounts of bone formation by osteoblasts. In addition to the weak nature of the bones, they tend to be thinner than normal, although growth may be relatively unaffected. Multiple fractures can lead to deformity. The sclerae of the eyes are typically a bluish colour and many cases also have a related defect in dentine structure, dentinogenesis imperfecta. This dentine is poorly attached to the overlying enamel and this can lead to rapid loss of the enamel and subsequent wear of the unprotected dentine. Patients may often therefore require extractions, and these need considerable care in their execution, although fracture of the jaw during such extraction is relatively uncommon.

Osteopetrosis

This inherited but very rare condition is sometimes known as marble bone disease because of the density of the bone that encroaches upon medullary spaces and may therefore compromise haemopoesis. The condition arises due to inactivity of osteoclasts. The problem can affect the jaws where the lack of vascularity of the tissue may lead to infection. The avascular bone makes eradication of infection by antibiotics difficult because adequate levels of such antibiotics may not be effective in the affected area because of the lack of blood supply. Similarly, surgical removal of affected bone can be followed by very poor healing and the risk of reinfection. Extractions may not only be difficult, therefore, but may also lead to infection. Reduction of the medullary spaces compromises haemopoesis, which then takes place in the liver and spleen. Regardless, anaemia is progressive without marrow transplantation.

Osteoporosis

This disorder is characterised by loss of bone density. The composition of the bone is normal and there are no demonstrable metabolic changes. Physiological bone loss

Table 36.4	Risk factors for osteoporosis
Physiological	*Pathological*
Ageing	Alcohol
Female sex	Corticosteroid drugs, Cushing's syndrome
Early menopause	Multiple myeloma ⎫
Immobility	Diabetes mellitus ⎬ rare
Underweight	Hypogonadism ⎱ causes
Childhood maturation failure	Thyrotoxicosis ⎭
	Smoking

with increasing age accounts for the apparent increasing prevalence of this disorder. The risk factors for osteoporosis are listed in Table 36.4.

Treatment is unsatisfactory. Prevention is preferred and hormone-replacement therapy (HRT) is effective in postmenopausal women. Patients with osteoporosis have increased alveolar resorption if they are edentulous.

Paget's disease

This disease can affect the jaws but is normally more of a problem in the weight-bearing bones. It is characterised by irregular resorption of bone with subsequent redeposition and it therefore disrupts normal bony architecture. During the resorptive phases, areas of bone may be severely resorbed, leading to distortion under normal weight bearing function. There may be pain in the bones, large vascular regions in the medullary spaces and consequent problems in cardiac function due to 'pooling' of blood in these areas. In the formative phase, occlusion of bony foramina can prove a problem and the relative avascularity following redeposition of bone can then make infection in bone more difficult to manage. Paget's disease is essentially a disease of the elderly, although a juvenile form is recognised.

Clinical appearance

The skull can enlarge, as can the jaws and in particular the maxilla. Deformity can result from vertebral column and lower limbs being unable to deal with the forces and deforming as a result. This deformation led to Paget's disease being known as 'osteitis deformans', but this term is now rarely used. Enlargement of the jaws, where they are affected, may result in loss of fit of prostheses and the teeth themselves may show excessive deposits of cement known as hypercementosis.

Diagnosis

Blood samples may show very high levels of alkaline phosphatase with normal values for calcium and phosphate. Radiographs show patchy areas of radiolucency interspersed with radio-opaque density. The descriptive term 'cotton wool' has been used to describe these changes and is an accurate reflection of the radiographic changes seen. Bone biopsy may show irregular areas of resorption or evidence of previous resorption in the form of reversal lines. These are heavily staining haematoxilin lines, which denote the boundary of previous resorptive activity.

Management

In the general management of Paget's disease, bisphosphonates are the usual form of treatment. These drugs appear to have a direct effect on hydroxyapatite crystals, which make the bone less receptive to resorptive activity and hence reduce the rate of turnover. Dental problems may be encountered in the form of excessive bleeding if the area of the jaw affected is undergoing active resorption, and infection can be a complication where the bone has reformed and become relatively avascular. Added to these problems may be hypercementosis of the roots resulting in large-rooted teeth that may be difficult to extract conventionally. Prophylactic antibiotics are often prescribed for extractions if the bone is sclerotic and areas of exposed bone such as prominent interdental or interradicular septa should be trimmed and covered by soft tissues with appropriate suturing.

Rickets

Rickets arises as a result of defective calcium and phosphorus metabolism during bone growth. After cessation of bone growth the condition causes osteomalacia. It may occur in three ways (Table 36.5).

Biochemistry reveals a low normal calcium and phosphate (both maintained by parathyroid activity) and an increased bone alkaline phosphatase level. Treatment is with oral vitamin D.

Scurvy

Scurvy is caused by vitamin C deficiency. This is now not seen in clinical practice but, historically, caused bone defects due to defective collagen formation, which also caused bone pains due to periosteal haemorrhage.

Table 36.5 Vitamin D deficiency	
Reduced intake/ absorption	Poor dietary content of vitamin D Fat malabsorption – steatorrhoea
Skin synthesis impaired	Lack of exposure to sunlight Pigmented skin
Metabolism abnormal	Impaired renal activation of 25-hydroxyvitamin D to 1,25-dihydroxy vitamin D; e.g. chronic renal failure Interference by anticonvulsant drugs

37 Dental implants

Introduction

Dental implants are now increasingly used to attach crowns, bridges or dentures by anchorage to bone. Extra-oral implants are also available for attaching facial prostheses such as artificial ears or noses, and for bone anchored hearing aids.

Placement of implants requires careful patient selection and treatment planning. Although the surgical techniques are straightforward, they are exacting and practitioners should only embark on implant treatment after appropriate training and experience.

Types of implant

Early implants were unreliable because the attachment to bone was by a layer of connective tissue. A variety of pins, screws and blades were tried but epithelial downgrowth frequently led to rejection. The resulting loss of alveolar bone led to an even more difficult restorative problem.

Subperiosteal implants were less damaging but required a general anaesthetic to expose the bone surface for impression taking. Chrome–cobalt frames were constructed in the laboratory and a further anaesthetic was then required for insertion. They were often in function for many years but epithelial downgrowth usually resulted in failure. Removal of failed implants was difficult due extensive scar tissue.

Transmandibular implants appeared to have some advantages but an extraoral incision was required and the surgical technique was demanding. They were obviously unsuitable for routine use as they required specialist expertise and hospital facilities.

The progression to modern implantology followed the discovery of osseointegration, with the predictable success of titanium implants. Osseointegration implies

Table 37.1   Osseointegrated dental implants
Osseointegration
Indications for implant treatment
Patient selection
Treatment planning
Surgical technique
Augmentation of bone
Complications
Success rates

contact between the implant surface and bone without any intervening connective tissue layer. It is, in fact, an ankylosis of implant to bone and some prefer the term 'functional ankylosis'. The bone does not recognise the implant as a foreign body, which becomes, in effect, part of the bone. Thus an osseointegrated implant forms a direct bone anchorage for a prosthesis.

Osseointegration is therefore a prerequisite to successful implant placement and a consideration of the requirements for this is followed by a description of the indications for implant placement in dentistry. Discussion of patient selection and treatment planning will be followed by a description of the surgical techniques involved in implant placement including augmentation techniques, complications and a consideration of success rates (Table 37.1).

Osseointegration

The requirements for successful osseointegration of an implant are listed in Table 37.2. Suitable implant materials are discussed below.

Implant materials

Ideally, an implant should be non-toxic, biocompatible, strong and aesthetic.

Table 37.2   Requirements for osseointegration

Suitable implant material
Minimal surgical trauma
Primary implant stability
Adequate bone volume and quality
Delayed loading (healing phase)

Metals such as nickel and chromium used in stainless steel are corroded in living tissue and taken into the bloodstream. There is concern about possible neurotoxicity. Titanium is also absorbed and may be detected in tissues at very low concentrations, but there is no evidence of toxicity.

Implant materials can be biotolerated, bioinert or bioactive. Stainless steel, chrome cobalt and other alloys are tolerated by bone but are linked by a connective tissue layer rather than an intimate bond. Titanium implants make direct contact with bone but are regarded as bioinert because there is no chemical bond. Bioactive materials such as calcium phosphate and hydroxyapatite allow a true chemical bond to develop as the bone surface remodels.

The material should be able to withstand occlusal forces and be capable of accurate machining into cylinders with screw threads for initial stability in bone, and with suitable abutment connections. Unfortunately, a bioactive material with adequate mechanical properties has not yet been developed.

Surface characteristics can modify the properties of the material. Correct pore size is important in osseointegration of ceramics. Surface roughness may affect the reaction of tissues to implants enhancing osseointegration as well as increasing the surface area in contact with bone.

Titanium

Titanium is the best material available at present. It is a highly reactive metal that oxidises in the atmosphere to form an inert surface layer of titanium oxide. It has good mechanical properties and can be machined. Implant fractures can occur but these are minimised by careful implant design and avoidance of a traumatic occlusion. A disadvantage of titanium is its grey colour, which may be visible at crown margins if there is recession and may discolour thin mucosa. The surface can be polished and anodised and surface roughness can be achieved by addition or subtraction processes. In plasma coating, titanium powder is sprayed onto the implant as an inert

gas at high temperature in an electric arc. Plasma-sprayed implants have a much greater surface area and mechanical resistance to rotational forces. Abrasion of the surface with titanium pellets or grit blasting and acid etching may also achieve similar effects. Some workers claim that these surface modifications promote a chemical and mechanical attachment to bone. Rough surfaces exposed to the mouth will be difficult to keep clean and plaque formation will result in peri-implant disease. Transmucosal elements and abutments are therefore made smooth. A 'gingival' cuff attachment is achieved by reorientation of connective tissue fibres and possibly by adhesion of epithelial cells.

Ceramic

Ceramic implants had good biological and aesthetic properties but lacked mechanical strength. In practice the incidence of implant fracture was unacceptable and they have been discontinued. It is possible that better ceramics will be developed.

Hydroxyapatite

Hydroxyapatite can be used as a coating on titanium implants because it is osteoinductive. It enhances, and reduces the time for, osseointegration. It is also used in particle or block form to augment bone for placement of implants. It does have mechanical weakness and disruption of the surface occurs in function, although these microfractures do not seem to result in loss of implants. Fractures can also occur at the interface between hydroxyapatite and titanium.

Implant system

Many implant systems are available and many factors need to be considered when making a choice. These are listed in Table 37.3.

Surgical principles

Initially an implant bed must be prepared by drilling a hole in the bone to receive the implant. It is essential to minimise tissue damage when preparing the implant bed. Mucoperiosteal flaps should be well designed, carefully reflected and gently retracted, so that healing is optimal. Healthy soft tissue cover enhances osseointegration by providing a barrier to infection and restoration of blood

Table 37.3 Criteria affecting choice of implant system
Use commercially pure titanium
Components proven to withstand masticatory load
Physiological response of bone when loaded
One- or two-stage system
Type of surface, i.e. plain, plasma sprayed, roughened or hydroxyapatite coated
Plain cylinder, or threaded ± self-tapping
Diameter and length
Efficiency of drill system
Immediate or delayed loading
Suitability of abutments

Table 37.4 Bone drilling for osseointegration
Use sharp drills (single or limited use)
Use purpose designed drills
Use drills of smaller diameters first, rather than one-stage cutting
Use slow drill speeds (<2000 rpm)
Use cooling with copious chilled saline
Avoid clogging of drill channels – repeated withdrawal
Thread tapping or self-tapping systems are available

Table 37.5 Methods of improving implant success in the maxilla
Use additional implants to share load
Use connecting bars for bracing
Use maximum length of implant
Consider augmentation of ridge bone
Consider sinus lift to extend available ridge
Reduce occlusal table and eliminate traumatic occlusion
Allow more time for osseointegration

supply. With transmucosal systems, soft tissue is sutured around the implant neck and a good seal is even more important.

Bone preparation is carried out with the minimum heat production so that, as far as possible, the osteocytes near the bone surface remain vital. If there is bone damage the inflammatory reaction will produce a fibrous repair resulting in a connective tissue layer between implant and bone rather than osseointegration.

The requirements that must be taken into account when drilling bone to receive an implant are listed in Table 37.4.

Primary implant stability

The implant bed should be prepared accurately to conform to the shape of the implant, so that there is maximum contact with healthy bone. This good congruence also results in primary implant stability, which is essential during the healing phase.

Screw threads are often used as they increase primary stability, enhance resistance to occlusal forces and increase surface area.

Bone quality and quantity

Blood supply is essential for bone vitality so the maxilla might be thought to be better suited for implant placement. In fact, there is a significantly better success rate in the mandible, which is likely to have a poorer blood supply especially in the older edentulous patient. It seems, therefore, that a firmer bone structure is an advantage. The cortical plate in the maxilla is often thin or absent and the cancellous bone is crumbly.

The pattern of bone resorption and anatomical structures in the maxilla also cause problems. Resorption causes bone loss from the anterior and crestal surfaces, often leaving a narrow ridge in a retruded and high position. Thus there is less bone and the implants have to be placed in a poor position. The superstructures may then be placed in a compromised position. The occlusal load on the implants may therefore be beyond physiological tolerances.

Implants can still successfully be placed in the maxilla if allowance is made to avoid exceeding the above limitations by the methods listed in Table 37.5.

Resorption in the mandible does not alter the antero-posterior implant position but there can be severe loss of bone height. The alveolar bone has often been completely resorbed and there is a pencil-thin mandible. Augmentation is rarely required, even in this situation, and two implants may be sufficient to stabilise a lower denture. This is fortunate, as denture instability is more of a problem in the mandible.

Blood supply may be compromised by radiotherapy but, although this causes more failures in the mandible, there is still a reasonable success rate. In the maxilla there are many more failures after radiotherapy. A course of preoperative and postoperative hyperbaric oxygen therapy, if available, may improve success in the maxilla but is not usually needed in the mandible.

Table 37.6	Classification of bone quality
I	Cortical bone predominant
II	Dense cancellous bone and thick cortical bone
III	Dense cancellous bone and thin cortical bone
IV	Porous cancellous bone and thin cortical bone

Table 37.7	Indications for implant treatment
	Difficult edentulous cases
	Long span bridges
	Free end saddles
	Single tooth replacement
	Special indications

The quality of bone available is also important and this can be assessed using the classification listed in Table 37.6.

Healing phase

It is a fundamental requirement that undue loading is avoided until osseointegration has occurred. This is one of the main differences compared to previous implant practice where there was immediate loading and osseointegration rarely occurred.

In the mandible, 3 or 4 months are required for osseointegration, whereas in the maxilla 6 months is allowed. These rules have been relaxed in the anterior mandible only. If bone quality is good, depth is adequate and four or five (or possibly fewer) implants are placed, the superstructure may be fitted immediately. Theoretically, function encourages bone formation and there is some evidence that controlled loading could be beneficial. This is difficult to control in practice at present.

Indications for implant treatment

The availability of implants has expanded treatment options for a number of restorative problems highlighted in Table 37.7.

Difficult edentulous cases

Poor retention of a mandibular prosthesis not only interferes with eating but also inhibits social contact, as patients are afraid that the denture will dislodge in speech or mastication. The attached mucosal ridge may be little more than 1 mm wide and the sulcus mucosa is prone to pain or ulceration. Severe resorption often results in prominent genial tubercles or exteriorisation of the mental nerves so that provision of a comfortable denture is impossible. An implant-supported fixed prosthesis restores function and confidence. An implant-supported removable denture is a simple, cheaper and effective option. Two implants with stud attachments or a bar can be sufficient to stabilise a denture, which is then mainly tissue borne. Implants are always placed between the mental foramina in edentulous cases.

Retention problems occur in the maxilla, although less frequently because the hard palate gives better support and retention for a conventional denture. Resorption can lead to a flabby ridge and retrusion. Implants placed in the anterior maxilla will aid retention and stability but poor bone quality requires placement of as many implants as possible and a bar may be required for bracing.

Patients who are unable to tolerate a denture, due to gagging, or who are unwilling to wear a removable appliance, can benefit from an implant-born bridge, although the lip will not be as well supported as with a denture flange. This problem should be explained to the patient, who may then prefer a conventional denture.

If the patient decides on implant treatment, ridge augmentation may be necessary, especially in the maxilla. The available bone can also be increased by a sinus lift where a bone graft or synthetic material is placed in the maxillary antrum.

Long span bridges

Implants can be used where the span is too long for a conventional bridge or when abutment teeth are compromised by bone loss, short roots or extensive restoration.

In the maxilla, there may be limiting factors such as inadequate or poor quality bone. Resorption may result in an unfavourable position or angulation of the implant, necessitating a long clinical crown or placement of the restoration well in front of the ridge. These aesthetic problems are noticeable with a short upper lip. Lip contour may be not be as good as that obtained by a denture flange. Augmentation should be considered as in edentulous cases.

In the mandible, the pattern of bone resorption is less of a problem and the main constraint is the proximity of the inferior alveolar or mental nerves.

Free end saddles

Replacement of mandibular molars is difficult with conventional dentures. There is a risk of mental anaesthesia when placing implants in the posterior mandible so it is essential to allow a good safety margin when calculating implant length. Drill tips do not conform exactly to the shape of the implant so allowance must be made for the additional depth of the implant bed. The maxillary antrum limits implant placement in the posterior maxilla.

Single tooth replacement

It can be simple and cost effective to replace an incisor tooth with an implant when there is adequate bone. If there is a diastema, the difficulties in construction of an adhesive bridge or partial denture are avoided. Also, preparation of adjacent teeth is avoided and there are no denture clasps. Unfortunately, the pattern of bone resorption can result in an unfavourable path of implant emergence in the maxilla (especially if there is a history of previous replantation or transplantation of a canine or incisor). If there is crowding, the nasopalatine canal can be large enough to prevent implant placement. This can sometimes be overcome by restoration of ridge form by bone augmentation.

Special indications

Implants may also be indicated under special circumstances that are not dental in nature. These are listed in Table 37.8.

Patient selection

Patient selection is important when planning implant treatment to avoid a poor outcome and complications.

Clinical history and examination

The clinical history and examination will reveal the patient's caries and periodontal disease experience. Patient compliance can be an important indication of suitability. It is also important to ascertain the patient's expectations of treatment.

Table 37.8 Special indications for implant treatment
Wind instrument players or singers Denture intolerance due to gagging Psychological aversion to dentures Xerostomia, e.g. Sjögren's syndrome Physical disability (e.g. cerebral palsy, stroke or myasthenia gravis)

Table 37.9 Medical problems compromising implant success
Cardiac disease Haematological disease Immunological disease Bone disorders Other systemic disease Oral disease

Medical history

A detailed consideration of the patient's medical history is essential because several conditions can compromise implant success by interfering with healing, or increasing the risk of infection (Table 37.9).

Cardiac disease

Severe cardiac problems can present risk but many patients with mild disease can benefit from implants. Simple questions about exercise tolerance give an indication of the patient's ability to withstand a surgical procedure. Implant failure is more likely in a patient with severe debilitation. Patients who are at risk of endocarditis may be suitable but regular monitoring and radiographs are advisable, and any failing implant should be removed without delay. Implants are contraindicated in patients who have had a recent myocardial infarct, a valve replacement, are in cardiac failure or who have had previous bacterial endocarditis.

Haematological disease

Treated or mild anaemias should not prevent implant treatment. Patients with haemophilia and other significant factor deficiencies would not normally be suitable. Warfarin therapy is a relative contraindication, but surgery may be possible in selected cases with careful monitoring of the international normalized ratio (INR).

Immunological problems

Prolonged corticosteroid therapy can present a risk but the patient can be given steroid cover. Implant survival may be reduced in patients on corticosteroids and this should be balanced against the potential benefit to the patient. Patients on chemotherapy and those with severe immune deficiency should not be considered. Drug addiction depresses immune responses and implies poor compliance. Smoking has an adverse effect on implant survival and patients should be strongly advised to cease. Smoking most probably reduces the success rate by significantly reducing the bony blood supply, especially to the mandible.

Bone disorders

Most bone diseases are a contraindication. Osteoporosis is especially common in older females but the jaws are less affected and implants can still be successfully placed.

If a patient has undergone radiotherapy there will be a poor success rate in the maxilla although hyperbaric oxygen (HBO) has been used with some success. Fewer problems are encountered in the mandible and HBO is not essential.

Other systemic diseases

Many other medical conditions, such as renal or liver disease, can compromise treatment and consultation with the patient's physician is advisable if in doubt. Individuals with well-controlled diabetes can be accepted, although they have a greater risk of peri-implant disease. Patients with psychiatric disorders should be accepted with caution, especially if they attribute their problems to dental disorders.

Oral disease

It is important to ensure that the patient has a stable periodontal condition and low caries rate at the time of assessment, although many patients require implant treatment as a result of previous neglect. Mucosal disorders should be eliminated as far as possible. Bone quality and availability should be assessed (Table 37.6).

Treatment planning

Apart from appropriate patient selection, successful treatment planning requires consideration of the available bone and space within the mouth (Table 37.10) and the associated anatomical structures (Table 37.11). Treatment planning also needs to be informed by appropriate radiographic examination and examination of articulated study casts.

Radiographic examination

Conventional radiography, including an orthpantomograph (OPT) and periapical or lateral views where relevant, is necessary. The OPT is most useful because it indicates vertical bone height and the position of all relevant bone cavities and nerve canals. It is important to make allowance for distortion and magnification when using an OPT. Transparent overlays are available but more accuracy can be obtained by inserting a base plate with standard metal balls or strips of gutta percha over the planned implant positions before taking the radiograph. This latter method enables exact calculation of available bone when implants are to be placed close to the inferior alveolar nerve or other important structures.

Serial tomograms or computerised tomography (CT) scans may also be used where detailed mapping of available bone and anatomical structures is required. CT scans are not always readily available and they involve a

Table 37.10 Available bone and space for implants
6- or 7-mm ridge width (i.e. implant diameter + 2 mm)
Proximity of adjacent teeth or foramina (incisive, mental)
Adequate distance between implants for superstructure
Depth of bone
Safety margin for inferior alveolar nerve, floor of nose and maxillary antrum
Undercuts
Sufficient intermaxillary space for superstructure

Table 37.11 Anatomical structures important in implant treatment planning
Maxilla
floor of nose
maxillary antrum
nasopalatine foramen
Mandible
inferior alveolar nerve
mental nerve

much higher radiation dose. Scatter due to metal restorations can render the image unusable. CT images can be very helpful but can be disappointing unless the radiologist is familiar with dental requirements and software.

Magnetic resonance imaging (MRI) is becoming more readily available. It has no radiation dose and the only known hazard is with ferrous metals in the magnetic field. It is likely to replace CT scanning and – eventually – most other X-ray investigations. New machines will be less likely to induce claustrophobia and noise levels are now significantly reduced.

Study casts

Study casts are invaluable for demonstrating treatment options. Duplicates can be used for a diagnostic wax-up so that tooth position can be planned. A template can then be constructed with indicator holes drilled as an aid to the surgeon, so that implants are placed in the optimum position at operation.

Other treatment options

After considering the factors relating to patient selection and treatment planning, restorative options should be considered (Table 37.12).

Surgical technique

Flap design

Mucoperiosteal flaps are usually taken along the crest of the ridge. Relieving incisions may be short, as it is not usually necessary to expose all the alveolar bone. If there are adjacent teeth it may be necessary to release the interdental papilla. Flaps should be handled carefully as poor healing could compromise osseointegration.

With two-stage implants where the implant is buried, it used to be common practice to keep the incision away

Table 37.12   Treatment options
Removable partial denture
Fixed bridge
Complete denture
Implant-supported denture
Implant-supported bridge
No prosthesis

from the crest so that the suture line was not directly over the implant. This was technically more difficult and is now less popular because of the risk of haematoma formation or flap necrosis.

When augmentation procedures are planned, a bevelled flap is taken so that mucosal cover of the membrane or graft is achieved. A bevelled flap taken from the palatal aspect can also be used to improve the bulk of buccal interdental papilla when uncovering a buried implant at the second stage.

Bone drilling

Purpose-made sharp drills are essential. Many manufacturers advise single use and supply prepacked sterile drill kits. It is essential to have an accurate indication of drill speed so that overheating is avoided by keeping below 2000 rpm. Thermal damage is also minimised by incremental drill stages up to the final diameter. Thread tapping, where required, may be hand driven or by very slow drilling, preferably using a drill with a torque controller. Copious irrigation with chilled saline solution is essential. Drills must be withdrawn frequently to allow cooling and prevent clogging of the drill channels. It is important to maintain drill direction, or the implant bed will be inaccurate.

Countersinking is used where the system requires the cover screw to be buried or where the transmucosal element is to be submerged to improve aesthetics.

Insertion

Decontaminated and sterilised implants are individually packed in vials. Titanium forceps are used if handling of the implant is required, but this is not normally necessary due to the design of manufacturer's delivery system. A fixture mount may be included in the package or attached by the operator.

The implant should be placed with as little contamination as possible. Good flap retraction will reduce contamination by saliva and epithelial surfaces. The method of insertion varies but most implants are screwed in either by hand or using a drill with a torque controller. Irrigation is used to prevent overheating. Excessive force should not be used because heat will be generated, and there is also a danger of damage to the implant or cold welding it onto the fixture mount.

A cover screw is placed and the soft tissues are sutured over or around the fixture according to the system in use.

With two-stage systems, where the implant and cover screw are covered by mucosa, it is important to ensure that the cover screw is seated properly, as soft tissue or bone formation below the cover screw can be difficult to remove from the implant face at the second stage.

Abutment connection

Two-stage implants have to be uncovered to allow abutment placement. This is done through a small incision on the crest of the ridge or by removing a circle of mucosa using a punch. Bone may have grown over the cover screw and this is removed using the manufacturer's bone mill. Instruments are also available to remove any bone that has formed on the implant face because of a loose cover screw. The implant face must not be damaged during bone removal as the junction with the abutment is accurately machined. A portal of entry for micro-organisms would cause problems with infection later.

A suitable abutment is chosen and screwed in, taking care that it is seated correctly and avoiding crossed threads. Selection of a suitable abutment at this stage can be difficult because the soft tissue level will vary as the mucosal cuff matures. Alternatively, a healing abutment can be placed and the final abutment is selected once the soft tissues have healed.

Augmentation of bone

When there is insufficient width or height of bone it may be possible to gain additional bone either before or at the time of implant placement.

Various methods of bone augmentation can be used, including onlay grafts, guided bone regeneration, sinus lift procedures or ridge expansion. Bone graft materials may be in block or granular form (Table 37.13).

Table 37.13   Bone graft materials
Autograft: patient's own bone, e.g. iliac crest, tibia or intraoral
Allograft: human donor (not used due to risk of cross-infection)
Xenograft: calcified matrix derived from biological material, e.g. bovine bone or coral (no risk of cross-infection due to removal of protein?)
Synthetic material: e.g. hydroxyapatite, tricalcium phosphate, glass

Onlay grafts

Blocks of bone may be used for extensive defects. Cortical bone taken from the patient's iliac crest or calvarium is preferred but harvest involves major surgery and the risk of donor site morbidity. Implants are placed some months later when the graft has taken.

Immediate placement is also advocated, as early loading may reduce resorption and the patient is spared a second operation. However, there may be an increased risk of loss of fixtures and bone due to infection.

A reliable substitute for autologous block bone is still awaited.

Guided bone regeneration

Healing by osteoblasts produces bone but, when a blood clot is organised by fibroblasts, collagen formation is predominant and scar tissue is formed. When a suitable membrane is placed over bone, however, fibroblasts are excluded and angiogenesis and osteogenesis occur in the cavity below. This is the basis of guided bone regeneration.

Membranes can be non-resorbable (e.g. polytetrafluorethylene) or resorbable (e.g. collagen). The shape of the cavity can be maintained by using a reinforced membrane. Alternatively, the membrane can be supported with bone, bone substitute or a mixture of both. Small steel posts may also be used as supports. The periphery of the membrane is stabilised by screws or pins, which can also be resorbable. Recent developments with the use of bone morphogenic proteins may revolutionise bone augmentation in the future.

Sinus lift procedure

There is often insufficient bone height in the posterior maxilla due to bone resorption and the presence of the maxillary antrum. Onlay bone grafts are prone to failure and may be unsuitable due to lack of intermaxillary space. The sinus lift procedure creates additional alveolar bone height within the antral space.

The antral lining is exposed by removing a window of bone on the buccal aspect via a buccal mucoperiosteal flap. The antral lining is carefully elevated intact and is supported by bone-grafting material. It is also possible to leave the bony window attached to the antral lining and support both with graft material or implants. Immediate implant placement is only advised if there is sufficient bone for primary implant stability (about 6 mm in height).

An alternative is to approach the antral floor using osteotomes to enlarge a bur hole on the crest of the ridge. The antral lining can then be lifted and supported by bone graft material. When there is sufficient bone for primary implant stability the lining can be lifted through an implant preparation. If the preparation is stopped just short of the antral floor the cortical plate can be tapped upwards with the lining. The cortical plate and the implant then provide support for the lining.

Ridge expansion

Where there is sufficient bone depth but the ridge is too narrow, the implant bed may be prepared by bone expansion, provided that there is a cancellous layer between the cortical plates. The crest of the ridge is exposed leaving the rest of the alveolar bone attached to mucoperiosteum. The ridge is widened by D-shaped and round osteotomes between the cortical plates prior to drilling.

Success rates

The patient's appreciation is a very good indicator of success but objective criteria are required to monitor the effectiveness of osseointegrated implants (Table 37.14). Various criteria have been suggested but the most reliable way to obtain comparable data is to record removal rates. Cumulative survival rates are based on an actuarial calculation that allows for the fact that implants in a series will have been present for differing times. It is reasonable to expect that, in the maxilla, 90% of implants will survive for 10 years. In the mandible a 95% 10-year survival is expected.

A number of adverse events may complicate implant placement (Table 37.15). Avoidance of these complications can only be achieved by careful planning and an exacting surgical technique based on sound training and experience.

Table 37.14   Criteria for evaluation of success

Patient satisfaction
Survival
Suitable position
Mobility
Amount of bone loss
Health of adjacent soft tissues – pocketing and
    inflammation
Infections or radiographic evidence of peri-implant bone
    pathology
Operative complications e.g. damage to nerves or
    adjacent teeth

Table 37.15   Complications of implant treatment

Intraoperative
    implant in poor position
    damage to mucosa and adjacent teeth
    bone damage, i.e. lateral perforation, fracture of
        alveolar bone or mandibular fracture
    perforation into adjacent areas, e.g. lower border of
        mandible, nasal cavity or maxillary antrum
    nerve damage, e.g. inferior alveolar nerve
    loose implant due to incorrect drilling
    contamination of implant or bone
    implant damage, e.g. crossed thread or surface defect
    primary haemorrhage – especially floor of mouth,
        possible airway compromise
Postoperative
    pain
    swelling
    reactionary or secondary haemorrhage
    infection of peri-implant soft tissue or bone
    exposed or loose cover screws
Late
    mucosal recession
    bone resorption
    mobility
    implant fracture

38 Cryosurgery and laser surgery

Introduction

Conventional surgery has used the scalpel to cut or excise tissue during surgical procedures. The scalpel, however, has limitations as a surgical tool. When an area of tissue is excised haemorrhage may be difficult to control and a skin graft or flap may be needed to cover the defect or prevent scarring. Cutting or coagulating diathermy cause damage to the adjacent tissues. The physical effects of cold and lasers offer alternative methods of removing or devitalising tissue. They work in different ways and they will be considered in turn.

Cryosurgery

Cryosurgery relies on the fact that rapid freezing and thawing of tissues cause cell death and necrosis. Cryosurgery is thought to cause ice crystals in and around cells, causing disruption of cell membranes and contents. These effects are enhanced by rapid freeze and thaw cycles. Blood flow to the area is reduced so that a larger and colder 'iceball' is achieved at the next application. Vascular damage also results in ischaemic necrosis. Immune mechanisms may be altered with beneficial or adverse effects.

Oral lesions are often surrounded by abnormal mucosa. The operator must therefore consider the effects of cryosurgery at the edges of treated area. If there is epithelial dysplasia it is possible that cryosurgery could potentiate malignant change.

Uses of cryosurgery

Cryosurgery can be used in a number of conditions and in several is the treatment of choice (Table 38.1).

Freezing can be used to treat surface lesions such as warts or small tumours. It is particularly suitable for

Table 38.1   Uses of cryosurgery
Ablation of warts and small tumours
Ablation of haemangiomas
Treatment of bony cavities
Blocking of nerves

haemangiomas around the mouth. Several applications may be required but cryosurgery has the advantage that there is no haemorrhage and the surface may be left intact. Viral warts necrose and vascular lesions regress. There is often significant oedema but postoperative pain is unusual. With a deeper freeze the mucosa or skin may necrose, but re-epithelialisation occurs as the lesion sloughs away and healing is usually good with minimal scarring.

Bone cavities may be treated to reduce recurrence of lesions such as odontogenic keratocysts or central giant cell granulomata. The bone is devitalised but still remains functional until it is replaced by vital tissue. In the mandible the inferior alveolar nerve may be spared as nerves regenerate surprisingly well after freezing.

Cryosurgery is also used to treat painful nerve lesions because nerves can be blocked without causing the secondary neuralgia that often follows nerve section, avulsion or alcohol blocks. Pain relief lasts for several months but repeat treatments are often required. The evidence-base for this application of cryosurgery is lacking but it has a place when conventional treatments are ineffective. Infraorbital, mental or inferior alveolar nerves can be treated after surgical exposure. An intraoral approach is used. The most common condition treated in this way is trigeminal neuralgia that no longer responds to therapy with drugs such as carbamazepine, or when drug side-effects are severe. Neurosurgical options should always be kept in mind. The surgical management of trigeminal neuralgia is discussed in Chapter 19.

Cryosurgery has been advocated for ablation of malignant tumours either as a curative procedure or for palliation. Incomplete ablation of the lesion is unacceptable and could easily occur, as it is not possible to predict accurately the extent of tissue destruction. Moreover, case reports of accelerated tumour growth following incomplete treatment raise the possibility that host immune response is compromised. Malignant and premalignant lesions are therefore better treated by other methods.

Cryoprobes

Dermatologists apply liquid nitrogen to skin lesions using a stick but a more precise method is needed for the mouth. A cryoprobe is a surgical instrument with a cold tip. The temperature is determined by the boiling point of the refrigerant liquid. The freezing effect may be achieved by evaporation at normal pressure, as with liquid nitrogen applied directly with a stick or spray, or within the probe tip. Other probe tips rely on the Joule Thompson effect, where a pressurised gas is forced through a small orifice. The refrigerant properties of the various liquid systems are listed in Table 38.2.

Nitrous oxide units are commonly available in hospitals and are suitable for most oral applications. They work from a nitrous oxide cylinder so they are always ready for use. Liquid nitrogen machines are much more powerful but must be filled with liquid nitrogen on each occasion. This can be inconvenient for routine use and handling a liquid at $-196°C$ is hazardous.

Probe tips come in a variety of shapes and sizes. Flat or dome-shaped tips from 3 to 10 mm are useful in the mouth (Fig. 38.1). Long, narrow, insulated probes are available for freezing nerves.

Cryosurgery techniques

Under local anaesthesia the probe is applied to the lesion and switched on. The probe is held firmly onto the lesion until an ice-ball forms and freezing is continued. The time of application will usually be about 1 min. The probe should not be pulled away because it will be adherent to the lesion. For vascular lesions, the effect is enhanced by compressing the lesion with the probe, which decreases blood flow. On turning the machine off there should be a rapid thaw and the probe is released.

One or two further applications are made after 1 min to allow a complete thaw. Experience is necessary to

Table 38.2 Refrigerant properties of liquid cryoprobe systems		
Type	Boiling point	Surface temperature
Liquid nitrogen probe	$-196°C$	$-150°C$
Nitrous oxide probe	$-89°C$	$-75°C$
Carbon dioxide probe	$-78°C$	$-50°C$
Liquid nitrogen spray	$-196°C$	$-196°C$

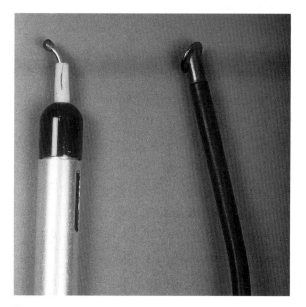

Fig. 38.1 A variety of shapes and sizes of cryoprobe tips.

judge the amount of treatment and the extent of the freeze. The size of the ice-ball produced in a glass of water gives an indication of the effects on tissue temperature but the blood supply will modify this effect in living tissue.

If necessary, a specimen can be obtained for histopathology while the lesion is frozen. Haemostasis would then be required and, of course, there would be a surface defect. Freezing fixes the tissue temporarily before transfer to formal saline so that good sections are possible.

Some liquid nitrogen units have the option of probe or spray freezing. The latter is a very effective tool for use on wide areas or uneven surfaces. It produces a very rapid deep freeze and is more effective than the probe for freezing large soft tissue lesions.

When treating a bone cavity after curettage of a lesion, a water-soluble gel may be used to aid contact with the bone surface and, in this situation, a liquid nitrogen unit

Table 38.3 Advantages and disadvantages of cryosurgery
Advantages
no haemorrhage
minimal postoperative pain
good recovery of nerve function
minimal scarring
bone structure maintained
blood vessel recovery
adjacent normal tissues recover
excellent for haemangiomas
possible treatment of painful nerve lesions
Disadvantages
cannot be used to cut tissues
difficulty in assessing extent of treatment
excessive swelling (could endanger airway)
effects at the periphery (dysplastic changes can be potentiated)
whole lesion not available for pathology
tumour growth may be accelerated
not effective for lymphangiomas

would be necessary to provide an adequate effect. A liquid nitrogen spray would be preferable because it produces a much faster and deeper freeze.

Care must be taken to retract and protect mucosal flaps and adjacent soft tissues, especially with liquid nitrogen machines.

It is also possible to freeze a resected portion of mandibular bone after tumour ablation and replace it to restore continuity without the need to use a bone graft. The bone section is placed in a container of liquid nitrogen. This method is not often used because it is possible that some cells from the original lesion could survive. The most common reason for removal of full thickness mandible is squamous cell carcinoma, and such a risk would not be acceptable.

Advantages and disadvantages of cryosurgery

Cryosurgery is the preferred treatment for some conditions but it has certain drawbacks. The advantages and disadvantages of cryosurgery are listed in Table 38.3.

Lasers

'Laser' is an acronym for 'Light Amplification by Stimulated Emission of Radiation'. The properties of laser light depend on wavelength. A CO_2 laser at 10.6 μm wavelength produces invisible light that is absorbed by water and biological tissues and destroys them on contact. An argon laser produces visible light at around 0.5 μm; this passes through water but is absorbed by pigments such as melanin or haemoglobin. It may be used in eye surgery because it will not damage the lens or eye contents but acts on the retinal surface in treating conditions such as diabetic retinopathy or a detached retina. Surgical lasers are usually designed for cutting, coagulation and ablation of tissue. When a CO_2 laser beam meets the target tissue its energy is converted into heat. Cell structure is destroyed by expansion as water boils. Denaturation of proteins also occurs but the laser lesion deepens mainly as a result of cell disintegration at its surface. The result is a very narrow layer of tissue damage below the treated area and better healing.

Light waves from a normal source do not produce a powerful cutting beam because they emerge randomly at various wavelengths. Laser light, however, is spatially and temporally coherent. This means that the waves are all of the same wavelength (monochromatic) and are in parallel, so that none of the energy from the light source is lost by interference. Compare a 60-watt light bulb producing light and heat with a 60-watt laser beam that would cut through steel.

Laser light has many similar properties to ordinary light. It is reflected by mirror surfaces. At some wavelengths it will travel along an optic fibre or be refracted in a lens or prism. These effects are used to deliver the light to the probe tip or operating microscope and to focus it on the object. Alternatively, a fibre delivers the energy by contact or proximity with the target. When the beam is invisible, as with the CO_2 laser, a red aiming beam is often provided.

Output may be in a continuous wave or pulsed. Pulses are single or repeated typically with a duration of 0.1 s or less. Pulses of less than 1 μs are produced in Q-switched lasers, which deliver very high energy without generating excessive heat.

Tissue effects may be photoablative (molecular disruption), photothermal (cutting or coagulation), photomechanical (tissue disruption) or photochemical (photodynamic therapy). Low power lasers have been used to enhance healing, promote blood clotting and relieve pain, although these effects still require controlled clinical trials to exclude a placebo effect.

If a laser beam strikes a shiny surface it may be reflected and burn healthy tissue, the operator or others nearby. Laser beams travel without loss of intensity, so even if the beam is focused it may cause damage at a

Table 38.4 **Precautions required when using lasers**
Non-reflective instruments (achieved by sand blasting)
Protective goggles
Wet swabs to protect tissues
Restricted access to laser area, warning lights and notices
Training and certification of users
Armoured or reflective endotraccheal tubes (+ inflation of cuffs with water)
Avoidance of inflammable skin prepping solutions
Smoke evacuation (+ face mask)

distance. Moreover, it will continue to cut deeper into the wound as long as it is applied An anaesthetic tube can easily be pierced, resulting in ignition of anaesthetic gases within the lungs, which is usually fatal.

There is also concern about the potential effects of plume or surgical smoke produced by electrosurgery and lasers. Toxic chemicals are produced when tissue is burned. Blood aerosols and viruses such as human papilloma virus in the laser plume are thought to be capable of transmitting disease. A surgeon's mask alone does not provide adequate protection. High-volume aspiration (similar to that on dental units but with special filters) is recommended.

In view of these hazards to patient and operator special precautions are needed and these are listed in Table 38.4.

Oral surgical applications

The CO_2 laser is most useful and is readily available in general hospitals. At present, the most frequent indications are soft tissue lesions where the extent of the excision prevents primary closure, and where skin grafting was previously required to prevent scarring.

White patches and premalignant lesions

Biopsy is essential to determine the diagnosis and degree of epithelial dysplasia. Nutritional deficiencies such as iron or vitamin B_{12} should be treated. Patients must be strongly advised to give up smoking. If lesions do not respond and excision is required, the CO_2 laser is a good option.

Erythroplakia and premalignant leukoplakia

These are treated similarly. Mildly dysplastic superficial lesions can be treated by ablation. Severely dysplastic lesions need a deeper excision and it is then advisable to use the laser as a knife so that the whole lesion can be sent for histopathology.

Erosive lichen planus

Erosive lichen planus that does not respond to any other treatment is occasionally treated by laser with some success, but this is best considered as a last resort kept for patients with severe symptoms.

Denture-induced hyperplasia

This is a common condition that is very suitable for laser treatment, especially if it is extensive. The denture should be adjusted and left out as much as possible for several weeks so that extent of surgery can be decided.

Squamous cell carcinoma

The CO_2 laser is used in the resection of malignant tumours, such as squamous cell carcinoma. Small tumours in the floor of mouth can be completely resected with a wide margin.

Other lesions

The submandibular ducts can be divided with little chance of postoperative salivary obstruction. Small tongue lesions can be excised with the laser alone, except that larger blood vessels can be troublesome. When excising large tumours the laser can be used selectively for dividing tongue or treating areas of field change beyond the excision margin.

Types of laser

Several types of laser are available (Table 38.5). These will be discussed below.

Carbon dioxide

The CO_2 laser has ideal properties for soft tissue surgery. It removes lesions with minimal damage to underlying tissue. There is less inflammation and oedema and little scarring, so that wide areas can be treated without the need for skin or mucosal grafts. Small blood vessels (<0.5 mm) are coagulated so that haemostasis is rarely

Table 38.5   Therapeutic lasers

Type (and mode)	Wavelength and colour	Uses
Excimer (pulsed)	0.190–0.351 μm invisible UV	Skin lesions, corneal surgery, angioplasty, tooth surface conditioning
Argon (continuous wave)	0.488 μm blue and 0.515 μm green	Vascular lesions, intraocular surgery, blood coagulation, middle ear lesions, composite curing
KTP (pulsed) (fibreoptic delivery)	0.532 μm green	Telangiectasia and coagulation of larger vessels, tonsillectomy, urethral strictures, bladder surgery, salivary duct strictures
Tuneable dye laser (continuous wave or pulsed)	0.504 – 0.632 μm variable	Vascular lesions, tattoo removal, photodynamic therapy, ?dentine sensitivity and other dental uses
Helium–neon (continuous wave)	0.633 μm red	Aiming beams and pointers, laser Doppler flowmetry, caries diagnosis, stimulation of wound healing
Diode lasers (pulsed)	0.650–950 μm	Pain relief, biostimulation, tooth whitening
Neodymium:YAG (continuous wave, pulsed or Q-switched)	1.06 μm invisible infrared	Tumour removal in oral surgery, gynaecology, bleeding peptic ulcers, fissure sealing, caries, dentine hypersensitivity, dentine, enamel and bone cutting, varicose veins (long pulse), analgesia (low power laser)
Holmium:YAG (pulsed) (fibreoptic delivery)	2.100 μm invisible infrared	Ureter and bladder surgery, lithotripsy, myocardial revascularisation, dacrocystorhinostomy
Erbium:YAG (pulsed)	2.94 μm invisible infrared	Skin resurfacing, caries removal, enamel, dentine and ?bone cutting
Carbon dioxide (continuous wave, pulsed or Q-switched)	10.6 μm invisible infrared	Tumour removal in gynaecology, ENT and oral surgery, denture-induced hyperplasia, skin resurfacing, gingival surgery, implant exposure, fissure sealing, caries, scaling of root surfaces, ?dentine, enamel and bone cutting

required. Unlike cryosurgery, no potentiation of malignant change has been observed. Scanning technology enables a focused beam to adopt a pattern for resurfacing procedures such as wrinkle removal where it is claimed that tissue is vaporised before any thermal damage or carbonisation occurs.

The specific advantages of a CO_2 laser are listed in Table 38.6.

Simple procedures can be quickly carried out under local anaesthesia. The lasered area is left raw and haemostasis is rarely needed. Carbonisation during treatment leaves black particles on the surface. A greyish layer about 2 mm thick forms on the surface due to coagulation of exudate. This eschar is lost as re-epithelialisation proceeds beneath. The surface is restored after 1 or 2 weeks and further improvement continues in succeeding months.

Table 38.6   Advantages of the carbon dioxide laser

Excision of wide areas with minimal scarring
Haemostasis, i.e. bloodless field
No significant swelling (airway not compromised)
Moderate postoperative pain
Safe on malignant and pre-malignant lesions
Extent of excision visible
Skin graft not needed

Neodymium:YAG

The neodymium:YAG (or Nd:YAG) laser units are also used on soft tissue. 'YAG' is yttrium aluminium garnet, which is added to the neodymium lasing medium. Surface lesions can be ablated as with the CO_2 laser. When different settings are used, however, deeper penetration is possible (e.g. in the treatment of endometriosis).

Argon

The argon laser produces visible light that is absorbed by pigments such as melanin. It is suitable for retinal surgery and is particularly effective in diabetic retinopathy. It may also be used for vascular lesions such as port-wine naevus, and is effective in removing some tattoos.

Helium–neon

Helium–neon (He–Ne) lasers produce a low-power, red, aiming beam for some invisible lasers and are useful pointers in the lecture theatre.

Dye lasers

Dye lasers can be tuned to selected wavelengths for treatment of various types of vascular naevus according to their colour. They are used similarly in tattoo removal, although removal of green pigment is not achieved by this, or any other, laser. In photodynamic therapy they may be used to switch on a cytotoxic drug at the site of a malignant tumour.

KTP lasers

KTP lasers produce a green light that is used for treating telangiectasia and pigmented lesions; they are used for bladder surgery and urethral strictures. In ENT surgery, KTP lasers are used for tonsillectomy, sinus surgery and tear-duct surgery. Their versatility is partly due to the delivery system, which uses optic fibres of 1 mm or less in diameter. KTP lasers have the potential for treating parotid or submandibular duct strictures.

Other lasers

A laser may be set to produce a continuous wave or a pulsed output. Very short pulses allow high energy levels to be achieved without generation of excessive heat. Wider surgical applications are then possible. Carbon dioxide and erbium:YAG lasers are being developed to cut enamel dentine and bone.

Index

307